An Organ of Murder

Critical Issues in Health and Medicine

Edited by Rima D. Apple, University of Wisconsin–Madison and Janet Golden, Rutgers University–Camden

Growing criticism of the U.S. healthcare system is coming from consumers, politicians, the media, activists, and healthcare professionals. Critical Issues in Health and Medicine is a collection of books that explores these contemporary dilemmas from a variety of perspectives, among them political, legal, historical, sociological, and comparative, and with attention to crucial dimensions such as race, gender, ethnicity, sexuality, and culture.

For a list of titles in the series, see the last page of the book.

An Organ of Murder

Crime, Violence, and Phrenology in Nineteenth-Century America

Courtney E. Thompson

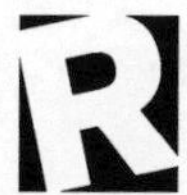

Rutgers University Press

New Brunswick, Camden, and Newark, New Jersey, and London

Library of Congress Cataloging-in-Publication Data

Names: Thompson, Courtney E., author.
Title: An organ of murder : crime, violence, and phrenology in nineteenth-century America / Courtney E. Thompson.
Description: New Brunswick, New Jersey : Rutgers University Press, [2021] |
Series: Critical issues in health and medicine | Includes bibliographical references and index.
Identifiers: LCCN 2020020801 | ISBN 9781978813069 (paperback ; alk. paper) | ISBN 9781978813076 (cloth ; alk. paper) | ISBN 9781978813083 (epub) | ISBN 9781978813090 (mobi) | ISBN 9781978813106 (pdf)
Subjects: LCSH: Phrenology—United States—History—19th century. | Criminal anthropology—United States—History—19th century. | Criminal psychology—United States—History—19th century | Criminology—United States—History—19th century.
Classification: LCC HV6059 .T46 2021 | DDC 364.2/4—dc23
LC record available at https://lccn.loc.gov/2020020801

A British Cataloging-in-Publication record for this book is available from the British Library.

∞ The paper used in this publication meets the requirements of the American National Standard for Information Sciences—Permanence of Paper for Printed Library Materials, ANSI Z39.48-1992.

www.rutgersuniversitypress.org

Manufactured in the United States of America

For Scott

Contents

Illustrations

An Organ of Murder

Introduction

Through a Mirror, Darkly

The phrenologist Lorenzo Fowler had a meeting scheduled for an autumn day in 1849. Rather than viewing his subject in the comfort of his office, he ventured out onto the streets of New York City. He traveled half a mile from Clinton Hall to the New York Halls of Justice and House of Detention, colloquially known as the Tombs, where the warden, who had written to invite the phrenologist on this occasion, welcomed him to the institution. Perhaps he received a tour of the prison with the warden, but the main event was the set of "test examinations" conducted by Fowler on three prisoners. The warden maintained a "studied silence" as Fowler examined each of his subjects in turn, writing down his descriptions of their characters and phrenological characteristics. Only then were the identities and the charges against these prisoners revealed, with the correspondence between these data and their crimes standing as proof of the "triumphant success of phrenological truth."[1]

When one imagines the phrenological encounter, one often thinks first of a client paying for a reading as a combination of self-help and amusement, an image that is part of our cultural lexicon, captured in popular imagery and satirical accounts. Fowler's trip to the prison at first glance appears to be an inverted image, a dark mirror to the phrenological visit. Few would suspect that at the same time as phrenologists were being paid to examine men, women, and children in their offices and in tours of the country, they were also paying close attention to and examining another population: convicted criminals in prisons. Indeed, the criminal was more essential for the development of phrenological theory and practice than the paying client, central to both the self-conception of the phrenologist and the development and articulation of phrenological theory.

Phrenology, the science of reading the shape of the skull to interpret and predict powers of mind and character, has a rich history and historiography.[2] As early as 1933, Robert Riegel argued that, "contrary to common belief, phrenology did not originate as the scheme of money-making fakers, but from the study of able men using the best scientific methods of their day."[3] The scientific nature of phrenology, and its place within the history of science, has been well established by historians. Beginning in the 1970s, scholars including Geoffrey Cantor, Roger Cooter, and Steven Shapin closely analyzed the social structures, cultural meaning, and scientific status of phrenology, particularly in the British context. Their debates about the development and meaning of phrenology, its social and intellectual status, and its techniques continued to inform historians of science over the next fifty years.

Why have historians of science and medicine returned again and again to phrenology? The same features that draw historians account in part for the fascination it held for practitioners, commentators, and clients nearly two centuries ago. Phrenology was capacious in its meanings, porous in its boundaries, flexible in its interpretations, and adaptive to various applications. Phrenology was a mirror reflecting that which observers most desired—or most feared—to see, in themselves, in others, in science, and in society. As such, historians have also contemplated this prismatic mirror, analyzing the various images it has produced, considering how phrenology reflected and refracted social concerns about topics like gender, race, reform, education, and the nature of scientific inquiry itself.

The mirror of phrenology also offers another, darker side. While many historians have remarked on the utopian side of phrenology—its reformist ethos and applications, its uses by clients for self-improvement, and so forth—phrenology also reflected a negative image of such utopian visions. Phrenology not only promised to perfect or improve the human race, but simultaneously suggested that not all minds were capable of perfection or improvement. Phrenology was not just an amusing pastime, nor was it only a matter of theoretical debate for elite scientists about the nature of science itself. There were real stakes to this debate and these practices, particularly for those at the bottom rungs of society.

An Organ of Murder examines the ways in which the criminal and criminality became central objects of phrenological research, theory, and public discourse from its origins in Gall's *Schädellehre* (doctrine of the skull) at the turn of the nineteenth century to its efflorescence and decline in midcentury American practical phrenology. I argue that a primary theme associated with phrenology at each stage of its history was a focus on the problem of crime and the criminal. In the United States, phrenology shaped the production of medicolegal knowledge around crime, the treatment of the criminal, and sociocultural expectations about the causes of crime. Phrenologists made the criminal a central figure in their work and thus a primary tool for the articulation and dissemination of their science. The criminal was the research and demonstration subject par excellence for the spread of phrenology, and the courtroom, the prison, and the gallows were essential spaces for the staging of scientific expertise.

In particular, phrenological ideas helped to construct ways of *looking* alongside modes of *language* for identifying, understanding, and analyzing criminals and their actions. These ways of seeing and describing were subsequently translated from the realm of phrenology into both popular and elite conceptions of criminal behavior.[4] Decades before the "invention" of criminal anthropology by Cesare Lombroso in the 1870s, phrenologists were using visual evidence of facial and cranial anatomy to explain the potential of individuals for violence and criminality, and this discourse also inflected popular uses of visual judgment. Phrenological language around the causes and nature of criminality not only structured mid-nineteenth-century medicolegal approaches to the problem of violent crime but continues to hold a place in our modern lexicon. These two vocabularies—lexical and visual—enabled criminal profiling *avant la lettre*. Both phrenological language and images of criminality remain a ghost in the machinery of the contemporary carceral state.

This study is centered on the nineteenth-century United States, with a focus on the decades of the 1830s through the 1850s. These decades were crucial for the development of phrenology in the United States, including the rise of phrenology as an elite intellectual pursuit among learned professionals, the emergence of practical phrenology and decline of elite phrenology, and the heyday of practical phrenology in America, set against the political, social, and cultural currents of the antebellum period. This book draws a distinction between two cohorts of phrenologists and their respective eras of influence in America. First, I identify a group of educated and professional men—particularly physicians, lawyers, and professors—who orchestrated the introduction of phrenology into American intellectual circles during the 1820s and 1830s. These men established the earliest phrenological societies and journals in the United States, and they sought in phrenology a body of knowledge that could be applied to their respective professional fields (especially medicine), even as these professional fields experienced challenges to their expert status in this period.[5] In contrast to these phrenological enthusiasts stood another group, proponents of a new variety of phrenology that was emerging by the early 1840s: practical phrenologists, as they named themselves, were phrenologists by trade. Rather than attempting to speak to an educated elite, they instead focused on a popular audience as itinerant lecturers who "read" heads for a fee. After the decline of elite phrenology by the beginning of the 1840s, this group of practical phrenologists became the face of phrenology in the United States, contributing to longstanding misapprehensions about the nature of phrenology in the nineteenth century.

Much has been written about phrenology in Europe and in Britain, due to its Continental origins and the role of Scottish and English phrenologists in popularizing the science in the first two decades of the nineteenth century. In the United States, the profound enthusiasm of early adopters matched that of British phrenologists, and the midcentury turn to practical phrenology made the science all the more prevalent and culturally influential in America. Within this context, phrenological approaches to crime and punishment—whether practical, rhetorical, or cultural—were put to use and became common currency. For example, in the United States, prison officials frequently invited phrenologists into prisons, and phrenologists and phrenological enthusiasts were called to serve as expert witnesses on the stand. Phrenology from its inception spoke to the problems of crime, but the applications of the science to this problem were more successful and longer-lived in the United States. The unique circumstances by which American phrenology was adopted, promulgated, and popularized contributed to its ability to move from theory to practice, especially in the realms of law and penology.

As with many histories of nineteenth-century science and medicine, this story about American phrenology must be told through a partially transnational lens: American phrenology could not have existed without its Continental and British progenitors. American phrenological enthusiasts, practical phrenologists, and phrenological clients alike responded throughout the century to intercontinental crosscurrents, and this transnational movement of ideas, people, objects, texts, and capital is a central part of my study. Further, the engagements of American phrenologists with European scientific developments are also part of this story, particularly how phrenologists reacted to late nineteenth-century innovations in criminal theory.

Little attention has been paid to the role of phrenology in American criminal jurisprudence and penology.[6] This book demonstrates that phrenology—both elite phrenological enthusiasm and practical phrenology—had much to say about these subjects, influencing the development of various approaches to crime in American medicine, law, and culture. In particular, I illuminate the concurrent development of approaches to medical jurisprudence in 1830s America and the rise of elite phrenological enthusiasm in medicolegal circles in this period. This book demonstrates the deep-seated commitment to and influence of phrenological theory among medicolegal experts, especially Isaac Ray, and thus locates phrenology in the history of medical jurisprudence and the insanity defense.[7]

This project also decenters the traditional history of criminology, which has located its origins in 1870s Continental positivism, by positioning phrenology as more than a precursor to theories of the criminal mind.[8] The majority of the history of criminology has focused on the post-1870s positivist moment, instigated by the Italian criminal anthropologist Cesare Lombroso's theories of degeneracy, which in turn were inspired by Charles Darwin's theories of heredity.[9] I suggest that phrenological criminology as it developed within American phrenology and popular culture was a coherent and consistent set of theories and practices that predated the "invention" of criminology in the 1870s.

By tracing the long-lasting influence of phrenological language and imagery in American culture, law, and medicine, as well as the practical applications of phrenology in courts and prisons, I complicate considerations of phrenology in American history. I demonstrate that the elite intellectuals of the 1830s were as influential in medicolegal arenas as the practical phrenologists of midcentury proved to be in popular culture, and moreover that both groups were invested in issues of crime and punishment as a means for demonstrating the utility of phrenology and advancing their own claims to expertise over criminal matters. This project thus intervenes in the history of phrenology, exploring its influence in American medicolegal thought, particularly with regard to questions of criminal insanity and medical jurisprudence, as well as in the history of criminology, penology, and popular culture.

Phrenology was not just a scientific curiosity or a precursor to positivist criminology, but rather a robust system of criminal science in its own right. This work traces the long-lasting influence of phrenological visual culture and language in American culture, law, and medicine, as well as the practical uses of phrenology in courts, prisons, and daily life. I further demonstrate the seriousness with which educated phrenological enthusiasts took up phrenology in the early nineteenth-century United States, with particular attention to the utility they found in phrenology for solving the problem of crime. As I argue in this book, the early adopters of phrenology in Jacksonian America were physicians, professors, and legal experts, and their embrace of this science constituted what I term a "phrenological impulse." This desire to apply phrenological theories, language, and practices to find practical solutions to social problems had a profound and enduring effect on the development of medical jurisprudence, theories of criminal insanity, and approaches to prison reform in nineteenth-century America. This book extends and reconsiders the history of medical jurisprudence and criminal science, along with the history of phrenology. In so doing, I consider the making of expert knowledge within, and the relationships between, the realms of medicine, law, and scientific practice in nineteenth-century America, as well as the place of both elite and popular science in American culture.

An Organ of Murder is organized chronologically, moving from the first decades of the nineteenth century through the turn of the twentieth century. Chapter 1 re-examines the history of the origins of phrenology in Continental Europe and the United Kingdom between the turn of the century and the 1820s, focusing on the role of criminals and the prison in the development of early phrenological theory. This chapter begins with a reconsideration of Franz Joseph Gall and Johann Gaspar Spurzheim, demonstrating the extent to which the prison was used as a laboratory for the articulation of phrenological theory. Next, I discuss the interventions of the Combe brothers, particularly George Combe's writings on the nature of criminal responsibility. This chapter concludes with a discussion of the criminal theory contained within phrenology: the identification of an "organ of murder" and the language of the criminal propensities. I describe how these organs were "read" visually on the head, and how the language of organs and propensities became tied to the problem of crime. This chapter establishes the extent to which criminals and penal spaces were foundational for and essential to phrenology.

Chapter 2 addresses the introduction of phrenology to the United States in the 1820s and the early 1830s as well as the connections built across the Atlantic between two different phrenological communities. The chapter first discusses the founding of the first phrenological societies in the United States and the work of the earliest converts, particularly Charles Caldwell. I then turn to a transatlantic debate about the validity of phrenology, which focused on the skulls and characters of famous murderers, especially Burke and Hare, and in which American phrenological knowledge was mobilized as part of a British dispute. I next retrace the journey of Spurzheim to the United States, which directly resulted in the founding of the Boston Phrenological Society. This organization would become the locus of phrenological enthusiasm in the United States, as these elite, educated, urban professionals saw in phrenology the potential to undergird their expertise in their given fields. Finally, I explore the phrenological cabinets of the Boston and Edinburgh societies, discussing the extent to which they incorporated criminality into their cabinets and the transatlantic networks required to build these spaces.

Chapters 3 and 4 cover the development of American phrenology between the 1830s and the 1850s in two sites, the courtroom and the prison, and among two cohorts of phrenological adherents, elite phrenological enthusiasts and practical phrenologists. Chapter 3 focuses on the uses of phrenological theory and language in the realm of medical jurisprudence between the mid-1830s and the 1850s. Phrenology emerged in this period as one possibility for crafting medicolegal expertise, particularly on the topic of criminal insanity. This chapter begins by contextualizing medical jurisprudence in early America; at the same time that phrenology was gaining ground in the United States, theories of medical jurisprudence were in flux. I next turn to Isaac Ray, a central figure in the development of theories of medical jurisprudence in the United States, and the work of other phrenological enthusiasts in the realm of medical jurisprudence. Ray's work, particularly *A Treatise on the Medical Jurisprudence of Insanity* (1838), helped to introduce phrenological language and ideas into American courtrooms. This chapter concludes with an exploration of court cases in which attorneys, judges, and expert witnesses made implicit or explicit use of phrenological theories. These cases of "phrenology on trial" suggest both the uses of phrenology for the building of medicolegal expertise and the extent to which phrenological language around the propensities was incorporated into medicolegal theories about the nature of criminal responsibility.

Chapter 4 explores the relationship between American phrenology and the penal system from the mid-1830s through the 1850s. This chapter engages with practical phrenology, focusing on the tension between the anti–capital punishment and reformist ideology broadly promoted by practical phrenologists and the simultaneous necessity of the prison and the gallows for the production of phrenological materials and capital. This chapter begins with an overview of the context of the reformist impulse in American culture and the variation of practical phrenology promoted by the Fowler brothers. Next, the chapter discusses visits by American phrenologists to prisons, which they used as testing sites to promote the truth of their science, and the extent to which phrenologists participated in pre- and post-execution examinations of convicts. The chapter concludes by exploring the inherent tension between discourse and practice: phrenologists decried the horrors of capital punishment but required access to the heads and skulls that were its fruits.

Chapter 5 focuses on the midcentury popular culture of practical phrenology in the home and the urban landscape. I relate the popularity of phrenological messages about criminal potential to broader social anxieties about strangers, immigration, mobility, and danger in the antebellum city and discourses about policing. This chapter first develops the dichotomy between "good" and "bad" heads, which juxtaposed great men and notorious villains and was prevalent in popular phrenological writing. Next, I explore how this lesson was interpreted for daily use, especially anxieties about self-improvement and childrearing. Beyond practical uses of the maxims of phrenology, this chapter also addresses fictional fantasies of the perfect predictive abilities that "phrenological detectives" used to catch criminals before (or shortly after) the act. This chapter concludes with a brief exploration of the racialization of criminality in the postbellum period, discussing the extent to which phrenology participated in this shifting narrative about criminal types. The chapter also reflects on the ways in which phrenological ways of seeing inflected both self-knowledge and mid-century attempts to know others in a "world of strangers."

Chapter 6 turns to the final third of the nineteenth century, reconsidering the development of new fields of criminal science through the lens of phrenological reception. This chapter begins with a discussion of the development of the neuro disciplines as framed within a dichotomy of "old" and "new" phrenology, exploring how phrenologists and critics alike interpreted the genealogy of these sciences. The next two sections address the criminal sciences of Cesare Lombroso and Alphonse Bertillon respectively, focusing in particular on the continuities between these "new" sciences and phrenological tradition, and on the ways in which phrenologists responded to these developments, viewing them as an extension of their own practices.

The epilogue considers the afterlives of this phrenological impulse in the twentieth and twenty-first centuries, as well as the phrenological futures inspired by the traces of this epistemology. I discuss the demise of the phrenological profession and the last case of phrenology in court: the 1928 murder trial of Eula Mae Thompson in Georgia. I then address recent developments in criminology, particularly attempts to identify a "criminal gene" and the use of functional magnetic resonance imaging (fMRI) to identify the criminal mind. The epilogue considers the longevity of phrenological language and images of the criminal, suggesting that phrenological concepts continue to inflect how we think about, describe, and attempt to solve crime in the present day.

Chapter 1

Origins and Organs

The plot of the 1824 English play *The Phrenologist* focuses on the romantic pairings of George Wonder and Captain Percy, dashing young men in pursuit of the affections of two young ladies, Rhodanne Fairlake and Eliza Wonder. Rhodanne and Eliza are the ward and daughter of the buffoonish antagonists, Sir Thomas Wonder and General Alfight, who intend to keep the young ladies as their own wives. The young men, having escaped the debtors' prison in which their uncles had arranged their imprisonment, decide to avenge themselves on Sir Thomas and General Alfight by disguising themselves "as teachers of the new science of Phrenology," in order to make fools of the older men and steal away the young ladies.[1] Phrenology, in this short play, provides a means for amusement and petty revenge, as well as a mechanism through which this complex matrimonial contest can be decided.

At first glance, "The farce of all farces is surely Phrenology," as one song in the play proclaims.[2] Yet the low stakes and silly premise of *The Phrenologist* aside, this farce nevertheless suggests serious potential consequences for the uses of phrenology, particularly in the realm of crime and punishment. In between the encounters between the would-be lovers, Sir Thomas adopts the principles of phrenology and begins to apply them to his patrimony. In Scene III, Sir Thomas, now a fervent convert to phrenology, examines the head of an accused murderer brought into his study. Sir Thomas declares that, according to his reading of the prisoner's head: "This poor, harmless, inoffensive young man never broke any thing in his life; he has no organ of destructiveness."[3] When the prisoner himself claims responsibility for his actions, Sir Thomas argues that the prisoner's own organ of lying was causing him to act in this way, and that he had no organ of murder at all. Sir Thomas determines, based on "the organs of murder, malice, destructiveness, and lying" on the skull of the deceased victim, that "the case is clear; he is in the conspiracy, and has killed himself to get this inoffensive man hung."[4] Later in the play, Sir Thomas reveals the grand plans his phrenological study has inspired: two acts of parliament related to jurisprudence, which would require that "every judge, magistrate, police officer, constable, and all persons concerned in the preservation of his Majesty's peace shall be Phrenologists."[5] Further, "the judges being convinced of their guilt on a phrenological investigation, shall order a skilful surgeon to cut out the offending organ."[6] This farce had a sharp edge.

Even within the light context of a farce, *The Phrenologist* suggests the darker potential of phrenology to be used as a tool to exert social control, to assess culpability and criminality, and to determine punishment and imprisonment. Few phrenologists had ambitions for phrenology as extravagant as Sir Thomas, who proposed a system of phrenological hegemony over crime and punishment. And yet, the potential for phrenology to serve such a significant social and political role was an object of interest—one that inspired enthusiasm, criticism, and satire alike—among both phrenologists and their opponents. In *The Phrenologist*, the idea of phrenology as a mechanism for crime and punishment was played for laughs, but some phrenological enthusiasts saw in phrenology real potential for solving such complex social problems.

This chapter explores the origins of phrenology in the Continental context, as well as its translation into the Anglophone world via the United Kingdom. I illuminate the origins of a phrenological approach to crime, which I argue was foundational to the discipline of criminal science and essential to the enthusiasm for phrenology in Britain and particularly in the United States. From its origins, phrenology was prefigured with concerns about criminal minds and behaviors, and its conception of crime was essential to its spread, its mobilization within elite circles, and, as in the case of *The Phrenologist*, its wider circulation in popular culture. While phrenological criminology would achieve its pinnacle within the American context, it developed in response to conversations set into motion by European phrenologists. Later chapters will unpack the ways in which phrenological enthusiasm in the United States was predicated on the applicability of phrenology to crime; this chapter focuses on the development of the theoretical underpinnings of a phrenological criminology in the Continental and British contexts.

Continental Craniology

Franz Joseph Gall was a physician and an anatomist before he became known as the founder of the new science of what he termed *Schädellehre* (doctrine of the skull), or *organologie*—which was later transmuted to "organology" or "craniology" before becoming "phrenology."[7] Born in 1758 in the village of Tiefenbronn in an area that would become part of the Grand Duchy of Baden, Germany, Gall studied first in Baden Baden and then Bruchsal before beginning medical studies in 1777 in Strasbourg.[8] He continued his medical studies in Vienna, receiving his medical doctorate there in 1785 and establishing a private practice in the city.[9] His anatomical studies and reading, particularly of philosopher Johann Gottfried von Herder, inspired his early publications and developing theories of mind and cerebral localization, and by 1792 or 1793 Gall began to develop his theory of organs corresponding with innate faculties.[10] In the late 1790s, Gall began lecturing and publishing on the subject in Austria, before his lectures were deemed to be subversive by the state, due to their materialistic implications for morality and religion. His lectures were banned in December of 1801, which paradoxically increased the public knowledge about and popularity of his system.[11]

Beginning in 1805, Gall staged a triumphant tour through Europe before settling in Paris in 1807, by which point he had become a minor medical celebrity.[12] Gall was well received in Paris and remained there until his death in 1828. Shortly after his move to Paris, he published the first book of his four-volume *Anatomie et physiologie du système nerveux en général, et du cerveau en particulier*,[13] eventually followed by a more accessible account of his localization theories, *Sur les fonctions du cerveau et sur celles de chacune des parties* (1822–1825).[14] Along the road to Paris, Gall was joined by an assistant, the German physician Johann Gaspar Spurzheim, with whom he collaborated on *Anatomie et physiologie*.[15]

Gall's theory of "craniology" was based on a few simple tenets. Craniology proposed that the brain, the organ of the mind, was an aggregate of mental organs that were localized into specific functions. Further, the relative size of these organs could be used to assess the power of that organ, and the shape of the skull external to the organ could be used to assess the power of that organ and hence the mental faculties.[16] The final tenet of craniology—that the disposition of the skull, especially its "bumps," indicated power of mind—is most commonly recalled today, but craniology also broadly articulated a theory of localization of mental capacities well before anatomical localization efforts in the mid-nineteenth century.[17] However, Gall's craniology was not, in spite of his training, primarily influenced by his anatomical and physiological research. While the new science drew on the credibility his education provided, it was based on Gall's correlation of his subject's self-descriptions of their characters with his manual examination of their skulls.[18]

One of the earliest features of phrenological practice was the phrenological visit to the prison. Gall and Spurzheim initiated this practice in the early years of the science, and it was replicated by leading practitioners as they worked to find a place for their science. Although phrenology drew its credibility from the association with anatomy and physiology, Gall's experimental method was primarily subjective and impressionistic.[19] He invited diverse individuals into his house to take personal histories exploring the characters of his subjects.[20] Only then would he examine the head, tracking the shape of the skull to correspond with each individual's self-reported character. These individual examinations would have been time-consuming. Larger groups of individuals were also needed for study, and it was here that institutions, chiefly the prison, became useful research sites.

In 1805, Gall visited the prisons of Berlin and Spandau in order to examine hundreds of convicts.[21] According to contemporaneous accounts, among these prisoners he found the "organs of Secretiveness and Acquisitiveness predominated . . . sometimes so strikingly apparent, that at a glance the thief might be distinguished from the other criminals," as well as large organs of Destructiveness in others.[22] In prison visits, he "gave the most convincing proofs of his ability to discover such malefactors, as were among the prisoners."[23] Among the hundreds of convicts Gall viewed at these prisons, he found so many with the "organ of thieving" that "no innocent person was found," and in others he identified "the organ of murder" as well.[24] Newspapers confirmed Gall's remarkable abilities, observing that his analysis "uniformly corresponded with the register of their crimes."[25] Other accounts described more focused displays of virtuosity, as in one article that described Gall examining six anonymous skulls, in all of which he discovered the organ of theft; the skulls were confirmed after the fact to have belonged to a gang of robbers.[26]

Such "practical test[s] of the truth of this system," conducted on the heads of convicts, were framed by contemporary commentators as the defining moment of craniology.[27] Even books and essays that expressed skepticism about phrenology nevertheless framed these prison trips as an essential moment in which phrenology was tested and the doctrine formed: "It was at Berlin, and the fortress of Spandau, where they first put their doctrine to the test of experiment, by its application to congregated multitudes."[28] Even if this author expressed skepticism at these findings, he nevertheless represented these prison trips as essential experiments.

By entering the prison, Gall was able to examine hundreds of subjects in a single visit, and he had, by virtue of the prison registers and the reports of their crimes, detailed accounts of the prisoners' characters that he could compare with their skulls. These spaces were also sources for material capital, particularly the criminal skulls he acquired from prison authorities.[29] These prison visits were research trips, where the volume of captive heads and characters available to Gall rendered the prison a laboratory for the production of knowledge about the correspondences between heads and characters. Thus, the basis of both phrenological criminal theory and phrenological theory more generally was predicated on findings from within the prison, as were later defenses of the science staged within prisons, as I discuss in chapter 4.

Gall continued this research in prisons in Berne and Fribourg, in Switzerland, and Celle and Torgau, in Germany, as well as other prisons—sites that served as laboratories for the further development of his science and for proofs of the same.[30] Spurzheim followed his mentor's path into the prison, though his visits were much farther afield. Spurzheim's early visits to prisons, workhouses, and hospitals were a part of his extended tours throughout England, Scotland, and Ireland, more representative of a kind of tourism than an experimental exercise, as his letters to his later wife suggest.[31] Despite this, reports of Spurzheim's prison visits framed them as demonstrations of virtuosity in culling criminal minds from a mass of subjects. During an 1827 visit by Spurzheim to Hull, England, for example, he visited a charity hall, a refuge for the insane, a grammar school, and the town jail, where he inspected the inmates with precision and showmanship: "On entering the felons' side, his eye passed rapidly over the greater number of them, but rested upon two or three individuals, whom he inspected with magical rapidity, and instantaneously seized the peculiarity of their characters. This facility was the most surprising; for even those who had a quantity of hair on the head, he placed his hand or hands over the four regions, and his conclusions proved astonishingly correct."[32] The rapid eye of the phrenologist alone was sufficient to render judgment within the prison, followed by a manual examination that reinforced the assessment gleaned at a glance.

Phrenology, as Spurzheim would rename it, was not the first attempt to create a science of the mind or self.[33] The most clear historical analogue and antecedent to phrenology was physiognomy, a science often confused with phrenology or taught in tandem to it, even by phrenologists themselves.[34] Physiognomy has a long genealogy, dating to Aristotle, but it had largely declined over the centuries from a high art or science to a superstitious practice of the masses, associated with palmistry and fortunetelling.[35] Most publications on the subject of physiognomy during the centuries before Gall's birth categorized physiognomy alongside astrology, chiromancy, and related practices for reading faces and fates.[36] This changed somewhat with the reimagining of physiognomy in the 1770s by Swiss minister Johann Caspar Lavater, who reframed the practice as simultaneously an art and a science for the educated gentleman. His lavish and heavily illustrated *Essays on Physiognomy* elevated physiognomy out of the vulgate and into refined society, even as Lavater himself became a celebrity.[37] Lavater also made strong claims as to the scientific nature of his endeavor, illustrating for example the importance of angles and the mathematic division of the features of the face; but as a nonscientist, Lavater's claims could only stretch so far.[38] When Gall's new craniology appeared on the scene with a seemingly anatomical and scientific basis for his assessment of character, along with explanations for the causes of these faculties, craniology/phrenology proved more compelling than the older physiognomy.

Gall's system also did more to compartmentalize character. By focusing on discrete faculties or organs of mind, Gall enabled a more precise assessment of character and intellect. The implications of the science were at times problematic, especially the association with materialism. The science could not be divorced from its association with social, philosophical, political, and religious questions, critiques, and concerns, rendering it a lightning rod for controversy and a capacious receptacle for greater significance.[39] In the hands of both its supporters and its critics, phrenology *meant* something—it suggested something either great or troubling with regard to mankind, and the interpretation was in the eye of the beholder. Even the founders of the discipline, Gall and Spurzheim, were not in accord. Gall conceived of his science as an instrument for the use of the elite to govern the unenlightened masses, based in a belief in the immutability of human nature.[40] Spurzheim had a more utopian outlook, believing that phrenology could be used to perfect—not govern—the human race.[41] These disagreements, among others, led to the schism between the two and influenced the shape of the iteration of phrenology that later crossed the Atlantic.

In the popular sphere, Spurzheim's utopianism triumphed. Perhaps his point of view was more palatable, as he argued in his own publications that there were no "bad" organs, only the abuse of organs.[42] Spurzheim, however, was also a born promoter, motivated by a desire to seek fame and fortune.[43] His role in popularizing phrenology, particularly in the Anglo-American world, elevated him to such an extent that his status sometimes obscured the role of Gall in the development of the science. Spurzheim's extensive tours in the United Kingdom, his brief trip to the United States, and his many English-language publications on phrenology would make him a key spokesman for phrenology in the English-speaking world.

The Brothers Combe and Criminal Responsibility

On the heels of a personal and intellectual break with Gall, Spurzheim journeyed to the United Kingdom in 1814 for an extended tour throughout the country. Over the next three years, he hopped from city to city, acting as both an ambassador for the fledgling science and a tourist, visiting various institutions for his amusement and edification.[44] During his trip he published his first English text, *The Physiognomical System of Drs. Gall and Spurzheim*, the primacy of which was surely helped by the fact that Gall's *Anatomie et physiologie* was not translated into English until 1835.[45] He also lectured extensively on the subject, though his lectures rarely drew large crowds. Reception of these theories was stymied in part by the xenophobia engendered by the recent Napoleonic Wars, as well as negative reviews of his book published in the *Edinburgh Review*.[46]

Edinburgh, however, would soon become a center not only for the critique of phrenology in the United Kingdom but for its defense, largely due to the efforts of George Combe, a Scottish lawyer, and his brother, Andrew Combe, a physician.[47] George Combe was converted to the new science while attending Spurzheim's lectures in Edinburgh and became one of its most assertive popularizers. The Combe brothers, together with a few friends, established the world's first phrenological society, the Edinburgh Phrenological Society, in 1820.[48] Within six years, the Society claimed 120 members, most of whom were professional and educated men, and within another decade the United Kingdom would host twenty-nine such societies modeled on the Edinburgh example.[49] The Edinburgh Society also published the first phrenological periodical, *The Phrenological Journal and Miscellany*, as well as the *Transactions of the Phrenological Society*, which primarily published papers given at the society's meetings.

George Combe, a lawyer by training, had different motivating concerns, assumptions, and educational background than Spurzheim or Gall, which inflected the phrenology he popularized. In particular, Combe was invested philosophically with the idea of natural law and its effect on human responsibility, concerns which would come to fruition in his 1828 phrenological text *The Constitution of Man Considered in Relation to External Objects*, which became a global best seller.[50] Combe moved away from the overly anatomical accounts of Spurzheim and Gall into moral philosophy, reframing a very old idea—human happiness depended upon the laws of nature, the violation of which leads to unhappiness—through the use of phrenology as analytical tool.[51] The expansion and explication of the phrenological faculties in this text, some of which had clear connections to lawful and unlawful behavior, pointed the way for the application of phrenology not only to questions of moral responsibility, but also, potentially, to matters of crime and punishment.[52] *The Constitution of Man* addressed both punishment and the causes of crime, and Combe expanded on these themes in later publications, such as his 1853 work, *Remarks on the Principles of Criminal Legislation and the Practice of Prison Discipline.*

Combe's approach to phrenology was preoccupied with questions of natural law, including the nature of crime and punishment.[53] He argued in later revised and expanded editions of *The Constitution of Man* that "every crime proceeds from an abuse of some faculty or other," and further that these abuses stemmed from overly active faculties, from great excitement due to external causes, and from ignorance as to the uses and abuses of the faculties.[54] Most importantly, Combe argued that these causes "exist *independently of the will of the offender*."[55] He advocated for a replacement of what he termed the "animal system" of crime and punishment, which was harsh and in which few measures, except terror, were taken to prevent crime, with a new moral system, which would be more cognizant of the causes of crime and more measured in its response. In Combe's proposed moral system, once a "tendency to abuse the faculties appeared in any individual, instant means of prevention would be resorted to."[56] What these preventative measures might have been was somewhat unclear, but Combe was emphatic that in his system the causes of criminal behavior would be removed.[57] The terms he used to separate the two systems—"animal" and "moral"—mirrored a common division of the phrenological organs, the low, "animal" propensities, versus the high moral and intellectual faculties. Combe's system focused not on criminal behavior or lawbreaking per se but on tendencies to abuse the (phrenological) faculties that would lead to these behaviors.

Combe further critiqued execution as another kind of abuse of the faculties, as an example of the violence of animal law. Within the moral and intellectual system for which he advocated, the causes of crime must first be understood in order for the effects to be avoided. Combe was arguing for a more compassionate approach to crime, as well as for the importance of education and rehabilitation of criminals, rather than merely punishment. Anticipating critiques of his proposed moral system, especially concerns that "punishment would be abrogated and crime encouraged," Combe answered sharply that the call for more suffering than needed proceeded from "the yet untamed barbarism of our own minds."[58] Combe's chapter on punishment was not just an extension of phrenological theory into the realm of the criminal, but also introduced a new, compassionate, and liberal way of thinking about both the causes of crime and appropriate means of punishment.

The Constitution of Man, republished in several editions in both the United Kingdom and in the United States, became in some ways more representative of the doctrines of phrenology than the more technical and anatomical texts originally published by Spurzheim and Gall. While the German physicians were continually lionized as the fathers of the science, it was Combe's gloss that formed the basis for popular understanding and commentary in the Anglo-American world. In this way, Combe's language of law and his interest in crime and punishment became a central part of phrenological discourse. Combe also penned further texts on the subject, including *Remarks on the Principles of Criminal Legislation and the Practice of Prison Discipline*, which was republished as a serial in the *American Journal of Phrenology* in the 1850s and excerpted in part in other periodicals, including the American prison reform journal, *The Prisoner's Friend*.[59] American law journals, including the *American Jurist*, also excerpted Combe's writings on prison discipline and criminal insanity.[60] By the 1850s, Combe's position on the matter had become more prescriptive, narrowing to focus in particular on reforming the criminal, and eschewing practices including execution, transportation, and penal servitude. However, for some criminals, especially recidivists and murderers, indefinite imprisonment remained an option: some criminals, particularly murderers, were "not fit to be afterwards trusted with liberty," and should be "confined, held to labor, and instructed; but cut off from all hope of ever again breathing the free air of social life."[61] Criminals should be treated with sympathy and educated, Combe argued, but some criminals could not be reformed into proper members of society.

Combe's early observations on crime and punishment, though expanded upon in his later writings of the 1840s and 1850s, were foundational for such discourse within the transatlantic phrenological community, which developed these ideas into what amounted to a reformist and even nearly utopian platform, especially in the American context.[62] George Combe directed the entry of phrenological theory into the realm of penology and jurisprudence: if Gall and Spurzheim used the prison as a laboratory or research site, Combe opened the door to consider the practical applications of phrenological knowledge about crime to questions of penal discipline, legal culpability, and jurisprudence. Additionally, Andrew Combe, his physician brother, published extensively on matters of mental illness, and his work *Mental Derangement* (1831), which made use of phrenological theory, influenced contemporaneous discussions of mental illness and moral responsibility in criminal insanity.[63]

The Combe brothers shifted the focus of phrenology in the British context, orienting it toward moral, social, and religious problems and the practical application of phrenological tenets, and away from the anatomical foundations that Gall and Spurzheim had stressed.[64] This reorientation was reflected in the *Phrenological Journal* and the *Transactions*, the twin mouthpieces of the Edinburgh Phrenological Society. While much of the *Phrenological Journal*, at least at first, was occupied with the threats and critiques of antiphrenologists and focused on defending the new science, from the first issue it published essays that used criminal skulls and questions of crime as central areas of inquiry. Similarly, the first edition of the *Transactions* included an extended discussion of the lives and deeds of three murderers and a report on convicts within a prison, with respect to their phrenological characters, as presented by George Combe and others.[65] Throughout the 1820s and into the 1830s, other writers in *The Phrenological Journal and Miscellany* discussed visits to prisons and examinations of convicts, modeled after Gall, or considered the role that phrenology could play in reforming criminal legislation, among other practical matters of social interest.[66] A new agenda for phrenology had been set: it would be promoted through a shared language focused on crime.

An Organ of Murder

Phrenologists developed both a visual language and a lexicon within their science to indicate and describe criminal potential. The foundations of the discipline were predicated, in part, on divisions and faculties of mind that explained criminal behaviors. Each partitioned space on the skull, as depicted in the phrenological bust in figure 1, stood for an "organ" within this system, with each "organ" representing a particular trait; these in turn were organized into sets, such as the "animal," "intellectual," or "moral" powers of mind. The number of organs changed over the course of the century to include a greater variety of organs: Gall had originally identified twenty-seven organs, which Spurzheim later expanded to thirty-three, and Combe added to this once again, ending up with thirty-five organs, which would become the generally accepted number throughout the century.[67]

Images of the phrenological bust, with its inscribed organs, were common in printed texts on phrenology, and busts were also available for purchase for the cabinets of enthusiasts. Phrenological writings and popular accounts in newspapers and other periodicals frequently used the names of these organs with little explanation for what the name indicated, suggesting that there was an expected familiarity or literacy on the part of the reader with the organs, their location, and the implications of their indicated size. The general outlines and

PHRENOLOGICAL HEAD. 405

No. 7, Destructiveness—Executiveness; thoroughness and severity. *Excess:* Cruelty; vindictiveness. *Deficiency:* Inefficiency; a lack of fortitude under trial.

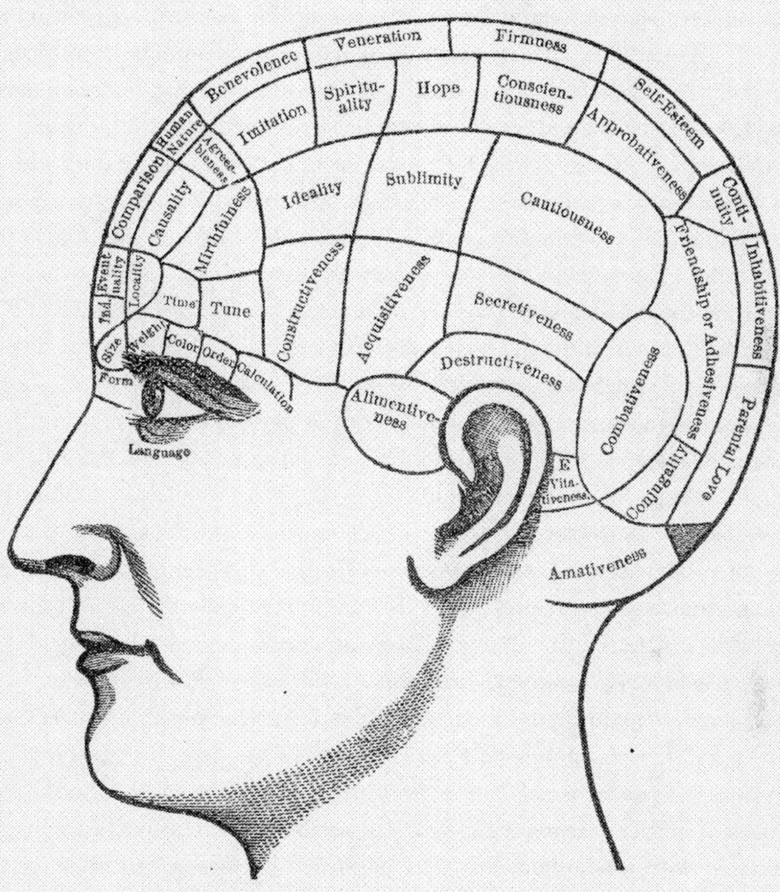

PHRENOLOGICAL HEAD.

THIS IS REGARDED AS THE MOST CORRECT INDICATION OF THE POSITION OF THE PHRENOLOGICAL ORGANS AND THEIR RELATIVE SIZE AND FORM.

No. 8, Alimentiveness—Desire for food; appetite. *Excess:* Gluttony· intemperance. *Deficiency:* Want of appetite; indifference in regard to food.

Figure 1. Phrenological head. Credit: Wellcome Collection. Attribution 4.0 International (CC BY 4.0).

mechanics of this system and its organs would not have needed much explanation for the nineteenth-century American reader.

The most important set of organs related to the criminal type was that associated with the "animal" or "selfish" propensities, a set of organs that broadly circled the ear.[68] Most significant was the organ that came to be known as "Destructiveness," located just above the ear. In Gall's earliest writings on the subject, he identified this as the organ of *Würgsinn*, stemming from *würgen*, which can be translated as the action of strangling, throttling, or choking.[69] In other texts discussing Gall, it was given instead as the organ of *Mordsinn*, from the German word for murder.[70] In his writings, Gall expanded on the nature of this organ, which he observed would, in normal expression, relate to the slaying of animals, but in unnatural moments to homicide.[71] While Gall argued that having this organ would not necessarily make someone a murderer, early translators of and commentators on his texts expressed some dismay at his easy inclusion of an "organ of murder," choosing instead to translate this organ into English as the organ of slaughter.[72] Spurzheim and Combe, publishing in the United Kingdom, aside from expanding the number of organs of the skull, also replaced these terms with the more neutral "Destructiveness." In a similar vein, the originally identified *Diebessinn*[73] or *Eigenthumssinn*[74]—the organ of theft that Gall saw in the skulls of so many convicts—became, in English, "Acquisitiveness."

Destructiveness became the essential organ for the identification of criminals, particularly murderers, even if it was linguistically distanced from the more problematic implications of *Würgsinn* and *Mordsinn*. The renaming of these particular organs was celebrated by British writers as an improvement on the science: "in giving to the powers names indicating a general feeling and propensity and not an impulse to a particular act. Thus, in place of an organ of Theft and of Murder, we have now the organs of Acquisitiveness and Destructiveness."[75] While this renaming project—attributed primarily to Spurzheim's influence, though popularized by Combe—may have functioned linguistically to remove determinism or materialism from the phrenological system, expectations remained about the existence of these organs on the skulls of criminals, especially Destructiveness. Large Destructiveness did not necessarily mean that an individual would be a murderer or a criminal—Spurzheim himself exhibited large Destructiveness, according to Combe[76]—but the notable murderers and criminals reported on by phrenologists possessed this organ in abundance.

The organ of Destructiveness was located just above the ear, and Acquisitiveness, Secretiveness, and Combativeness, the other organs commonly associated with the criminal, were arrayed in a semicircle above this organ along the sides of the head in a region of the "animal propensities," roughly in the area of the temporal bone. Throughout the nineteenth century, European and American phrenologists produced a genre of phrenological writing focusing on the phrenological characteristics of famous criminals, and these organs figured prominently in these accounts. Read together, these profiles of criminals reveal shared expectations for consistent characteristics for criminal subjects, even though they ostensibly represented the specific characteristics of infamous individuals. Along with the enlargement of Destructiveness and the nearby organs, most murderers also exhibited smaller organs in the moral and religious sentiments—which included Conscientiousness, Integrity, Veneration, Benevolence, Hope, and so forth—located across the crown of the head.

While many phrenologists would protest that correlation did not imply causation, the majority of the murderers that they profiled exhibited the predicted set of characteristics, with large "animal" propensities and low moral and intellectual qualities. One phrenologist's brief account of a murderer's skull was characteristic of both the findings and the common attitude: "It has the worst possible combination of organs, and all of a monstrous size. Amativeness, Secretiveness, Acquisitiveness, Destructiveness, and Combativeness, are prodigious; Conscientiousness and Veneration seem as if they were planed out; and the whole crown of the head is at least an inch lower than a head of such capacity ought to be. It has every indication of a wicked and innately immoral man."[77] Other accounts of the phrenological characteristics of criminals reinforced this image. In every case where a murderer's Destructiveness was noted, it was described as "large," "very large," "extremely large," "enormously large," "enormously developed," "excessively large," and so forth.[78] In nearly all of these cases, Secretiveness and Acquisitiveness were described and assessed alongside Destructiveness, and Combativeness and Alimentiveness (appetite or gluttony) were frequently added to this litany as well. When described numerically, these characteristics were given the highest or near-highest scores by the phrenologist, typically a six or seven out of a possible seven.[79] How these numbers were achieved or descriptive assessments made were never fully explained to the reader. As Fenneke Sysling has observed, while these charts were intended to "suggest objectivity and measurability," they were filled not with measurements but "a more subjective indication of size, which was then expressed quantitatively."[80] Of the remaining organs, Cautiousness, Benevolence, Veneration, Firmness, Conscientiousness, and Self-Esteem, organs that are primarily arrayed along the crown of the head, were most commonly accounted for, with Conscientiousness and Benevolence typically measuring as deficient in particular. Intentionally or not,

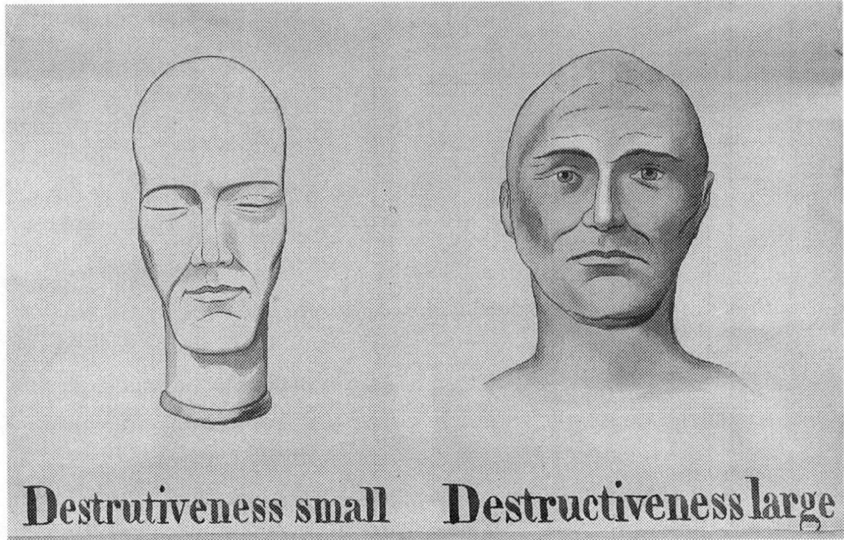

Figure 2. Phrenological poster depicting small and large Destructiveness. Fowler & Wells, Portrait Posters for Physiognomy Lectures, poster 1. Beinecke Rare Book and Manuscript Library, Yale University.

phrenologists were reading the same defects and excesses of organs into their murderous subjects: a composite image was emerging of not just *a* criminal but *the* criminal.

The composite image of a criminal viewed face-on would be wide above the ears and to the sides of the head, with a flatness or narrowness to the crown, as illustrated by figure 2. This image, a poster from a mid-nineteenth-century American phrenological lecture, was labeled solely as a representation of the organ of Destructiveness, but the transformation to the head depending on the size of this single organ indicates its significance for the reading of skulls and the elucidation of types. Given the metonymic use of Destructiveness for the set of animal propensities, this comparative illustration suggests the differences between "good" and "bad" heads—perhaps even the criminal type and its antithesis. Large Destructiveness coded for the entire set of animal propensities, which together often signaled a violent and criminal mind: "The animal propensities, when abused, produce all the varieties of felony which scourge and disgrace the human race."[81]

Complicating this narrative, however, is the identity of the two individuals depicted in figure 2. The specific illustrations, though not named in this panel, can be identified from other phrenological writings as Gosse ("Destrutiveness [*sic*] small") and Black Hawk ("Destructiveness large").[82] The portrait and biography of the Sauk leader Black Hawk (1767–1838) was used throughout the century to represent large Destructiveness.[83] However, Black Hawk's Destructiveness and other large animal organs were often read in an ambiguous and sometimes complementary light: "These organs, when large, or very large, always give great energy and force of character, and, in a savage state, would give cruelty, cunning, and revenge; would make an Indian the bold and desperate warrior, and tend to raise such a one to be a leader, or chief."[84] Further, "the brain of Black Hawk is so balanced as could scarcely fail to render him distinguished, amid the circumstances and influences which exist in a savage state."[85]

Black Hawk was framed in phrenological writings not as a "bad head" or a criminal, suggesting that expectations of criminality did not directly relate to racial characteristics in the phrenological system, and that animal propensities would be read in different ways depending on the status and ethnicity of the subject in question.[86] Like criminals, nonwhite subjects, especially Indigenous Americans, were frequently described with recourse to the animal organs. However, the excess of these organs usually was used to predict savage or warlike behavior, sometimes held up as a positive attribute, as opposed to criminality. The animal organs, when used to discuss Indigenous Americans and certain other nonwhite groups, usually signified savagery and a lack of civilization, not criminality; violence, but not murder.[87]

This racial relativism within phrenology indicates both the subjectivity at the heart of the phrenological enterprise as well as the fact that criminality, if not violence writ large, was not specifically racialized, at least in the first two thirds of the nineteenth century in the United States. While some of the criminals discussed by phrenologists were nonwhite, most of the famous murderers found to have excessive Destructiveness were of European descent. When African American criminals were discussed in phrenological journals, for example, their race was rarely used as an explanatory framework for their criminality. The message was often ambiguous. One article on a "notorious murderer," George Wilson, described the man as having an "animal temperament," large in the region of the animal propensities around the ears, and having committed his crime with "barbarous cruelty."[88] In many ways this description of Wilson echoed the discussions of other murderers of the era, and his racial background was never discussed in the text; it is only the inclusion of an illustration of his bust that reveals that Wilson was likely of African descent. Were Wilson's purported notoriety, barbarism, and animality due to his race? If not for the image, such a connection could not be made even implicitly, since the language was not distinct from that used to describe criminals of European descent.

If anything, American phrenologists, particularly practical phrenologists like the Fowler brothers, exhibited particular care in their discussion of African American criminals, following a broader attempt to construct and circulate images of the "good negro" as part of their discourse, which was motivated in part by abolitionist politics.[89] Compare, for example, the descriptions of the skulls and characters of two murderers, published one year apart in the same journal. First, the description of a murderer of European descent, John Haggerty:

> His head was large, measuring twenty-three inches; but the integuments were very abundant, and the skull three times the usual thickness; so that the amount of brain was not over the average. . . . The great mass of brain lies behind a line drawn from the ear up, and in the base of the brain; consequently the animal organs, and those more intimately connected with them, were very predominant. All things considered, he was very much of an animal. . . . It is a desperate, dangerously shaped head, poorly balanced, with a powerful body to stimulate a powerful animal, selfish mind, with comparatively weak moral and intellectual brain.[90]

Second, the description of George, an enslaved man who murdered his enslaver:

> It is a better than ordinary negro skull, remarkably thin . . . and is a better than ordinary negro's development. . . . His developments of intellect and taste more than excelled the majority of his race, and his investigating and applying qualities would have made him a proficient under fair advantages. It was remarked of him by D. Wilson, that if he were to read law two months, he would beat any lawyer in the county. . . . His governing faculties were his selfish propensities, and the strength of his brain was found in the region of ACQUISITIVENESS, DESTRUCTIVENESS, SECRETIVENESS, CAUTIOUSNESS, and FIRMNESS.[91]

The two skulls had the same overall shape and defects—overdevelopment of the selfish or animal propensities—yet the interpretation of the meaning of these signs differed markedly. The discussion of George did mobilize race but elevated him as an exemplar of his race—it was not inevitable that he would be a criminal or behave violently at all. In comparison, Haggerty was an "animal," with a "desperate, dangerously shaped head."

Haggerty's own ethnicity may complicate this analysis even further: he was described as "white" at several points in the record of the trial, which will be discussed further in the third chapter, but was also described by his own attorney as a "native of Ireland."[92] As Matthew Jacobson has demonstrated, Irish immigrants, among others, represented "whiteness of different color," a challenge to strong boundaries between racial categories.[93] By the 1840s, physical and physiognomic characteristics marked the Irish as a racial type associated with negative stereotypes. Haggerty's racial status, his "whiteness," was itself fluid and uncertain.[94] In the same way that race may have played a role in the discussion of Wilson without any direct or explicit reference, ideas about ethnicity may also have factored into Haggerty's phrenological profile, even though it did not mention his Irish origins. These uncertainties around ethnicity aside, the animal propensities were read differently depending on other identity markers.

Circumspection with regard to criminals of African descent, in particular, may relate to the abolitionist leanings of many popular phrenologists. *The American Phrenological Journal*, in which this account of George appeared, promoted abolition among other progressive reform movements, and those articles that discussed the characteristics of people of African descent moved between promoting stereotypes of lower capacity, especially for intelligence, and suggesting that there was more potential than generally acknowledged. Sometimes individuals of African descent were mobilized as positive exemplars: Eustache Belin, an enslaved man who famously warned his enslaver and helped him escape from the violence of the Haitian Revolution, was described as "eminently distinguished for the qualities of virtue and benevolence," held up throughout the century by phrenologists as an exceptional individual.[95] In another article, an illustration of Eustache was used as a positive example of small Destructiveness in comparison with a white murderer, suggesting that racial characteristics were not necessarily criminal characteristics, similar to the three-part comparison of Gall, Eustache, and murderer Chauffron in figure 3.[96]

Comparisons between criminals, whether cross-racial or not, reinforced the connection between particular organs and behaviors. Phrenologists compared and contrasted the measurements of murderers, primarily through measurements taken by caliper.[97] Sets of murderers (or convicts or other criminals) were considered collectively and comparatively, separate from other categories of humanity. The murderous mind was sufficiently consistent that one might indeed construct a specific, physical profile of the head—and hence the mind—of a murderer, down to the quarter inch. Such a profile, in the nineteenth century, might have been used to predict the actions of a criminal, and prevent them even before they acted. This was the promise of phrenology: the predictive powers of physiognomy made specific, measurable, and useful in the fight against crime.

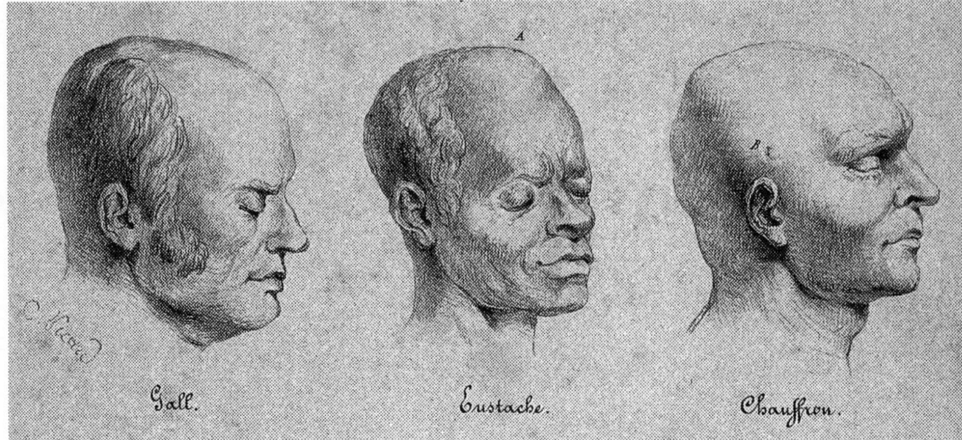

Figure 3. Three portraits shown for their phrenological exemplarity: Gall, Eustache, and Chauffron. Lithograph by C. Picard, 1842, after J. P. Thenot. Credit: Wellcome Collection. Attribution 4.0 International (CC BY 4.0).

A Language of Propensity

Beyond the specific organs and the visual lessons they conveyed to the interested observer, phrenology also promoted a unique language of crime around the term "propensity." The term itself, relative to patterns or inclinations of behavior, seems to have been borrowed from translations of Philippe Pinel's writings on insanity at the turn of the nineteenth century. The term used in these original French texts was "penchant," more commonly translated as "tendency." English translations in this period chose to use "propensity" instead, and it is possible that Spurzheim was influenced by both Pinel and the English translations of these texts, as he cited Pinel extensively on the subject of insanity and chose to use this word exclusively.[98] Spurzheim applied the idea assiduously to his own work on the organs and his explanation of behavior. For example, as Nicole Hahn Rafter has explained, the language of propensity was particularly pervasive in his chapter on "The Organ of the Propensity to Destroy, or of Destructiveness," from his *Physiognomical System*, which is suggestive of the applicability of phrenological theory to crime.[99] However, this chapter and Spurzheim's use elsewhere in his published works also indicates the enthusiasm with which he took up the language of propensity and mobilized it for the benefit of phrenology. Moreover, the term "propensity" was not applied to all organs: only the "animal" organs were typically referred to as propensities, while other groups of organs were usually referred to collectively as faculties.[100]

Contemporary and later commentators connected Spurzheim's writings to the introduction of the language of propensity into phrenological discourse, although much of this discussion was focused on the softening of the language and materialism of Gall's theories. For example, in an 1824 supplement to the *Encyclopædia Britannica*, an article on "Cranioscopy" reflected on the theories of phrenology at length, including a detailed account of each of the organs using the language of propensity. Destructiveness was listed as the "propensity to destroy in general, but more especially to destroy life."[101] The article noted that Gall had initially "called this faculty *murder*; but Dr. Spurzheim thinks it produces the propensity to destroy in general."[102] In the *Encyclopædia Londinensis* published in the following year, this information was reproduced nearly verbatim.[103] This same description of the organs, including that of Destructiveness, which included this language of propensity and identified Spurzheim as the originator of this language, was reproduced in various books and newspapers throughout the ensuing decades.[104]

In the United States, the same representation of phrenological theories was common by the 1830s, with the language of propensity in particular reserved for violent criminal behaviors. Increasingly, commentators inferred a connection between the organ, the propensity, and criminal acts, sometimes as part of a single definition: "DESTRUCTIVENESS. *Propensity to destroy, exterminate, and inflict pain.*"[105] In an explanation of each of the organs of phrenology in the *Mechanics' Magazine* in 1834, for example, Destructiveness was characterized by "Cruelty. Barbarity, sanguinary disposition, propensity to murder," and Acquisitiveness was described in part as "Covetousness, propensity to steal. Theft. Usury."[106] Other early accounts of phrenology in the United States focused in particular on Destructiveness. One article in the *Boston Traveler*, which discussed a recent publication of Spurzheim, included an explanation of the organ of Destructiveness, described in part as a "propensity to kill."[107] Another account from 1838 in the *Salem Gazette* reflected on a recent lecture by Combe in Boston on "the organ of *Destructiveness*, or a propensity to kill."[108] Combe enhanced this lecture with the use of skulls from his collection: to illustrate the organ, he exclusively used the skulls of murderers. "Destructiveness, or propensity to destroy," an oft-repeated phrase combining the two ideas, reinforced the notion of this particular organ in connection with a specific action, easily analogized to—or baldly stated to be—murder.[109]

Similar connections were made in other accounts between the organ of Acquisitiveness and a "propensity for stealing," which, alongside other propensities to vice, was considered to be one of the "strongest evidences in favor of the truth of the doctrine of Phrenology."[110] Even when commentators carefully distinguished between the "propensity to steal" and the "propensity to acquire or accumulate" in relation to this organ, they maintained the language of propensity.[111] These connections were likely reinforced by the commonly retold stories of Gall's visits to view convicts in the prisons of Spandau and Berlin, which introduced the idea of an "organ of theft" and, in so doing, drew a clear connection between the organ, the behavior, and the crime.

To be clear, "propensity" was not a word invented or discovered by Spurzheim or other phrenologists; it was in common usage by the time of these publications. In these writings, "propensity" built a linguistic bridge connecting phrenology, on the one hand, and the problem of violent criminality on the other. The constant usage of the term in phrenological texts throughout the century in both Britain and the United States forged an association between propensity, phrenology, and particular kinds of behaviors—a language that comprised the problem (crime), its origin (the phrenological organ or organs), and the solution (the system of phrenology). Further, this language provided a shared framework that lent scientific credibility to the various sciences that used this language, including phrenology as well as other developing psychological and hereditarian notions of criminality.

From its first introduction into the English vernacular, phrenological theory, especially around the organs associated with criminal behavior, was rife with the language of propensity. This language also allowed phrenological frameworks for thinking about crime to spread in a coded or implicit way. When commentators throughout the century indicated that a criminal exhibited a "propensity to destroy," a "propensity to murder," a "propensity to steal," and so forth, they were using phrenological language and concepts to explain and discuss criminal behaviors, even if they no longer had recourse to specific organs like Destructiveness or if they eschewed phrenology altogether. Other scientific figures, including Pinel, James Cowles Prichard, and Benjamin Rush, also made use of this language, but replication of their theories using this language was much less common, and in Prichard's case, postdated phrenological usage.[112] Rush had in fact coined the term "phrenology," which came to be representative of Gall and Spurzheim's theory of mind, not his own; it is not difficult to see how another term originating with other thinkers similarly came to be primarily associated with phrenology.[113]

Newspaper accounts and medical texts together reinforced the association between phrenological tenets and the language of propensity with regard to crime. "Although we may not be inclined to accede to all the speculations of the phrenologists," one writer observed in *The Medico-Chirurgical Review*, it was nonetheless "most assuredly to them that the merit belongs of first boldly canvassing the subject" of a "horrid propensity to commit murder."[114] Phrases like the "propensity to steal" and "propensity to murder," along with the visual identification of the organs of murder and theft, became part of an American scientific vernacular used to explain crime. This language of propensity and visual language of organs, mobilized by phrenological enthusiasts and nonphrenologists alike, allowed for continuity within scientific approaches to the criminal throughout the nineteenth century.

From its origins in Continental craniology, the criminal was an essential object for the development of phrenological theory. Gall and Spurzheim made use of the prison as a research site, using the bodies and skulls of convicts to develop and promote their theories of character and its correspondence with organs. The "organ of murder" was one of the best-studied organs within the phrenological canon, signaling its centrality to phrenological theory. Even as such language was replaced, a new, subtler way of looking at and speaking about skulls emerged and spread—a language of propensity that would inflect discussions of criminality throughout the nineteenth century.

In the play that opened this chapter, the question Sir Thomas asked Percy in order to determine the culprit responsible for the murder—"Has he the organs of murder, malice, destructiveness, and lying?"[115]—was certainly intended to poke fun at the pretensions of phrenologists, as were his far-reaching parliamentary acts, which would have made phrenologists of all members of the court and constabulary. But for some, such a question was not one to be taken lightly, and such proposals pointed the way toward practical solutions to the problems of crime. It was not in the more contested British context that phrenology would find an expression of this potential, but in the United States, where phrenology moved closer to Sir Thomas's vision of the practical applications of phrenology to crime than anywhere else.

Chapter 2

Transatlantic Societies and Skulls

Reporting on the affairs of her family and friends in Kensington, Pennsylvania, in December of 1823, a young American woman wrote a gossipy letter to her friend Anne Nelson, in which she recounted the pretensions of her visiting cousin, Francis, who "thinks that he can be a Poet-Sculpter-Painter [*sic*] or any thing in short that he pleases."[1] She highlighted, with some mirth, Francis's search for the perfect woman to marry: "for a great beauty she must be—with a grecian face—wide shoulders & hips—flesh sufficiently solid & all the proper bumps on her head—for he is a great believer, you must know, in this science of Phenology-Crainology [*sic*]."[2] Francis already inspected his servants in the same way, rejecting at least one for the shape of his forehead.[3] As early as 1823, average Americans were accessing phrenological concepts and putting them into practice. This young woman might have found her cousin's adherence to the science to be foolhardier than not, but the risible Francis might have been ahead of the curve.

Cousin Francis's adoption of phrenology was right on the heels—and near the site—of early American adherents. As early as 1805, articles began to appear on the pages of American newspapers and magazines describing a remarkable new science, "Dr. Gall's system of Craniology," and the "singularity of [the] opinions," of the German medical celebrity.[4] They reported on the banning of Gall's lectures in his native land, his subsequent popularity with a growing circle of followers, the early successes of the new science and its founder, and the general outlines of its principles.[5] The new science—alternately referred to as craniology, craniometry and, eventually, phrenology—seemed poised to elicit the same "profound admiration" in eager American readers as in its European disciples.[6] Early American reports on this foreign science further focused on one particular aspect of Gall's research and teachings: its application to and use of criminal minds, and Gall's prison visits.[7]

By the 1820s and early 1830s, conversations and controversies bridged American and British phrenologists into a shared community focused in particular on the question of the applicability of phrenology to crime. American and British phrenological enthusiasts together constituted a transatlantic network. These fruitful connections sometimes fueled controversy on either side of the Atlantic, but they were essential to the building of a shared intellectual community that saw in phrenology a path to expertise in various fields. This community, drawn particularly from American and British urban centers, mutually supported the efforts of phrenological societies to build social, intellectual, and material capital through the circulation of texts, objects, and people.[8] In this, they followed earlier, colonial-era patterns of transatlantic participation in the making of knowledge about medicine and health.[9] Through these connections and with a particular emphasis on criminal theory, phrenology made its way to the United States, where it helped to spur the development of phrenological enthusiasm among elite, mostly urban professionals—particularly physicians and lawyers. These phrenological enthusiasts, centered in northern cities (particularly Philadelphia, Washington, and especially Boston), eagerly adopted phrenological tenets, as translated through British print culture and promoted by luminaries like Spurzheim and Combe, and adapted the science for the young nation.

Building Transatlantic Phrenological Networks

Print culture was crucial to the transatlantic circulation of knowledge about phrenology; indeed, as James Poskett argues, "publication and reception were activities grounded in a global world of material exchange."[10] In Early Republic America, Philadelphia served as a nexus for the circulation of print and other materials about phrenology: by 1800, Philadelphia's book trade had grown to eighty-eight firms, making it the center of the American book trade, with New York and Boston in second and third place, respectively.[11] Even as the American book trade grew, however, it became more entangled in the London-based book trade. American print was decentralized, unregulated, and could not keep pace with demand, so British printers continued to direct the pace, shape, and priorities of the American book trade, providing a path for British and Continental authors and texts to make their way to the United States.[12]

The Philadelphia-based publisher Carey & Lea (after 1833, Carey, Lea, & Blanchard), founded by Henry Charles Carey and Isaac Lea in 1822, was the first

American publisher in the modern sense, directing the production of new books and reprints from acquisition through production and publicization.[13] They were the original publishers of James Fenimore Cooper's *The Last of the Mohicans*, with whom they had a long and profitable business relationship, and they later worked with other American authors, including Washington Irving, John Pendleton Kennedy, and Robert Ingersoll Lockwood.[14] Some relationships were less successful, as with John Neal, the novelist and phrenological enthusiast.[15] However, Carey & Lea was known in particular for its reprinting of British writers, especially novelists, including Jane Austen, Charles Dickens, Sir Walter Scott, and Mary Shelley,[16] as well as its broad list in the areas of science, medicine, law, and history.[17] Sometimes these two emphases came together, as with one of the first works published by the new firm in 1822: George Combe's *Essays on Phrenology*, edited and with a preliminary essay by John Bell, a Philadelphia-area physician.[18] The Careys published a number of phrenological works, both in translation and from American authors, becoming early adopters and promoters of phrenology in America.[19] A decade later, in 1838, a major and long-lasting phrenological journal, *The American Phrenological Journal and Miscellany*, originally directed primarily at a medical audience, would also begin publication in Philadelphia as well, through the publishing house of Adam Waldie.[20]

This transatlantic transmission of texts was often paired with the borrowing of other forums for the circulation of knowledge. In 1822, the same year in which Carey & Lea produced the first American edition of Combe's *Essays*, the first American phrenological society was founded in Philadelphia, only two years after the founding of the Edinburgh Phrenological Society. As Edinburgh was considered to be the "first among equals" among the centers of European medicine, it is perhaps not surprising that the example of this Society was borrowed by American medical men.[21] The aptly named Philip Syng Physick,[22] working alongside two other Philadelphia-area physicians, John Bell and Benjamin Coates, was the first president of what was then known as the Central Phrenological Society, a circle of prominent physicians.[23] With the first American phrenological society, medical luminaries preaching the gospel of phrenology, and a major publisher producing phrenological works, Philadelphia, already recognized as a leading center for American medicine, was poised to stand as the phrenological capital of America as well.[24]

The trio of Physick, Bell, and Coates would be replaced by other more peripatetic and prolific popularizers of phrenology—notably Dr. Charles Caldwell, a central figure for the early translation of phrenology to the United States. As a young man traveling through Europe, Caldwell heard Spurzheim lecture in

Paris, and after returning to America in 1821, he gave a series of lectures on the subject of phrenology to his medical students at Transylvania University in Kentucky, where he was a professor of medicine.[25] Caldwell repeated this class for his medical students at Transylvania and at the college of Louisville for several years. He then broadened his audience, giving popular lectures in Lexington, Louisville, and Nashville in Kentucky, and then later in Baltimore, Maryland, and Washington, DC, which precipitated the formation of phrenological societies in these cities and others throughout the 1820s and into the late 1830s.[26] Caldwell embodied the process of transatlantic phrenological adoption and dissemination.

Caldwell lectured, taught, and wrote on the doctrines of phrenology, penning the first phrenological text authored by an American, *Elements of Phrenology*, in 1824.[27] The book was intended by Caldwell not to amuse but to instruct—"Amusement is neither intended nor calculated to afford."[28] By writing this text for a scholarly medical audience, Caldwell set the stage for the early use of phrenology in America, where its reception would be focused among medical and other learned professionals. Other works followed, including the vehement *Phrenology Vindicated, and Antiphrenology Unmasked*; essays on the temperaments and on mental derangement; and an essay on penitentiary discipline and moral reform, among others on various medical matters.[29] Caldwell argued that phrenology was the science "the establishment of which no earthly power can resist," and for George Combe and other commentators of this era, it was Caldwell's valiant efforts to effect said establishment that linked him to the introduction of phrenology to America.[30] Combe, for example, esteemed him as "the American, who, above all others, has distinguished himself by his zeal and labours in favour of phrenology."[31] Combe was also inspired by Caldwell's writings on prison discipline in his revisions to *The Constitution of Man*, which informed his sixth chapter, on punishment.[32] Caldwell and his texts moved between British and American urban centers and the frontier, presaging the movement of phrenology itself.

Just as Caldwell's prolific publications and public profile sometimes obscured other pioneers in American phrenology, so too was Philadelphia's leading role in the establishment of phrenology in America soon to be displaced by another—Boston and its phrenological society, founded in 1832. Contemporaries like George Combe, as well as later historians, deemed the Boston Phrenological Society to be the most significant American phrenological circle, even though it was founded a full ten years after the phrenological society in Philadelphia and was preceded by at least one other phrenological society, in Washington, DC.[33] However, this focus on the Boston Phrenological Society and its origins has erased the interventions of earlier American societies into a transatlantic debate about the truth of phrenology and the place of criminal skulls as a focal point within the new science. Even as Americans were slowly being introduced to phrenological theories by Caldwell and others, early adopters of phrenology found themselves embroiled in a transatlantic controversy about the nature of phrenological knowledge and its application to criminality in particular.

Disputing Phrenology

The notorious William Burke and William Hare began a short-lived career of providing corpses for anatomical study in Edinburgh in 1827.[34] The first corpse they procured was that of a lodger in Hare's house; the body was taken from its coffin and sold to Dr. Robert Knox in November of 1827. The pair subsequently murdered sixteen people over the course of 1828 to the same ends, until their activities were uncovered. Burke, Hare, and both of their female partners were arrested and put on trial on Christmas Eve of 1828. Hare turned King's evidence and testified against Burke and his wife, Helen (Nelly) McDougal (or M'Dougal); the latter was found not guilty, but Burke was declared guilty and sentenced to be hanged. As a component of his sentence, the judge declared that Burke's body would be publicly dissected and preserved for posterity, a not uncommon punishment for criminals.[35]

The Burke and Hare murders, the trial, and Burke's execution all occurred in Edinburgh, the center of British phrenology.[36] Shortly after the execution, the Edinburgh *Phrenological Journal and Miscellany* featured an article on the phrenological developments of Burke and Hare, which had been read to the phrenological society in February of 1829.[37] After a lengthy disquisition on the nature of Burke's development, the author declared that "this case is highly instructive to the Phrenologist": "We have never taught, that a man cannot commit murder who has an organ of Benevolence, for every individual has all the organs; but that a man cannot commit cool murder without possessing Destructiveness largely developed, and here Destructiveness is very large. If it had been small, this case would have afforded a strong objection against that organ."[38] This infamous case provided further evidence for the correlation between particular organs and murderous behavior.

The Burke and Hare case became a focal point of a debate about the scientific validity and the social meaning of phrenology staged in print between Thomas Stone, medical student and antiphrenologist, and George Combe through 1829, a new episode of the decade-long Edinburgh phrenology debates.

In Geoffrey Cantor and Steven Shapin's dialogue about these debates, Cantor argued that "to all intents and purposes the Edinburgh debate over the scientific and philosophical basis of phrenology ended in 1828," as Combe and others hereafter moved from justifying the scientific basis of phrenology to considering the "social, political, and religious implications of phrenology."[39] Shapin disputed this dating of the "end" of this debate, seemingly chosen by Cantor as the year of the publication of Combe's *Constitution*. Moreover, Shapin asserted, "'social implications' *were* the debate, as much as technical issues were."[40] In this episode of the Edinburgh phrenology debates, the dispute between Stone and Combe, both the scientific justification *and* the social meaning of phrenology were at stake.[41]

Possibly inspired by the article in the *Phrenological Journal*, Stone opened this debate with a lecture read before the Royal Medical Society, for which he served as president, and subsequently published as a seventy-five-page treatise, which aimed to prove that phrenological theory was "in every respect as unfounded, and can as little be relied on, as any of those old physiognomical superstitions, of which they originally formed a part, and to which they are still essentially allied."[42] Stone used Burke and Hare to demonstrate the inadequacy of phrenological theory. Since phrenologists argued that "deliberate and selfish murderers possess always a large endowment of the alleged organ of destructiveness," then the skulls of Burke and Hare "should, on Phrenological principles, possess it exceedingly well developed."[43] Stone's examination of Burke's autopsy findings led him to conclude that "no such remarkable development was observable," and he included similar findings with regard to Hare, who he examined and measured himself.[44]

Stone's findings were not purely reliant on his examinations of Burke and Hare but were also based on studies of the heads of other criminals. To reinforce his argument, Stone appended six tables of measurements of various groups: all of the male crania in Spurzheim's collection; Englishmen; Scotsmen; Irishmen; thieves in an Edinburgh jail; and executed murderers from various anatomical museums.[45] Stone's approach was focused on data and measurement, and while he addressed many of the phrenological organs in his essay, his aim was to disprove the correspondence between Destructiveness and murder. He found that, contrary to phrenological doctrine, "the most atrocious murderers not only fail to possess a large endowment of the alleged organ of Destructiveness, but have it, very frequently, both *absolutely* and *relatively* below the average size."[46] Further, these same criminals often possessed high development of the "pretended organs of the moral sentiments."[47] In attacking the connection between Destructiveness and murder, as well as that between Acquisitiveness and theft, Stone attempted to demolish the central assumptions of phrenology itself.

George Combe, invoked with some disdain by Stone in his text, did not let this matter stand. First, in a letter to the editor of the *Edinburgh Weekly Journal* and then in a more direct *Answer to "Observations . . . ,"* Combe expressed his utter contempt for Stone, whose observations he deemed "so palpably ridiculous, that no man who understands the first elements of Phrenology . . . could have been deceived by them."[48] Combe argued that "it is easy for Mr Stone to mistify the public mind with measurements, and decimals, and assertions without foundation; but the eye and the hand will, in five minutes, refute a volume of such lucubrations."[49] In Combe's *Answer,* he was yet more pointed in his critique of Stone, attacking his method of measurement and bristling in particular at the charge of "dishonesty" of the phrenological method.[50] To this, Stone replied with his own *Rejoinder* to Combe's *Answer,* in which Stone gave a nearly line-by-line rebuttal to Combe's critiques of his *Observations.*

The back-and-forth between Stone and Combe turned on a few points. First, both authors were preoccupied with standards and methods of measurement. A chief device of Stone's attack on phrenology was the exactitude of his measurements and the mobilization of data on behalf of his argument. At the same time, Combe's argument rested in large part on contesting Stone's methodology, particularly his method of measuring the skull. Stone's rebuttal contended that he used the same principles of measurement as directed by Combe, expressing ironic surprise that "he now denounces this very mode of estimating its size as 'absolutely absurd and unintelligible!'"[51] This argument about methodology and measurement, however, primarily masked the underlying dispute, which was about the foundations of phrenology itself: the correspondence between crania and character. Moreover, the accusations on either side about truthfulness and deceit, and claims to trustworthiness and expertise, suggest the stakes of this debate—who could claim to be an expert, on what grounds, and in defense of *which* truth.

While to a certain extent the criminal subjects were merely the pretext for a larger debate about the validity of phrenology, the choice of criminals as case studies is telling. The focus on criminals in this debate over the truthfulness and utility of phrenological theory signals the centrality of the criminal to phrenology. Stone chose the criminal as a way to strike at the heart of phrenology. If one could disprove the connection between Destructiveness and the murderer as type, one could shake the foundations of the science. Moreover, while Burke and Hare were the inciting case study, Stone and Combe both were considering criminals more broadly, drawing from phrenological literature and other examples of infamous murderers, including those transmitted from afar.

In 1827, the Phrenological Society of Washington, DC, was only two years old when it published a short report by a Dr. J. A. Brereton, which comprised a phrenological analysis of the notorious Jacques Alexander Tardy, known as "Tardy the Pirate." Tardy was a celebrity criminal, albeit a fairly unsuccessful pirate. In 1827, he teamed up with three men—Jose Morando, Jose Hilario Casares, and Felix Barbeito—and together they boarded the brig *Crawford* in Cuba with plans to kill the officers and take the ship and its cargo as their own. On June 1, the conspirators attacked, killing all but three of the sailors. The conspirators then sailed to Norfolk, Virginia, where one of the survivors of the attack made his way ashore and revealed the murders. Tardy, knowing he would soon be discovered, committed suicide; Morando, Casares, and Barbeito were apprehended, put on trial before Chief Justice John Marshall (then serving on the Circuit Court of Raleigh, Virginia), found guilty, and hanged.[52]

Upon hearing of Tardy's demise, Brereton wrote to J. Everett, a surgeon of the U.S. Army stationed at Fort Monroe, near where Tardy had been interred, requesting Tardy's skull. This request was granted expediently, and Everett assured the phrenological society that the head was really that of Tardy: "I knew him and carefully examined him when dead—saw him buried, which was more than a mile from that of any other dead body."[53] The skull thus verified in its authenticity, Everett presented it to the Washington society, which prepared casts from it. The society found Tardy to have Destructiveness and Amativeness "very large" and Cautiousness "rather small." [54] Tardy's skull was also compared with those of fifteen other criminals executed for murder, based on caliper measurements, suggesting that this was a recognizable group that could be considered both comparatively and as a set. Brereton's report concluded that "Tardy, in his deportment, was harsh, uncouth and awkward," as well as "quarrelsome . . . particularly with his inferiors to whom he was overbearing and extremely severe."[55]

This report of Tardy included the measurements of the three co-conspirators in the matter of the *Crawford*, indicated by their aliases, Don Felix or Felix (Barbeito), Couro or Courro (Morando), and Pepe (Casares). In texts, the three Spaniards received much less attention than Tardy. As a celebrity pirate, it is not surprising he received the majority of the attention, but their nationality or ethnic identities likely played some role. Tardy's French nationality was often discussed with some dismay, as his "harsh, uncouth, and awkward" demeanor seemed to be counter to expected French behavior. Meanwhile, Felix, Courro, and Pepe were all Spaniards "of the darkest hue."[56] Perhaps some assumptions about ethnic identity and animality provided self-evident explanations for their behaviors, whereas Tardy's French-ness only raised questions. In most accounts of the *Crawford* affair, Tardy was framed as the mastermind, with the three Spaniards seemingly the brawn, not the brains, of the operation. Finally, Tardy's rather shocking suicide at the end of the crime—"'*he cut his own throat from ear to ear*'"[57]—and the loss of catharsis from him not being brought to justice likely prompted some of the fascination with Tardy. Even so, Brereton sent a report and casts of the skulls of all four of the men to Combe and the Edinburgh society.[58]

The skulls and the report provided by the Washington society provided fuel for the fire between Combe and Stone. Both cited the Washington report that appeared in *The Phrenological Journal and Miscellany*. In his first article, Stone borrowed Brereton's data on Pepe (though not Tardy), arguing that the organ of Destructiveness was mismeasured and misrepresented by the Washington society: "I do not pretend to know what sort of callipers are used in America . . . but of this I am satisfied, that the organ of Destructiveness has here been represented more than half an inch larger than it actually measures."[59] This discrepancy was suggested to him by Sir William Hamilton, an antiphrenologist, who observed that Pepe's skull was in fact particularly narrow in the span from Destructiveness to Destructiveness.[60] Stone concluded that "here, therefore, is the skull of a cold-blooded and execrable murderer, not only failing to possess a large organ of Destructiveness, but possessing it, according to *any* standard, absolutely and relatively below the average."[61]

While Stone addressed a number of other examples of criminals in his *Observations*, the Pepe case became a central point of the dispute between Stone and Combe. In Combe's *Answer*, while he deemed it "unnecessary to discuss Mr Stone's statements farther in detail," he was nonetheless "compelled" to defend the Washington society from accusations of incompetence.[62] Combe recapitulated the Tardy case and described the provenance of the skull of Pepe, charging Stone with having failed to measure it himself at the Phrenological Hall. Combe explained there were two skulls with the name of "Pepe"—only one was the murderer in question. Stone's error led him to use the wrong skull to draw his wrongheaded conclusions.

In Stone's point-by-point rebuttal of Combe, meanwhile, he devoted three pages to refuting these specific charges. He argued that the phrenological casts of hanged persons "being taken over the distended integuments, they are utterly *worthless*."[63] Stone averred that Destructiveness often measured "more on the *cast* than it did on the *head* during life," an indefensible and persistent limit to drawing conclusions about the heads of hanged murderers.[64] Stone's further defense was that the two alleged Pepes, in any event, were both murderers, Spaniards, and pirates, and so "how is Phrenology affected by the discovery of there having been *two* monsters of the name of Pepe?"[65] Stone disdained the phrenological project to the extent that he "should never dream of visiting the Phrenological Hall for the purpose of measuring casts," and so conversed directly with Professor Graham, the keeper of the skull of the "other" Pepe, which, despite a history of violence and murder, nevertheless conveyed the same measurements: a deficiency of Destructiveness. Thus, "instead of *one* Antiphrenological Pepe, there are now *two* Antiphrenological Pepes."[66]

The problem of Pepe exemplified a broader debate about the nature of phrenological truth, the means of phrenological measurement, and the correspondence between Destructiveness and murderous potential. The focal point of this debate was the immediate matter at hand, that of Burke and Hare. Yet this debate both was and wasn't about Pepe, or Burke and Hare, for that matter, but about the nature of phrenological truth and its utility in determining criminal responsibility.

This dispute demonstrates that American phrenological writers were not repeating or reprinting British and Continental phrenological texts in a purely receptive and passive mode. They were also producing new knowledge, including statistical data, and objects, like the casts of skulls, which were then transmitted to Britain, where they were adopted and mobilized. Further, the high stakes of this debate, which centered around Combe's authority, phrenology's validity, and Burke and Hare's culpability, demonstrate that American authors were esteemed to be of equal worth to sources and authorities closer to home. The Washington society was worthy of Combe's attention and defense, just as its data and the skulls it provided were essential to this dispute. The circulation of knowledge, skulls, and publications in this episode demonstrate the interconnectedness of the various societies and their role in communicating phrenological knowledge even as it was being developed. American phrenologists were not disconnected from British or Continental phrenology, but part of an ever-widening network of phrenologists. While American phrenological knowledge played only a minor part in this dispute, over the next decade, as phrenology came increasingly under siege in Combe's Edinburgh, a new cohort of elite, professional phrenological enthusiasts embraced the lessons of phrenology from a new epicenter: Boston.

Generating Phrenological Enthusiasm

Despite the uses of Washington data in the Stone/Combe controversy, or the early work of Caldwell and the Philadelphia phrenologists, the Boston

Phrenological Society has often been identified as the early heart of American phrenology, particularly for rigorous study of the science.[67] The preeminence of this society was enabled in part by its cultural context: it could not have developed or achieved the prominence it did if not for political and social currents within the city itself.

Boston, the "Athens of America," underwent profound change and growth in the decades following the Revolutionary War, and by the 1820s, New England community leaders "set out to establish Boston as the cultural standard by which national progress would henceforth be measured" through an extensive program of both formal urban renewal and charitable projects.[68] Philanthropic and reform efforts focused on remaking the city in an enlightened mold and promoting elite institutions, like Harvard University and Massachusetts General Hospital, as well as attending to problems of poverty, homelessness, intoxication, and crime, including penal reform.[69] At the same time, Boston elites consciously drew upon "City Upon a Hill" ideology, positioning themselves as intellectual and moral leaders of the young republic. Writers like Ralph Waldo Emerson, Nathaniel Hawthorne, and Henry David Thoreau were part of an American literary renaissance originating in New England, alongside the burgeoning Transcendental movement, which provided the critical mass of writers, philosophers, poets, and novelists that enabled Boston to claim its own artistic and intellectual elite.[70] By the 1840s and 1850s, Boston's intellectual culture had achieved "hegemony over the American mind," eclipsing the cultural and intellectual work occurring in other cities.[71]

By the 1830s, Boston was a growing, increasingly prosperous and influential city in flux, and its leaders and elites were invested in improvement, reform, and self-promotion as a model for the young country. The elites and intelligentsia of the city were, like those of other cities in Europe and the United States, developing forums and societies for the exclusive participation of these elites; commentators like Alexis de Tocqueville suggested that in this, Boston was the closest of the American cities to those of Europe.[72] However, Boston was distinct in at least two ways, according to Thomas H. O'Connor: first, Boston's elite was not exclusively comprised of academics or great poets and writers, but also welcomed physicians, lawyers, religious leaders, businessmen of varied industries, and women.[73] Second, there was a vested interest among this diverse intelligentsia to open the doors further to a general audience. Rather than hoard knowledge and resources for themselves, they wanted to make it possible for the lower classes to improve themselves.[74] Societies, academies, public lectures, and town lyceums were supported by print culture in the promotion of these new (and often uniquely American) forms of literature, philosophy, science, and other modes of knowledge production, often through the growth of circulating libraries.[75] Boston and New England were also the heart of the lyceum movement in the 1820s, which was focused on promoting practical knowledge among the working classes as a means to democratize knowledge.[76]

Boston was a fruitful place for the development of a new scientific society, the circulation of new scientific knowledge, and the promotion of theories that centered the reform of intransigent social issues. Phrenology, hotly contested in Edinburgh, would experience a more welcoming environment in Boston, where a broader public would also be able to access its print culture and its promoters. While the mode of phrenological enthusiasm promoted in Boston was primarily elite in nature, the openness of New England intellectual discourse also helped to sow the seeds for a broader embrace of phrenology among middle- and lower-class audiences.

The preeminence of the Boston Phrenological Society was also due to the auspicious nature of its founding, as it was tied directly to the life—and death—of one of the founders of the field, Johann Gaspar Spurzheim. In August of 1832, Spurzheim journeyed to the United States, the first trip by one of the founders to American soil. Spurzheim landed first in New York City and traveled to New Haven, Connecticut, where he was welcomed warmly by the president of Yale College, Benjamin Silliman, and participated in commencement.[77] From New Haven he traveled to Hartford, where Dr. Amariah Brigham served as his tour guide as he visited the Asylum for the Deaf and Dumb, the Connecticut State Prison, and the Retreat for the Insane.[78] By August 20, in the third week of his American tour, Spurzheim arrived in Boston, where he commenced a series of lectures at the Boston Athenæum before the popularity of his course compelled him to find a grander stage at the Masonic Temple and to add further lectures in Cambridge.[79] At the invitation of the president of Harvard, Josiah Quincy, he attended Harvard commencement and the meeting of the Phi Beta Kappa Society, and he also delivered a series of lectures to the medical faculty at Harvard and other professional men.[80] His packed Boston lecture schedule may have been his undoing: Spurzheim soon took ill and, after convalescence supported by his medical friends in Boston, passed away on November 10, 1832.[81] He was a month shy of fifty-six years of age.

Spurzheim's death was a momentous occasion in Boston. The day after his death, his friends convened to decide how to memorialize him. Quincy chaired this meeting, in which the group collectively made arrangements for the funeral and the distribution of his property.[82] The Boston Medical Association also convened a special session on November 14 to respond to the untimely death, voting unanimously to adopt a resolution that declared "that we view the decease of Dr. SPURZHEIM and the termination of his labors as a calamity to mankind, and, in a special manner, to this country," and directing the members of the organization to attend his funeral en masse.[83] On November 17, 1832, twelve physicians, led by John Collins Warren, Sr., and including Samuel Gridley Howe, examined and embalmed Spurzheim's body at Harvard Medical School, preserving the skull and brain for future study.[84] From the medical college, a well-attended public procession conveyed his body to a funeral held at Old South Church in Boston, with a funeral oration by Charles Follen, a Harvard professor of theology.[85] Finally, the body was interred in the Mount Auburn cemetery in Cambridge, the second person accorded the honor.[86] Nearly three thousand people attended these various ceremonies.[87]

Spurzheim's unexpected death "cast a gloom over the city," but it also served as a goad to the development of phrenology in America.[88] One month later, on December 31, 1832—the date of Spurzheim's birth—eminent men of Boston gathered in the Masonic Temple to found a new phrenological society.[89] Spurzheim's life and recent death were cited as the reason for the existence of the new society: "To his recent visit and labors amongst us, the existence of our Society is directly owing. In the midst of us he delivered his latest testimony in its favor; a testimony to which death has now set his seal, under circumstances calculated to bestow upon it a more than common interest."[90] Within three months, the new Boston Phrenological Society had ninety members, and by 1836 it claimed 127 members.[91] In 1834, the Society established the *Annals of Phrenology*, the first (albeit short-lived) phrenological periodical in America, which was, at first, primarily an organ for the republication of essays from the Edinburgh *Phrenological Journal and Miscellany*, as well as other journals like *The Lancet*, and a receptacle for the research conducted by members of the Boston Phrenological Society.[92] Phrenology was also promoted in the *Boston Medical and Surgical Journal*, the mouthpiece of Harvard Medical School and Massachusetts General Hospital, signaling the extent to which the Boston medical community supported phrenology.[93]

The recording secretary for the new Society was Nahum Capen, a lawyer who had been among those charged with the care of Spurzheim's personal effects after his death. Capen was also a publisher who had established Marsh, Capen & Lyon, the Boston publishing house that was responsible, along with Carey & Lea in Philadelphia, for some of the earliest American editions and translations of the works of Combe, Gall, and Spurzheim.[94] At the time of Spurzheim's death in 1832, Marsh, Capen & Lyon already offered four of Spurzheim's texts, and they rapidly expanded their phrenological offerings.[95] The publishing firm produced a number of phrenological texts by various writers throughout the 1830s and 1840s, as well as the *Annals of Phrenology*, and they also sold phrenological casts.[96] As with Carey & Lea, this publishing house helped to shepherd phrenology into a broader public, particularly by republishing works by the Combe brothers and Spurzheim for an American audience. The close ties between this publisher and the Society helped to further promote the publications and spread of phrenological texts.

The establishment of the Boston Phrenological Society coincided with a great groundswell of interest in phrenology in America, spurred in part by Spurzheim's death.[97] In an American edition of *The Constitution of Man*, Combe listed twelve new phrenological societies that had been founded in America by 1834, two years after Spurzheim's death, up from just three lone societies—Philadelphia, Washington, DC, and Boston.[98] The increase in the number of societies was a sign of rising interest in this period, but the geographic locations of these new societies also suggested a further shift: the locus of phrenological enthusiasm in America had become New England, with the Boston Phrenological Society at its center, due to the eminence of its members and their prolific publications, as well as its self-conscious connection to Spurzheim's legacy.[99] Not only did these new societies look to Boston as their guide, but several of them also asked Boston physicians and members of the Society to serve as officers and presidents (albeit in absentia) of these new societies.[100]

Phrenological enthusiasm was further transnational in nature—or even global, as James Poskett argues.[101] Caldwell, Spurzheim, and Combe all traveled back and forth between Europe and the United States, and Physick became the first American appointed to the French Académie royale de médecine.[102] Texts and objects, particularly skulls and casts of heads, moved between American and European metropoles. So too did letters, which "allowed phrenologists to connect apparently local issues to global politics."[103] Nahum Capen's papers provide a hint as to how this network operated and how far-flung its participants were.[104] These letters included correspondents from across the United States—a number from Boston and other Northeastern towns and cities, but also letters from South Carolina, Florida, Kentucky (from Charles Caldwell), Ohio, and Indiana. Capen's global correspondents included writers in Paris, Liverpool, Dublin, Copenhagen, London, Edinburgh, and a number of other British cities. Capen and other Boston phrenological enthusiasts participated in an ongoing, transnational conversation about the progress of their science.

Global or not, phrenological enthusiasm in the 1830s, especially around the locus of the Boston Phrenological Society, was certainly elite and medical in nature.[105] The original officers, for example, included Rev. John Pierpont, serving as president; Dr. Jonathan Barber, member of the London Royal College of

Surgeons and professor of elocution at Harvard University, as vice president; Dr. Samuel Gridley Howe, as corresponding secretary; Capen, lawyer and publisher, as corresponding secretary; and three physicians on its four-man council.[106] The Oneida Phrenological Society in New York, founded in 1835, had John McCall, a Boston physician, as its president, and included among its officers a professor at Hamilton College, a reverend, a physician, and two lawyers.[107] A decade earlier, the entrance of phrenology in America had similarly been shepherded by a group of physicians: Caldwell, Bell, Physick, and Coates. The status of these men in medical circles was not diminished by their association with phrenology, and if anything, grew in concert with the profile of phrenology. Physick, for example, was elected president of the Central Phrenological Society in 1822 while he was a professor of surgery at the University of Pennsylvania. Two years later, he was chosen to be the president of the Philadelphia Medical Society as well, a position he held until his death in 1838, and in 1825 he was appointed to the French Académie royale de médecine.[108] Coates and Bell, meanwhile, were both active members in the College of Physicians in Philadelphia.[109]

Students at medical schools also pursued phrenology as part of their medical curricula, with some even receiving their medical degrees based on theses on the subject. In 1830, for example, Leonard C. Taylor was conferred the degree of Doctor of Medicine at the University of Maryland, for a thesis on phrenology.[110] The following year, another medical student, Burwell R. Bobo, along with forty-one of his peers, became a Doctor of Medicine on the basis of his dissertation on "Phrenology as applied to Pathology and Surgery" at Transylvania University, in Lexington, Kentucky, where Charles Caldwell led the medical faculty.[111] Other men who received medical degrees on the basis of theses on phrenology included Samuel Harby, awarded the medical degree in 1832 from the medical college of Charleston College, Charleston, South Carolina; Francis H. Hamilton, awarded the medical degree in 1835 from the University of Pennsylvania medical department, Philadelphia, Pennsylvania; Martin Dunn, awarded the medical degree in 1837 from the College of Physicians and Surgeons of the Western District, Fairfield, New York; J. H. Worthington, awarded the medical degree in 1838 from Jefferson Medical College, Philadelphia, Pennsylvania; C. S. Kaufman, awarded the medical degree in 1841, from the Pennsylvania College medical department, Philadelphia, Pennsylvania; Miles M. Rogers, awarded the medical degree in 1842, from Geneva Medical College, Syracuse, New York; and J. F. McComb, awarded the medical degree in 1843 from the Medical College of the State of South Carolina, Charleston, South Carolina.[112] Professors like Caldwell also lectured to their medical students on the subject of phrenology, and other medical schools included courses on the subject in their curriculum, as at the Ohio Reformed Medical College.[113] Medical theses suggest that students incorporated phrenological theory and figures, especially Gall, into their theses on related subjects, especially those on the brain or insanity.[114] In this period, phrenology also sometimes received favorable commentary in medical journals and texts as well.[115]

Phrenological enthusiasts, particularly those with medical training, thought of their approach as distinct from so-called practical or popular phrenology and its practice of reading heads. "The most prevailing evil" for the progress of phrenology, a writer in the *Annals* argued, "is the practice of examining heads."[116] "There are individuals who make it their business, have their shops, and receive pay for their manipulations, so much *per* head!" the author complained, a practice he argued was degrading to the science and brought in only "superficial" (presumably popular, and nonintellectual) converts.[117] This author concluded that a rule for all phrenologists should be to examine "*no heads of living individuals of respectable standing*," an edict that allowed for prison examinations and similar practices.[118] This author was not alone in his protests against the scourge of reading heads and itinerant phrenologists, which were common objects of ire in this early period of phrenological adoption. This distinction was crucial to the self-fashioning of early adopters of phrenology, who were primarily concerned with "promoting Phrenology in a way more in accordance with scientific taste," and therefore attempted to distance themselves from those who adopted phrenology as a profession.[119]

In this attitude, American phrenological enthusiasts were much in accord with George Combe. Despite the fact that Combe framed his 1838–1840 trip through the United States as a "phrenological visit," generally speaking he refused offers to give single lectures, as opposed to courses of lectures, and thought poorly of itinerant lecturing on all subjects.[120] Combe argued that the progress of phrenology was impeded by such brief explorations of its doctrines. Similarly, he spoke with disdain of the growing cadre of "Practical Phrenologists" who "examine heads and write characters for fees."[121] Combe feared that the growing popularity of these practices would create "a strong feeling of disgust against Phrenology itself, in the minds of men of science and education."[122] In this, he proved to be prescient: by the 1840s, practical phrenologists, modeled in particular after the Fowler brothers, Orson Squire and Lorenzo Niles, became the primary exponents of the science, and the image of the phrenologist as one who examines heads for a fee became cemented in popular culture. However, at least in the 1830s, Combe and the Boston circle remained convinced that elite, scientific phrenology had an important place in the United States, and those who lectured on phrenology in the 1830s were as likely to be professors at institutions like Harvard University, like the Rev. James Walker, as itinerant practical phrenologists.[123]

George Combe's visit to the United States from 1838 through 1840 reinforced this growing interest among the professional classes in phrenology.[124] Combe's trip was taken in the spirit of Spurzheim's aborted earlier visit, and he began by following his mentor's footsteps, landing in New York and lecturing first in Boston before continuing on to other cities.[125] Combe's journey through the United States afforded him the ability to lecture extensively on the topic of phrenology. He was hosted and assisted in various cities by local physicians, like Bell and Brigham, and welcomed by physicians, professors, judges, and other notables in his visits to colleges, museums, prisons, asylums, hospitals, and other institutions. Combe's well-attended lectures and prior fame spurred interest in phrenology and contributed to the enthusiasm with which the science was increasingly met.

The enthusiasm with which Combe and his ideas were received, in turn, reinforced his status as an esteemed intellectual, at least in the United States. In 1836, when Combe was a candidate for the professorship of logic and metaphysics at the University of Edinburgh, a number of American individuals and groups wrote letters of support to Combe or the Boston Phrenological Society affirming their support of his candidacy.[126] The Massachusetts Medical Society, for example, wrote a letter to Combe proclaiming that "for the benefit of our fellow men, and for the reputation of the distinguished university of your city, we sincerely hope and trust that you will be the successful candidate for the office you have applied for."[127] This letter was signed by twelve physicians, including the professor of surgery of Harvard University, Dr. George Hayward. From Baltimore, a selection of six professors in medicine and the humanities from the University of Maryland, one professor from the Medical College of the State of South Carolina, the Secretary for the Maryland Academy of Sciences, a physician, and two counselors-at-law collectively signed an effusive endorsement of Combe's candidacy, "as a man of high minded powers and fine cultivation."[128] Another, similar letter was sent from Washington College in Hartford, Connecticut, signed by three professors, as well as Edward Terry, physician to the Connecticut Retreat for the Insane, and Amariah Brigham. This letter enthused that "Mr. Combe has unfolded the true science of the human mind; and the learning, candor & excellence of his writings show that he must be eminently qualified" for the post."[129] Other examples, in letters and in printed dedications to texts short and long, abound.[130]

The support of Combe in his candidacy for the position at Edinburgh, despite his loss of the position to Sir William Hamilton, suggests the strong connections between American and British phrenology, and the extent to which American phrenologists were not necessarily subordinate to British phrenologists. These supporters and phrenological enthusiasts had ties to elite institutions, given their status as learned intellectuals in various professions, and they shared their intellectual and social capital with their fellow enthusiasts abroad. Well wishes and publications, however, were not the only kinds of capital that were shared and transmitted across the Atlantic: material objects were also essential forms of capital used to support growing societies.

Collecting Criminals

In May of 1833, Amariah Brigham wrote from Hartford, Connecticut, to the then-secretary of the Boston Phrenological Society, Nahum Capen, offering an account of some skulls he hoped to procure from the local prison. Several men were currently on trial for murder and "two or more will undoubtedly be hung," and perhaps those skulls might be of some interest.[131] In the course of this letter, he reminisced about a phrenological excursion to the Hartford prison with Spurzheim. Brigham described how Spurzheim identified the two leaders of the conspiracy to commit murder—the very men Brigham expected would be hung. Spurzheim "begged" to examine the head of one particular conspirator minutely, and, on the basis of this examination, proclaimed that the convict was a "dangerous man—capable of doing any wickedness."[132] Although this was not a public proof of the truth of phrenology, this example was sufficient to impress both the warden of the prison and the young phrenological enthusiast, Brigham, and it was also discussed in later publications.[133]

Five months later, in September of 1833, Nathaniel Shurtleff had a hard trek from Boston to Hartford. On the first night of his trip, the young man was obliged to stay outside of Worcester, due to the lack of stagecoaches to take him to Connecticut. Luckily, the next day he found his way into a covered wagon, and hence into a chaise, then to the top of a stagecoach, and finally into another coach crowded with crying children and their harried mothers. At the end of this "troublesome time" and upon reaching Hartford, a valuable prize awaited: the casts of the heads of two criminals, procured for him and hence for the Society by Brigham.[134]

These casts (figures 4 and 5) can be identified as William Teller and Cæsar Reynolds based on the catalogue of the Boston Phrenological Society, which provides further details of the event.[135] Teller was the primary instigator of the

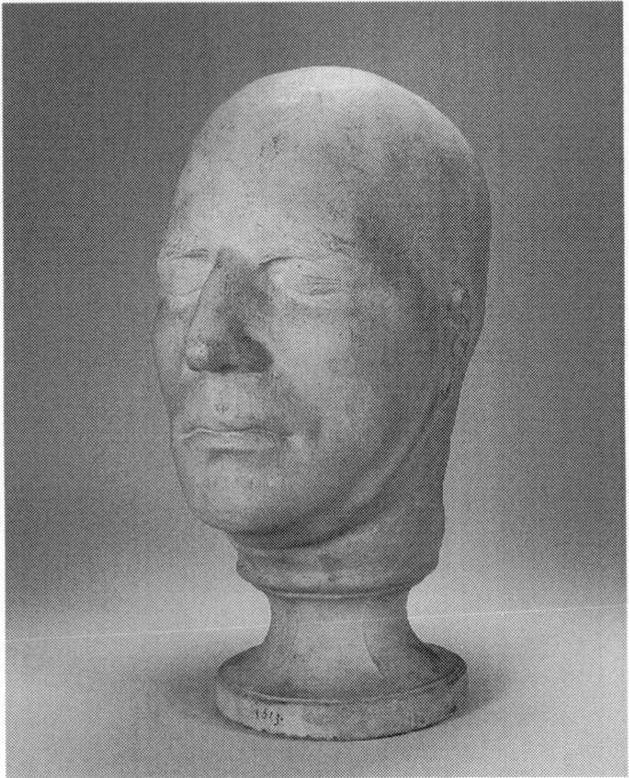

Figure 4. Phrenological cast of the head of William Teller, most likely cast by Nathaniel Shurtleff. Originally part of the Boston Phrenological Society cabinet. Warren Anatomical Museum in the Francis A. Countway Library of Medicine.

plan, but Reynolds, "under the influence of his destructive feelings, committed the murder."[136] In this case, the behavior of the two was interpreted using a racialized lens: Reynolds, who was Black, was described as "under the influence of his destructive feelings," compelled by his violent instincts, whereas Teller, who was white, was positioned as the mastermind of the scheme. The juxtaposition of the two—one with large animal organs, the other with larger reflective faculties—both descriptively and visually mimics the small and large Destructiveness illustration of figure 2, this time more overtly prefigured with racialized assumptions about qualities of mind and capabilities to plan and commit violent crime.[137]

The details provided in the catalogue for these and other specimens may have been the work of Shurtleff, the young man who procured these casts.

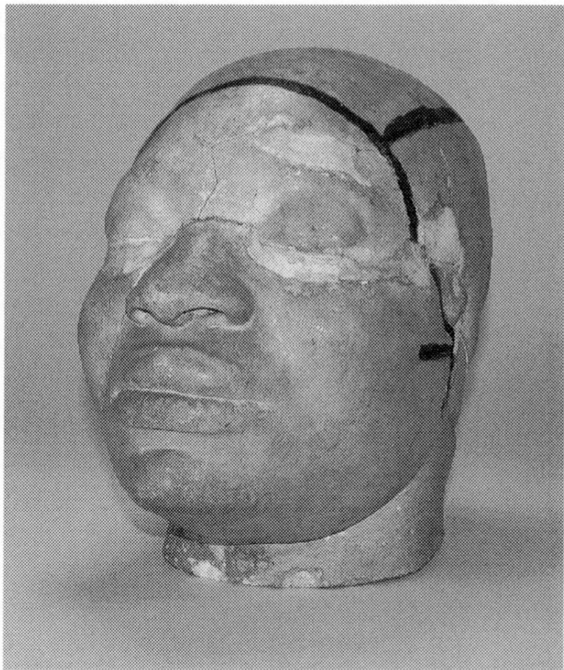

Figure 5. Phrenological cast of the head of Cæsar Reynolds, most likely cast by Nathaniel Shurtleff. Originally part of the Boston Phrenological Society cabinet. Warren Anatomical Museum in the Francis A. Countway Library of Medicine.

Decades later, in the 1860s, Shurtleff was elected the mayor of Boston, and he would also later become known for his antiquarian and historical works.[138] In 1833, however, he was just twenty-three years of age, a year away from receiving his medical degree at Harvard University, and dedicated to the phrenological cause.[139] As the curator for the cabinet of the Boston Phrenological Society, he was responsible for the care and creation of many of the casts held in this collection, along with his co-curator, H. T. Tukerman.[140] This cabinet had its origins in the cabinet of Spurzheim, as after his death, the Society absorbed his cabinet, a fortunate and timely acquisition.[141] Not content to rest with this founding collection, Society members worked hard to acquire ever more busts, casts, skulls, and death masks. By the time a catalogue of the cabinet was published in 1835, it comprised two subcollections: one, consisting of 286 numbered specimens, was attributed to Spurzheim and J. D. Holm, a London phrenologist; the second half of the collection, with a further 130 specimens, had been collected by the Society in the first three years of its existence, including Shurtleff's hard-won casts procured at Hartford.[142] Producing a phrenological cabinet was an exercise in both local and transatlantic networking, with skulls, casts, and busts passing from one phrenologist (or society) to the next.

The Society cast a broad net in its selection of heads for its cabinet, in order to capture the diversity of humanity. Perhaps the greatest number were casts of individuals who were exceptional in some way: so-called great men, such as Oliver Cromwell and Napoleon Bonaparte, as well as phrenological celebrities, like Gall and Spurzheim. But a number were esteemed as they related to particular phrenological organs, like writers, musicians, and artists of note, while others were unnamed or obscure but nonetheless exceptional, such as no. 232, "S. L. Kent. Can tell accurately how many yards of a carpet will cover any sized room," a useful talent indeed.[143] A not insignificant portion of the cabinet was devoted to "national types," or ethnic exemplars, especially Indigenous Americans. A section of the catalogue simply labeled "Nationals" included thirty-eight such specimens, ranging from "English form" and "Celtic" to "Jew," "Burmese," "Chinese," "Esquimaux," "Hindoo," "Highlander," and "African Negro."[144] Later additions to the cabinet raised the number of casts of national types to around seventy, with an emphasis on Indigenous notables, chiefs, and warriors from the Northeast. In this, the Society was both presaging and participating in the craniometric project of Samuel George Morton, the nineteenth-century pioneer of racial science and ethnography, whose own cabinet featured a similar variety of skulls, focusing on national and Indigenous types.[145]

Morton's *Crania Americana* was well received by the phrenologists of this era, particularly George Combe, who published an anonymous and exhaustive review of "the most extensive and valuable contribution to the natural history of man" in Benjamin Silliman's *American Journal of Science*.[146] Combe's participation in the development of the project and his promotion of the work was key to its embrace by phrenologists.[147] Morton had been a medical student at the University of Edinburgh in 1825 when Combe was a lecturer there, and it is possible that Morton became aware of phrenology during his studies.[148] Combe and Morton also became personally acquainted, first meeting in Morton's own cabinet in Philadelphia in 1838, where the two discussed Morton's collection and methods of measuring the skull.[149] Impressed with the collection and Morton's theories, Combe offered to write an appendix and to help advertise the book, including the anonymous review.[150]

While a clear distinction was usually made by contemporary commentators between Morton's science and phrenology—"He does not enter the field as a partisan, for or against Dr. Gall's doctrines," in Combe's words—his theories were nevertheless connected to and compared with phrenology in the reception of his work.[151] Combe corresponded with Morton during and after his travels in the United States, and the two also exchanged and borrowed skulls from one another's collections.[152] Both Morton and phrenological enthusiasts were interested in defining ethnic or "national" types in this period, and the Boston Phrenological Society was not unique in this emphasis. Indeed, Morton's collection of skulls was regarded as the "most extensive collection of crania in the United States" and even perhaps the world.[153] The Society could not have hoped to match Morton, at least in the collection of skulls of national types.

Similar to the ways in which "national" types were collected and partitioned in this collection, the catalogue of the Boston Phrenological Society also listed "Idiots" and "Insane" as distinct sets, with more individuals matching these descriptions added to the second part of the expanded collection. The numbers here were roughly equivalent: about twenty "idiots" and twenty "insane" individuals were included in the collection. Most were anonymous examples of a type: "Insane Woman," "Brain of a suicide," or "Idiot inferior to Ourang Outang."[154] Following directly from the "Nationals" section in the first half of the catalogue, these subheadings suggested that "idiots" and the "insane" were separate in some way from the rest of humanity. While other comparable casts appeared throughout the collection, the majority were categorized under these headings.

Criminals also featured throughout the catalogue. While not all individuals were labeled with biographical details including their crime, it is possible to identify nearly fifty of the casts as belonging to criminals, constituting at least 10 percent of the collection—less than the national or ethnic types but more than the "idiots" and "insane" combined.[155] Most of these criminals were identified with specific phrenological organs, especially Destructiveness (thirty casts, all criminals, including Burke and Hare), Amativeness (a rapist, an incestuous father, a sodomite and suicide, and an infanticide), and Acquisitiveness (three thieves and an arsonist), among others. The second part of the cabinet expanded this collection of criminals with recent cases, such as Gibbs the pirate, Antoine Le Blanc, and Major Mitchell, who will be discussed in the next chapter.

In this focus on the criminal, the Boston Phrenological Society was taking cues from the example of the Edinburgh Phrenological Society and from Gall's own cabinet. The first edition of the Edinburgh *Transactions* included a list of donations to the cabinet's holdings for 1824, which included the heads of some notable individuals as well as the casts or skulls for at least three murderers.[156] A catalogue of the Society's holdings from this period suggests a similarly broad collection of the various types of humanity, including the heads of more than twenty named murderers, with another cluster of twenty-four specimens simply listed as "murderers," as well as other assorted criminal types.[157] The catalogue also included a number of specimens of different nationalities or ethnicities. Similarly, Gall's collection, as reported in a five-part series published in the Edinburgh *Phrenological Journal and Miscellany*, included a number of murderers, robbers, assassins, poisoners, highwaymen, and other villainous figures, as well as many notable individuals and national types, among its 354 human specimens.[158] The diversity of these collections—and the prominent place of criminal types—may have set the expectations for the platonic ideal of the phrenological cabinet, enshrining the criminal within it.

However robust the cabinet of the Boston Phrenological Society might have been, the heyday of the Society itself was short-lived. The cabinet languished in obscurity for the better part of the decade of the 1840s, until the defunct Society, through former corresponding secretary Samuel Gridley Howe, gave its cabinet of skulls, busts, and portraits into the keeping of John Collins Warren Sr. in 1850. The cabinet became a foundational part of the still young Warren Anatomical Museum, instituted only two years earlier. Letters to Warren reveal that, at the time of donation, the Society was in a not insignificant amount of debt. The cabinet had been stowed away for some time in an attic, and it had diminished in size from the numbers of specimens described in the 1835 catalogue.[159] A copy of the *Catalogue* from the Warren Anatomical Museum, annotated to reflect both missing specimens and later additions, illustrates the extent to which the collection was in disrepair, with many pieces falling by the wayside in the intervening years.[160]

The Boston Phrenological Society may have closed its doors and abandoned its cabinet, but other phrenologists were collectors as well. The Fowler brothers, Orson and Lorenzo, and their associate Dr. Samuel Wells in New York, in the establishment of their phrenological rooms, also included a cabinet to which they added frequently throughout the decades after its founding. As early as the late 1830s, the Fowlers' cabinet was viewed by contemporaries as exceptional: "He has an extensive phrenological cabinet, which, in number, variety, and choiceness of specimens, exceeds, probably, any other in the country, unless it be that in the possession of the Boston Phrenological Society."[161] Within a decade, the Boston cabinet no longer stood as competition, and the Fowlers were able to present their collection as the premier phrenological collection in the United States.

The catalogue for the Fowlers and Wells cabinet, published in 1850, began auspiciously, listing the busts of George Washington, Benjamin Franklin, George Cuvier, and Shakespeare on the first page.[162] Within pages, however, the who's-who list of great men and women began to include murderers and other criminals of less well-known names, as, unlike the catalogue for the cabinet of the Boston Phrenological Society, this collection was not organized into subheadings or categories. Only the last names of many of the subjects were listed, but as common were such listings as no. 193: "Murderer. An Englishman."[163] A full accounting of a separate collection of skulls was not provided, though the catalogue noted that this collection embraced the skulls and busts of "Statesmen, Lawyers, Ministers, Mechanics, Mothers, Misers, Murderers, Maniacs, Thieves, Pirates, and Idiots."[164] The Fowler and Wells catalogue, published some twenty years after that of the Boston Phrenological Society, was not dissimilar in scope or types represented, if less well organized.

The effect of the phrenological cabinet, whether that of the Boston Phrenological Society or the Fowler brothers, was often striking: here were the highs and lows of humanity, arranged artfully on the shelf of the man of science, for his amusement and the viewer's edification. The phrenological cabinet was a macabre iteration of the scientific collector's cabinet, a popular practice in the nineteenth century for both scientists and enthusiastic amateurs.[165] Rather than displaying seashells, fossils, pressed plants, or scientific instruments, the phrenological cabinet presented a parade of skulls, death masks, and busts. While the technique of display would have been familiar to the nineteenth-century viewer, such a cabinet would also have served as a powerful and perhaps anxiety-inducing *memento mori*. The phrenological cabinet also conveyed a moral message regarding good and bad heads and deeds. This site emerged in this period as the final resting place for a criminal, the cabinet the terminus of the rake's path through the criminal justice system. From the courtroom to the prison to the gallows and postmortem, transported across seas and over many hundreds of miles, the criminal's final indignity was to serve as a literal object lesson within the phrenological cabinet.

American phrenology developed in interaction with Continental and particularly British phrenology as elite phrenological enthusiasts of this period communicated and shared knowledge, texts, objects, and capital in a widespread network that connected British and American metropoles. This perception of a shared community with common stakes contributed to the work of different phrenological elites to pool resources—whether skulls, data, or social status. National identity was set to the side in favor of a shared identity as phrenological experts.

Early adopters of phrenology in the United States, in particular, were not phrenologists per se, but rather phrenological enthusiasts. As members of other professions, especially medicine, and by and large learned and respected men in their disciplines and communities, these enthusiasts found in phrenology a useful body of knowledge that could be joined to their own fields of expertise. This phrenological impulse among members of different educated professions, especially medicine and law, stands as a significant legacy of phrenology in the United States, due to the influence of these phrenological enthusiasts on various fields of medicolegal import, including the development of medical jurisprudence, approaches to criminal insanity and prison reform, and popular and scientific discourses around criminality. The features of phrenology that made it particularly attractive to Americans in general, and medical and other professionals in particular, were those that seemed to respond to contemporaneous concerns for American society—including debates around education and social ills, especially insanity and crime.

Chapter 3

Phrenology on Trial

In 1834, John Neal, a young lawyer in Portland, Maine, was presented with an opportunity to defend the science of phrenology, to which he was a stalwart convert.[1] Decades later, Neal, a prolific author and reformer as well as a lawyer, reflected on his goals in this case, *State of Maine v. Mitchell*. He sought "the discovery of truth, the promotion of justice, and the enlargement of legal science."[2] By this he did not principally mean the liberation of Major Mitchell, his nine-year-old client but, rather, the defense of phrenology. As he observed: "It was high time that Phrenology and the believers in Phrenology should be put upon the stand."[3] This case, from Neal's perspective, was about phrenology, not Mitchell. It was the first—but not the last—time that phrenology appeared as part of expert testimony in American courts.[4]

Mitchell was tried for the maiming of another boy, seven-year-old David Crawford, and the defense focused on denying culpability by reason of mental instability. The centerpiece of Neal's defense was an injury to his head that Mitchell had received as an infant, which Neal argued explained the "strangeness of his conduct."[5] Neal had three physicians serve as expert witnesses in this case, all of whom commented on the state of Mitchell's skull (figure 6). Two of the physicians, Dr. Barrett and Dr. Mighels, referred to phrenologists in their testimony and declared that they were believers in the science.[6] After some back-and-forth with the prosecutor about the nature of this expert knowledge, the judge barred Neal and his experts from further use of phrenological theory. After deliberating for twenty minutes, the jury found Mitchell guilty of all charges and sentenced him to nine years of hard labor.

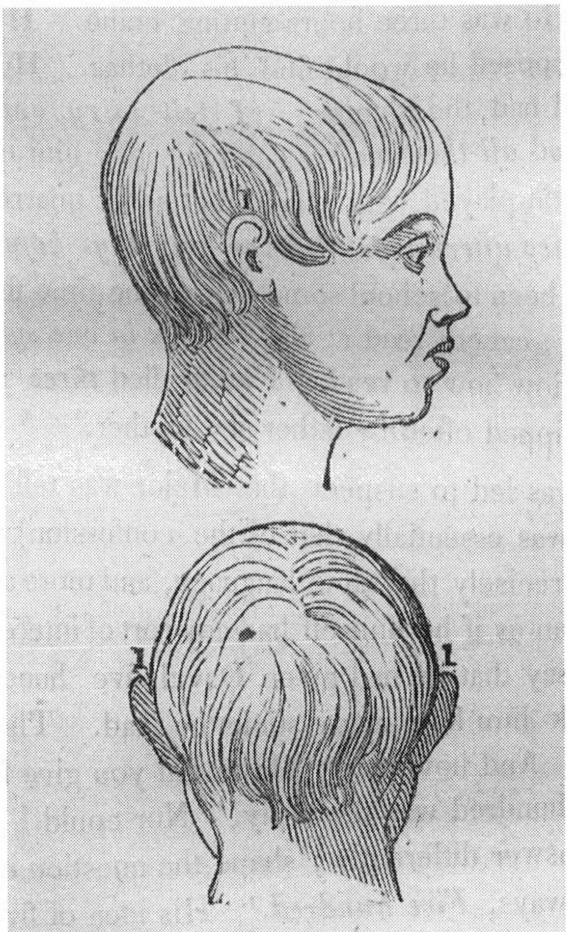

Figure 6. The profile of Major Mitchell, attributed to E. Seager. The numbers identifying the area just above the ear on each side of the head indicate the organ of Destructiveness. "Article IV. The Case of Major Mitchell," *Annals of Phrenology* 2, no. 3 (November 1835): 306. Yale University, Harvey Cushing/John Hay Whitney Medical Library.

Mitchell was not the only one on trial in this case: so too was phrenology, its status as a science, and its ability to be presented as acceptable evidence in a court of law. The Mitchell case, for phrenological enthusiasts, was an unfortunate failure of phrenology as medical jurisprudence. However, Neal read the case as a success: "Phrenology has been mentioned seriously in a court of justice without provoking laughter. Two most respectable physicians have acknowledged their belief in phrenology, as a science, *upon oath*."[7] For Neal, these factors were a sign of phrenology's rising fortunes as expert medical knowledge. As Neal further observed, there were other medical men waiting in the wings to bring phrenology to bear on medicolegal questions in courts of law. But medical professionals would first have to incorporate phrenological theory into their conceptions of medical expertise and medical jurisprudence. Phrenological expert witnessing and other explicit uses of the science were only one manifestation of the influence of phrenology on medicolegalism. Phrenological ideas and theories also permeated medicolegal discourse more subtly, through the adoption of phrenological language.

At the same moment in the 1830s and 1840s in the United States that legal scholars and physicians were defining the field of medical jurisprudence, they were also considering the potential for phrenology to contribute to the production of medicolegal knowledge in the courtroom. This medicolegal framing of the phrenological project made it a possible contender for courtroom usage. Beginning in the 1830s and well into the 1840s, the potential of phrenology to serve as medical knowledge for experts on the stand was tried—literally and figuratively—in courts of law and in medicolegal discourse. Phrenological ideas and language inflected both elite and popular understandings of the nature of criminality, particularly criminal insanity.

Why was phrenology useful to medical jurisprudence, for both medical and legal professionals? Medical jurisprudence in this period was on unstable ground due to the declining status of both the legal and medical professions, as well as uncertainty about the status and reliability of medical experts in the courtroom. This utility was only partially epistemological. The materialism of phrenology, which inspired censure when Gall first debuted his theories in Europe, was more appealing to medical and legal professionals in the United States, who sought a material grounding for explanations of the causes of criminality. The skull could provide tangible, visible evidence that could explain behaviors, which could in turn be easily demonstrated to nonexperts using phrenological images and language, especially those relating to the organ of Destructiveness and its attendant "propensity to murder." However, phrenology also provided a possible solution to the uncertain status of the two professions. As phrenology received favorable reception as an elite field of scientific inquiry, it provided a way to borrow expertise, authority, and trust. The short window in which phrenology was adopted, tested, and ultimately discarded represents the confluence of its heyday as elite science and the nadir of trust in medical jurisprudence.

In this chapter, I demonstrate the influence of phrenological thinking on the development of medical jurisprudence in the United States, especially around the question of criminal insanity. In the 1830s and 1840s, medicolegal experts were implicitly or explicitly influenced by the doctrine of phrenology. Some used phrenology explicitly on the stand, introducing phrenologists as expert witnesses, as in the case of Major Mitchell, or using phrenological knowledge and citing phrenologists in expert testimony or as a component of their defense. At the same time, phrenological ideas also spread through the courts in an implicit way through phrenological language and concepts, providing longevity for phrenology as a component of medicolegal expertise. This chapter thus evaluates both the implicit and explicit uses of phrenology as medicolegal expertise in the United States, demonstrating the legacy of a phrenological impulse in American legal medicine.

Negotiating Medical Jurisprudence in the Early Republic

The medicolegal realm in the early nineteenth-century United States was primarily characterized by three features: first, enthusiasm for and attention being paid to outlining what appeared to be a "new" discipline of medical jurisprudence; second, uncertainty as to the status of medical expertise and experts on the stand; and third, the permeability of the bounds of medical expertise, especially in the court. These features of medicolegalism were influenced by the uncertain status of members of the medical profession during this period, as well as the novelty of the field of medical jurisprudence, which had only recently become an object worthy of rigor and theory.[8]

Members of the professions, including both physicians and lawyers, were concerned with "declining power and status" in this period and with the legitimization of their fields of expertise.[9] In the early nineteenth century, the legal profession was still largely viewed as a kind of "handicraft," with legal training largely accomplished through apprenticeships, not unlike medicine.[10] While a few law schools did exist, it was not always clear *why* the law required higher study or higher status.[11] Law, like phrenology, was engaged in a process of self-legitimization.[12] American legal texts and journals, particularly *American Jurist*, also sometimes wrote favorably about the utility of phrenology.[13]

With regard to the medical profession, alternatives were emerging to orthodox medicine, particularly the Thomsonian movement and homeopathy.[14] These medical sects challenged both the claims to elite status and the economic fortunes of orthodox practitioners.[15] In the 1830s and the 1840s, the repeal of state medical licensing laws constituted another kind of stripping of professional privilege and reduced the disadvantages for irregular practitioners in pursuing medicine.[16] Moreover, the antistatus and antiprofessional ethos of the Jacksonian era increasingly turned the lay public against orthodox, trained practitioners.[17] Medical expertise was contested, embattled from without as well as within.

These challenges to the status of medical experts inflected a contemporaneous debate around medical jurisprudence, which had only recently become a central problem in the Anglo-American world. In the 1823 preface to his *Elements of Medical Jurisprudence*, American writer Theodric Romeyn Beck observed that as a student of medicine interested in the science of medical jurisprudence, he found that the English-language texts on the subject were limited to a single volume, most likely Samuel Farr's *Elements of Medical Jurisprudence* (1788), whereas Continental writings were largely inaccessible.[18] Beck's intention was to routinize and standardize medical knowledge in order to render it useful to "doubtful questions in courts of justice," and to note succinctly the "physiological, pathological, or chemical facts" necessary to a judicial case.[19] In the United States, Beck's work dominated the field until nearly midcentury, inspiring a wave of writing on medical jurisprudence from both medical and legal points of view.[20]

Due in part to Beck's opening salvo, physicians and jurists alike turned to the question of medical jurisprudence in the 1820s and 1830s.[21] Physicians writing on issues of medical jurisprudence were invested in finding a place for their practice within courts of law, believing that this was crucial to the future of the medical profession. James Mohr has traced the origins of medical jurisprudence in this early part of the century in order to identify some significant transformations: in the first half of the century, American medical schools gave medical jurisprudence an important place in their professional curricula and medicolegal problems stimulated research, but by the end of the century this attention had faded, driven in part by disillusionment and self-interest.[22] This early period, then, witnessed an important transformation in the role and profile of both medicolegal opinions and the medicolegal expert in the court of law.

In the 1830s, both legal and medical journals addressed the nature of medical expertise in legal spaces, underlining its problematic nature. Medical expertise, already at times unclear at the bedside, was increasingly also a contested feature of the courtroom. The medical expert, when placed on the stand, would often not only be forced to account for his expert reading of a particular case, but might also be examined on the basis of his role as a medical expert and the validity of medical knowledge writ large. As Beck had suggested, "in many instances, a legal decision depends on the testimony of medical witnesses," and it served as "a solid gain to the cause of justice" to improve the testimony of medical experts.[23]

Medical and legal authors approached the topic with different concerns. Jurists generally abdicated responsibility for developing systems of medical jurisprudence to the medical profession, but they frequently reflected on the problem of medical experts in the court. Beck's work was well received by the legal community, yet jurists continued to complain that "the science itself is one thing, the application of it another."[24] This was particularly troublesome because, as John Hooker Ashmun, professor of law at Harvard University, pointed out in the 1830s, in a large proportion of trials, "questions arise which can only be satisfactorily answered by a knowledge of some branches of Medical science," which required a medical expert.[25] Thus, the "testimony of medical men becomes often the turning point of decision."[26] Unfortunately, as Ashmun observed, "the members of that profession have never done themselves much credit in our courts. . . . Probably no class of men, certainly none of educated men, testify so unsatisfactorily."[27] This problem was ever at the forefront of legal discourse about medical experts. In 1841, nearly two decades after the publication of Beck's *Medical Jurisprudence*, one anonymous essayist in *American Jurist* observed sadly that, "medical men, even when possessing considerable reputation, make but a sorry figure on the witness-stand."[28] The fault for these failures of medical experts was often laid at the feet of the medical schools, in spite of the addition of courses of medical jurisprudence to the curricula of many medical schools and the publication of further texts on the subject.

And yet, medical experts continued to appear on the witness stand throughout this period, "sorry figures" or not.[29] Medical men took the stand in the early part of the century in an atmosphere of uncertainty. As phrenology was simultaneously drawing the attention of the medical community, it offered a potential way to shore up these claims to expertise. Joseph Chitty first explored this possibility in detail in his 1834 text, *A Practical Treatise on Medical Jurisprudence*. Chitty, an English lawyer, was a prolific writer of legal treatises and one of the first men to write on the subject of medical jurisprudence. In American medical colleges, Chitty's text was taught along with those of American writers like Beck.[30]

Chitty's *Practical Treatise* incorporated phrenological theory into the account of "The Nervous Function" in his ninth chapter. Throughout this chapter, Chitty repeatedly cited John Elliotson, an English physician and phrenologist who founded and served as president of the London Phrenological Society, as well as Gall. Chitty included a detailed account of phrenological doctrine, complete with plates depicting the phrenological organs. As a preface to this discussion, Chitty observed that Elliotson and Sir Everard Home, along with other physicians, were advocates of the doctrine that faculties and propensities of an individual could be ascertained through external examination, and that "*phrenology* or *craniology* is a science that may be studied with great practical utility."[31] Chitty further cited Elliotson, who argued that "phrenology may be of the highest use when in alleged criminals there may be suspicion of idiotism or insanity."[32] In particular, he suggested, the science might allow for the identification of madmen prior to execution, as they were not deserving of punishment. While Chitty observed that "certainly the doctrine of cranioscopy is not as yet admitted in the practice of law," he concluded that "If the sciences of cranioscopy and physiology could be brought to any *certain and unvarying result* it is obvious that they would be of the highest importance," influencing the law and its application, especially regarding criminals.[33] However, the present state of the science encompassed "too much uncertainty to induce any practical application of the doctrine."[34] While Elliotson's proposals were appealing, Chitty concluded that phrenology could not *yet* be applied practically in the medicolegal realm, despite its great potential.

In the same year that Chitty explored the hypothetical utility of phrenological knowledge for witnesses and judges alike in text, the case of *Maine v. Mitchell* put the practical application of phrenology to the test. The case of *Maine v. Mitchell* set the stage for two further developments in American medical jurisprudence. First, Isaac Ray, an eyewitness to the case, was inspired to consider phrenology as a possible source of expertise in cases of medical jurisprudence; Ray's adoption of some phrenological ideas and language allowed phrenological theories to spread in an often-unrecognized way from the late 1830s onward. Second, other lawyers, judges, and physicians, possibly following the example of *Mitchell*, were inspired to attempt to bring phrenology to bear on other court cases in following years in a more explicit, though ultimately unstable, use of phrenological knowledge.

Phrenological Enthusiasm and Medical Jurisprudence

Isaac Ray has been well explored in the history of psychiatry, as a physician, asylum superintendent, and founding member and president of the Association of Medical Superintendents of American Institutions for the Insane, the organization that would later become the American Psychiatric Association.[35] However, at the time of the Mitchell trial, Ray was a less well-known figure than his friend, John Neal. In the 1820s, it was the older Neal who served as mentor to the newly credentialed physician. Late in life, when Ray reflected on his time in Portland, he recalled Neal as one of the first friends he made there: "I have never ceased to think with feelings of lively interest + gratitude, of the kindness you showed me, + your constant + cheering encouragement."[36] Indeed, Ray told Neal, "I am indebted to no single individual so much as to you."[37]

Perhaps Ray attempted to demonstrate his indebtedness to Neal in the favorable account of the Mitchell trial he published anonymously in the *Annals of Phrenology*, the journal of the Boston Phrenological Society.[38] Ray argued that the Mitchell trial, presented by "one so competent for the purpose, as Mr. Neal," added to the "mass of evidence that is daily accumulating in favor of our science."[39] Ray had observed Mitchell before the trial and helped to prepare a phrenological reading of the young defendant, perhaps contributing to the defense.[40] While Ray applauded the "zeal and exertions" of Neal, he acknowledged that this was not an ideal case for the application of phrenology: "we could have wished a better case for the introduction of the light of Phrenology, into the dark passages of Criminal Law."[41] Ray expressed the belief that if the first case introduced had been more persuasive than the Mitchell case: "then would have been afforded an opportunity for a triumphant vindication of its utility, and an augury of its future stupendous influence."[42]

Ray was not alone in his hopes for the strong stand of phrenology in the realm of medical jurisprudence. In the United States, some of the early leading figures in phrenology were professors and authors on the subject of medical jurisprudence. John Bell, for example, one of the founders of the Central Phrenological Society in Philadelphia, was also a professor of medical jurisprudence.[43] Charles Caldwell, the early champion of phrenology, lectured on medical jurisprudence in Philadelphia, and continued to teach the subject at Transylvania University.[44] Caldwell saw the potential connection between phrenology and medical jurisprudence a year before Chitty's text was published. In his hundred-page-long defense of the science published as the first essay of the first issue of the first volume of the *Annals of Phrenology*, Caldwell observed that "Medical Jurisprudence is yet in a very defective condition" and "scarcely ranks among the sciences," and further that "Phrenology is the only source of *true* light in relation to it [medical jurisprudence]."[45] Caldwell's words placed medical jurisprudence squarely on the agenda for the Society's members and other phrenological enthusiasts. These arguments were in line with those of his medical and legal contemporaries, and his solution, phrenology, was a valid possibility for the development of medical jurisprudence, especially for the educated phrenological enthusiasts of the Boston circle.

Of equal importance were the ways in which phrenological enthusiasts considered the legal ramifications of the science. In this they were likely inspired by the legal background of George Combe. Combe's *Constitution*, while not directly addressing questions of medical jurisprudence, did consider phrenological knowledge in relation to law. His later works more assertively took on questions of criminal legislation and jurisprudence, and he addressed medical jurisprudence, including the works of Chitty and Ray, in his *Notes on the United States of North America*.[46] As both a lawyer and a phrenologist, Combe retained his status as a leading man of phrenology.

Other legal phrenological enthusiasts similarly worked to bridge these disciplines, with particular attention to medical jurisprudence. Aside from John Neal and the lawyers and law professors who supported Combe and his works, it was the lawyer and jurist Amos Dean who was the most prominent example of this kind of legal phrenological enthusiast.[47] Dean was an early adopter of phrenological practice who presented a course of lectures on phrenology in the early 1830s to the Young Men's Association for Mutual Improvement of the City of Albany, which he later published.[48] Dean also published a phrenologically inspired work entitled *The Philosophy of Human Life* with Marsh, Capen, Lyon and Webb in 1839, which was well received by the *American Phrenological Journal* (*APJ*).[49]

The *APJ* supported Dean throughout much of his career, proclaiming decades later that "The Albany Law School to-day, with Hon. Amos Dean at its head, has no superior,"[50] but their goodwill was probably bred in 1839, when Dean penned a series of detailed essays for the journal in which he explored the medical jurisprudence of insanity in three installments, incorporating phrenological theory into his account of the subject.[51] These publications suggest Dean's abiding interest in phrenology and his willingness to participate in this community. They also demonstrate that from the earliest development of phrenological networks in the United States, intellectual and textual space was devoted to issues of medical jurisprudence.[52] Dean founded Albany Medical College in 1838, where he taught medical jurisprudence even after Beck joined the faculty.[53] When the college was founded in 1838, it was George Combe, then on tour in America, whom Dean welcomed to campus to give the inaugural lecture.[54]

Over a decade later, in 1850, Dean published a text devoted to the subject, *The Principles of Medical Jurisprudence*, which became essential for teaching and understanding medical jurisprudence in the legal realm.[55] While phrenology was not overtly part of this project, the language of propensity pervaded the work, signaling Dean's continuing affinity for phrenological theory. Dean's deep commitment to phrenology and his role in developing phrenological thought on medicolegal issues rendered this work if not one of phrenology, then certainly one produced by a phrenological enthusiast.

In his articulation of the propensities in his *Principles of Medical Jurisprudence*, however, Dean was primarily following in the footsteps of Isaac Ray, who in 1838 had published *A Treatise on the Medical Jurisprudence of Insanity*. The confluence of insanity, medical jurisprudence, and phrenological theory was not accidental. Medicolegal scholars and phrenological enthusiasts alike considered phrenology to be particularly relevant in discussions about insanity. It was, however, in the United States that phrenological theories came to influence discourse around the insane criminal, due in part to the popularity of phrenological theories in elite medical and legal circles.

The Medical Jurisprudence of Insanity

Medical theorists in Europe and America turned their attention to the question of insanity around the turn of the nineteenth century, especially for forms of insanity related to the problem of criminal responsibility.[56] In 1801, French psychiatrist Philippe Pinel, working at the French hospital and asylum compounds of the Salpêtrière and the Bicêtre, coined the phrase *manie sans délire* to identify a form of nonintellectual insanity.[57] Pinel's students, Jean-Étienne Dominique Esquirol and Étienne-Jean Georget, though initially dismissing the concept of *manie sans délire*, eventually came to accept it and, in turn, to adapt it into the concept of *monomanie* or monomania.[58] Working around the same time, Gall and Spurzheim developed a related theory of mind, best represented in Spurzheim's *Observations on Deranged Manifestations of the Mind, or Insanity* (1817), which proposed the category of "partial insanity," an impairment of the moral organs of mind, but not the reasoning faculties.[59] Spurzheim's articulation of partial insanity suggested that the varieties of partial insanity were numerous, with the potential for as many kinds of insanity as there were powers of mind.[60] In 1835, these various threads were condensed into one theory of instability, that of "moral insanity," by James Cowles Prichard, an English physician, in his *Treatise on Insanity and Other Disorders Affecting the Mind*.[61] "Moral insanity" described a condition of mind in which the moral faculties were diseased, but the intellectual or rational faculties were not, such that these individuals would know that their actions were wrong but proceed regardless.[62]

Despite the seeming synergy of Prichard's moral insanity and phrenological theories about partial insanity and criminal propensities, Prichard was acknowledged as an antiphrenologist.[63] Phrenological writers commented on the wrongheadedness of his critiques and demonstrated that Prichard's work belied his antiphrenological stance. Prichard, they argued, despite all of his protesting, was really a phrenologist. In order to contest this "person of some eminence as a medical writer"—faint praise indeed—Andrew Combe stepped forward to "more clearly expose the conduct of a man, who deliberately shuts his eyes to truth, and gives currency to statements which he knows to be unjust, and to arguments which he knows to be invalid."[64] Combe declared Prichard to be one of the chief opponents of the doctrine: "If posterity shall deem determined opposition to the progress of Phrenology to be good service done to the cause of science, no man bids fairer to be remembered with honour than Dr. Prichard of Bristol."[65]

Despite the rancor between phrenological enthusiasts and antiphrenologists like Prichard, these individuals and their writings were often lumped together as one corpus of theories of criminal insanity. As one legal scholar remarked, it would be impossible for court or counsel to engage with cases of insanity without the facts of "*Simpson*, [Andrew] *Combe, Prichard, Pinel, Georget*," where both Simpson and Combe, known phrenological partisans, were associated with nonphrenologists, Pinel and Georget, and antiphrenologist Prichard.[66] Meanwhile, in witness statements on the stand on the subject of insanity, Spurzheim, Combe, and Gall were as likely to be cited as figures like Pinel and Esquirol, and often in the same breath. Thus, articles such as one found in the *Salem Gazette* in 1838 could be entitled "Moral Insanity," though addressing a lecture by George Combe on Destructiveness and murderous propensities.[67] Even in medical journals, this slippage occurred: the *Boston Medical and Surgical Journal* cited phrenological theory and Andrew Combe on the subject of insanity alongside Prichard.[68] In discussions about moral insanity and criminal responsibility, phrenology was equated with other forms of medical expertise, and these various explanations for criminal insanity were in conversation—and sometimes confusion—with one another.

Isaac Ray's *A Treatise on the Medical Jurisprudence of Insanity* (1838) took the concept of moral insanity as a unifying theme and became an essential text for the medicolegal framing of criminal insanity in the United States.[69] The *Treatise* was centered on the elaboration and synthesis of contemporaneous theories of insanity, making use of the concept of moral insanity as a challenge to the deficiencies of common law.[70] Ray became a primary resource for legal counsel, cited continually as an authority in court documents, legal commentaries, and popular accounts of famous cases featuring insanity, as well as texts on medical jurisprudence. Ray was also profoundly influenced by the doctrines of phrenology, translating phrenological texts for Marsh, Capen & Lyon in Boston, corresponding with leading phrenologists of the Boston Phrenological Society, and advising Neal in his defense of Mitchell, as well as authoring spirited defenses of phrenology for the *Boston Medical Magazine* and the *Christian Examiner*.[71]

As John Starrett Hughes has argued, Ray's early adoption and defense of phrenology were related to his conviction that phrenology was a Baconian endeavor, with regard to Gall and Spurzheim's anatomical studies and practices of observation.[72] However, as Hughes has claimed, by the late 1830s, when Ray wrote his *Treatise*, he had "completely sublimated his phrenological framework so that his attacks on common law doctrines of insanity would not be polluted by associated guilt," due to the declining reputation of phrenology in America.[73] Similarly, Kenneth J. Weiss has described Ray's early interest in phrenology as an "affair," asserting that "Ray stopped beating the drum for phrenology" around the time of the publication of the *Treatise*.[74] In effect, the increasing attacks on phrenology had soured his optimism with regard to the future of the science.[75] While Weiss and Hughes have framed the *Treatise* as a new chapter in Ray's professional development, I believe that phrenology was still subtly influencing his work.[76] Hughes notes—but dismisses—the numerous instances of Ray's use of the language of propensity, without connecting these language choices to the phrenological framework.[77] Whether intentional or not, the continued recourse to the language of propensity was a relic of Ray's earlier phrenological enthusiasm and study.

Ray's presentation of medical knowledge about the relationship between the brain and behavior was marked by its association with phrenological theory: "It is an undoubted truth, that the manifestations of the intellect, and those of the sentiments, propensities and passions, or generally, of the intellectual and affective powers, are connected with and dependent upon the brain."[78] The connection between brain and powers of mind would have appeared to a phrenological enthusiast to be a reference to the science, but the specific use of the categories of mental power—intellect, sentiments, propensities—referred more clearly to groups of known phrenological organs. This effect was underlined by Ray's citation of both Andrew Combe and Gall in this same section and elsewhere in the text, as well as the description of "faculties" (another word for organs).[79] Moreover, Ray's articulation of aspects of character made use of the same phrenological terminology, often incorporating the language of propensity, as in "various propensities, such as . . . destructiveness."[80] Elsewhere, Ray directly referenced the "animal propensities," the excessive activity of which he associated with imbecility.[81]

More specific examples of criminal propensities also appeared in the text. Ray described a "propensity to steal," for example, citing Pinel, Prichard, Spurzheim, and Gall.[82] He further discussed sexual propensities and propensities to incendiarism. Ray also described "the most important form of moral mania . . . a morbid activity of the *propensity to destroy*."[83] Ray cited Pinel as the originator of this concept, but also cited among its theorists "Gall and Spurzheim, Esquirol, Georget . . . [Andrew] Combe and Pritchard [*sic*]," among others.[84] Among the case studies Ray included in his exploration of this propensity, which he named homicidal insanity, were several cases from Gall's *Sur les fonctions du cerveau*;[85] another two cases were drawn from the Edinburgh *Phrenological Journal*.[86] In discussing homicidal insanity, Ray used phrases including "propensity to kill"[87] and "murderous propensity,"[88] observing that all such cases possess a common feature: "the *irresistible, motiveless impulse to destroy life*."[89] Such language would not have been out of place in a phrenological text.

Ray was not promoting a phrenological point of view in the *Treatise*, yet he made use of ideas and terms frequently tied to phrenology, providing them with the potential for further longevity in the medicolegal realm. For example, in his exploration of a case of homicidal insanity, he addressed phrenological theory obliquely: "whether we adopt an organ of destructiveness in the brain or not, it is to be assumed that the propensity to kill himself and the son arose from a morbid excitation of a certain part of the brain."[90] Whether the reader gave credence to an organ of Destructiveness—a purely phrenological concept—or not, he or she was directed to take into consideration such a thing as a "propensity to kill" related to a specific part of the brain. Ray avoided any clear association with and usage of more obvious phrenological theories, including the word "phrenology" itself, yet he continually made use of phrenological concepts and language.

Ray was considered by contemporaries to be inspired by phrenological theory, especially within the legal community. *American Jurist*, one enthusiastic supporter of Ray's theories, first published an essay by Ray on the "Criminal Law of Insanity" in 1835, three years before the *Treatise* was published.[91] When a commentator in the same journal took issue with the "correctness" of the views expressed in Ray's essay, the editors disputed this critique, pointing out that Ray had "evidently adopted the phrenological theory of insanity of Dr. Andrew Combe."[92] They went on to observe that phrenology was "now receiving the support of so many enlightened and scientific men . . . that it needs no defence at our hands."[93] Moreover, they argued that every lawyer "having the cause of humanity and science at heart" must acquaint himself with "the modern theory of insanity," which was based on phrenology and expounded by Ray.[94] In a second editorial, the journal further defended Ray's arguments, stating that "there is not a single position" for which "we cannot produce ample authority from the writings of Pinel, Gall, and Spurzheim, Esquirol, Georget, Marc, Hoffbauer, Haslam, Pritchard, Combe and Conolly . . . the most eminent names in this department of medical literature."[95] This series of essays demonstrates the legal embrace of Ray's phrenologically influenced theories and the acceptance of phrenological figures as medical experts.

If it was Ray, in 1835, who gained authority from appealing to phrenological experts, in court cases in the decades following the publication of his *Treatise*, the direction of authority would change. Phrenology was incorporated into court cases in the late 1830s through the 1850s by expert witnesses, judges, and attorneys alike, but Ray and his phrenologically influenced *Treatise* would be increasingly cited in these contexts, and with greater success than phrenology *qua* phrenology.

Phrenology in the Courtroom after *Mitchell*

After the failure of *Mitchell* in 1834, one might suppose that phrenological knowledge was easily dismissed from the legal repertoire. Yet phrenology made its way into American courtrooms over the course of the next two decades, borne by lawyers, judges, and expert witnesses alike, particularly in cases of criminal insanity. These explicit uses of phrenology and phrenological experts were few in number but nevertheless suggestive of the potential of the science to provide medicolegal expertise. Even after such explicit uses of phrenology fell out of practice, however, the implicit use of phrenological language, informed by Ray's *Treatise*, as well as Combe, Gall, and Spurzheim's writings, continued. Both explicit and implicit uses of phrenology in the courtroom were heralded by phrenological enthusiasts as successes supportive of phrenology.

Physicians who were phrenological enthusiasts and practical phrenologists sometimes served as expert witnesses, as in the 1847 case of John Haggerty (figure 7).[96] Haggerty, an Irish laborer, was tried in Lancaster, Pennsylvania for the murder of his neighbor, Melchoir Fordney.[97] Haggerty's trial, like that of Mitchell, represented the use of both the insanity defense and phrenology in American courtrooms.[98] John L. Thompson, one of the two members of Haggerty's defense team, opened his defense of his client with a claim to insanity, suggesting that the acts themselves showed that he was a "*raving maniac.*"[99] Thompson constructed a genealogy of this form of insanity, focusing, in particular, on an injury that Haggerty sustained twenty years earlier, as a new immigrant from Ireland to Montréal, Canada, where he served as a laborer. During his time in Montréal, he was struck by a cart and knocked unconscious. The result was a depression on the side of skull, which Thompson claimed caused permanent pressure on the brain: "chafing, irritating and producing unnatural excitement."[100]

In order to explain the location of this injury to the court, Thompson used phrenological language, explaining that the depression "passes over that portion

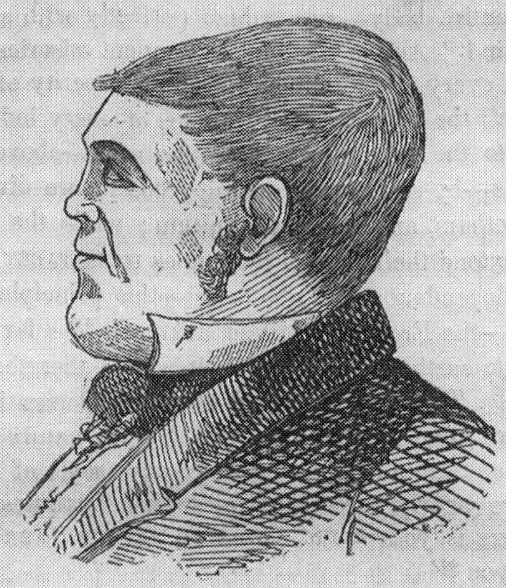

Figure 7. The profile of John Haggerty, from "Article XLII. John Haggerty, Murderer of Melchoir Fordney—Executed at Lancaster, PA., July 24, 1847," *American Phrenological Journal* 10, no. 7 (July 1848): 212. Yale University, Harvey Cushing/John Hay Whitney Medical Library.

of the brain which has been dedicated by Phrenologists, as the organs of Marvellousness, Conscientiousness and Hope, and terminates at Cautiousness."[101] For someone well-versed in phrenological theory, this would have been clear as a map of the location and spread of the injury; indeed, these directions allow the historian to approximate the location of the injury as well, using a phrenological bust. "But, however we may differ as to the merits of the science," Thompson continued, "no one can, for a moment doubt, that the effects of this blow have exercised a permanent and deplorable influence, over the thoughts, conduct and life of the unfortunate Prisoner."[102] This had the effect, Thompson concluded, of making him "RAVING MAD."[103]

The injury to the skull (and hence, to the brain) was linked directly to homicidal impulses and explained exclusively through the use of phrenological terminology and frameworks, in spite of the existence of other contemporary theories of insanity that would have explained this form of madness equally well.[104] The reference to phrenology may, at first, seem to denigrate the science ("while we may differ as to the merits of the science"), but Thompson's exclusive reliance on phrenological language and theory suggests faith in the theory. Moreover, the various players in this courtroom drama took phrenology very seriously.

As part of the defense, George Ford, the other defense attorney, called several physicians to testify as to the nature of Haggerty's skull injury. After the first two physicians testified, Dr. William B. Fahnestock, a phrenological enthusiast, was called to the stand. As a part of his testimony, he manually examined Haggerty's head. Fahnestock then used a phrenological bust to demonstrate the location and path of the injury. Echoing Thompson's opening remarks, Fahnestock indicated verbally and with the aid of the bust that the fracture "passes on the lower edge of Marvellousness or Wonder, Hope and Cautiousness. It passes also between Hope and Ideality."[105] At this point, the judge interjected with a question: "Does it [the fracture] pass near Destructiveness or Combativeness?" to which Fahnestock answered that it did not.[106]

Fahnestock's testimony was short yet suggestive of the relationship between phrenology and the courtroom, as well as the extent to which phrenology was taken seriously as a science. It also demonstrates the extent to which phrenological language, images, and concepts had become common knowledge by the 1840s. The lack of detailed explanations of his findings suggests an expectation of phrenological literacy on the part of the courtroom, just as Thompson's opening statement anticipated the ability of the listener to mentally map the location of the injury on an imagined phrenological bust. Indeed, when the judge put forth a question, it was not for an explanation of these findings or his methods, but a specific question regarding organs of mind not previously named. The judge himself demonstrated an understanding of phrenological principles, including the names of the organs. The focus of the judge on Destructiveness illustrates the strong association between that organ and murder in the public mind: the judge was asking if Haggerty fit the phrenological profile expected of a murderous mind. Further, the cross-examination by the attorney general did not dispute the status of phrenology or the nature of the evidence being presented, nor did he question Fahnestock's credentials. Despite the seeming legibility of this defense to all parties, however, Haggerty was found guilty and later hanged.[107]

The potential of phrenology to serve as expert knowledge in a court of law was only rarely put to the test, but it remained a potent possibility. A case several years later represents a successful application of phrenology in just such a matter. In an appeals case in Ohio in 1853, *Nancy Farrer v. State of Ohio*, in which the appellant was originally convicted for the murder of a child by poison, the case was appealed due to errors to the charge of the jury. The appeal focused primarily on the insufficient proof of Farrer's sanity, but it was the opinion of the court, which reversed the conviction and remanded the case to retrial, which incorporated phrenological evidence. In his decision, the presiding judge commented on the nature of medical jurisprudence and the role of phrenology within this system, echoing the Mitchell case: "We have no opinion to express on the claims of rival schools in medical jurisprudence. Whether phrenology is a science or a delusion, we shall not judicially undertake to pronounce. Whether medical science should be unalterably wedded to one established orthodox system, or progressive and eclectic in its character, we are not called upon to say."[108] In fact, the judge continued, it was not the business of the court at all what the main position of medical science might be, as "intelligent physicians of opposite faiths agree" on the state of the prisoner in this case.[109] "Medical men," collectively, and implicitly including those informed by phrenology, agreed on the nature of insanity in this case, and that was sufficient in the eyes of this court.[110]

Mirroring *Mitchell*, the judge had the final word not only on the case itself, but also on the nature of medical evidence. Here, however, the judge abdicated his role of passing judgment on medical evidence, whereas in *Mitchell*, the judge offered a clear opinion on what medical evidence was useful in courts of law. Phrenology was included as one of several "rival schools" of medical jurisprudence, and one that served equally well in this case. The judge cared nothing for the "quarrels of doctors"—including phrenologists—only for consensus, which he believed had been achieved in this instance.[111] Therefore, the appellant was to be judged as insane by any measure, the jury was improperly charged, and the conviction was overturned. There was no conflict between medical and legal knowledge, and phrenology could fit into this matrix, as far as it was useful to the court.

Aside from such explicit uses of phrenological knowledge and phrenologically inclined witnesses, phrenological language was frequently mobilized in courts of law during this period. In 1838, the Honorable Judge Joel Parker,[112] chief justice of the New Hampshire Court of Common Pleas, used phrenological terminology when charging a jury in a case related to the problem of insanity.[113] Parker's lengthy charge to the jury, which was published in full in three installments in the *New Hampshire Patriot and State Gazette*, was primarily composed of a discourse on the nature of insanity.[114] Parker observed that due to the way insanity was reported in public papers, as a last resort for desperate cases and used "for the purpose of aiding in the escape of criminals from justice," the defense itself was made "odious."[115] Parker argued that "a more thorough knowledge upon the subject of insanity itself" was needed.[116] He proceeded to lecture the jury on the causes and types of insanity, quoting at great length from Ray's *Treatise*, which had only been published earlier that year.[117]

Parker's primary focus was on the concept of "moral insanity," but the way he explained this concept was couched primarily in phrenological language: "an irresistible propensity to steal," "a morbid propensity to destroy," and so forth.[118] After reporting on the work of other physicians and asylum managers, including Dr. Samuel Bayard Woodward, superintendent of the State Lunatic Asylum in Worcester, Massachusetts, described elsewhere as an "avowed phrenologist,"[119] Parker again turned to Ray for defense of his exploration of "this frightful malady" in which "cases of irresistible impulse to kill may be connected with this imbecility or deficiency of mind."[120] Parker concluded this excursion into theories of insanity with a jeremiad against the "injustice" of confining individuals ill in this way to prisons, rather than treating them as patients and rehabilitating them.[121]

The phrenological community embraced Parker's charge as an example of the use of phrenology in criminal jurisprudence, as seen in the reporting on the case in the *APJ*.[122] The author remarked on Parker's use of the term "propensity," particularly the uses of "propensity to destroy," "propensity to steal," and propensities to other criminal behaviors, which were interpreted as clear references to phrenological concepts and organs.[123] George Combe also reported on this case in an 1840 address to the Association of the Phrenologists of Great Britain and Ireland, for which he served as president, and included it in his *Notes on the United States of North America* as well.[124] Combe explained that he was introduced to the case by Mr. Cushing, the editor of the *Law Journal*, who presented him with copies of the newspaper articles.[125] He stated that: "The whole charge is lucid, sound, and practical; and it is gratifying to a phrenologist to see the principles of his science brought thus practically to bear on the interests of a state, under the direction of one of its highest legal authorities."[126] For Combe, the use of phrenological language, especially the language around the propensities, and the citation of Woodward and Ray, indicated the embrace and utility of phrenological principles by the legal realm.

Parker's charge to the jury was not unique: admixtures of phrenological and nonphrenological theories, experts, and terminology persisted in courtrooms throughout the century. For example, phrenology appeared in an appeals case in 1840 in Mississippi, invoked by the counsel for the appellant in a matter regarding the disposition of a will, which the appellant, the son of the deceased, contested on the grounds that his father had been insane at the time of signing the will. The attorney for the appellant opened his case by arguing that "it is impossible to investigate this cause, without investigating, to some extent, the doctrine of the mind, and the effects of disease on the various organs of which it is composed."[127] He observed that it is a "conceded fact" that the brain consists of organs having different functions, and that this is something that "no man having any regard for his reputation in medical science" would dispute.[128] He continued: "But whether phrenology is or is not the only true physiology of the brain, and the brain the only sound basis of its pathology, we must of necessity refer principally to medical authors, in the discussion of the present case."[129] This might seem like a dismissal of phrenology at first glance, but included among these "medical authors" was one of the leading phrenologists of the era: Andrew Combe.[130] These arguments comprised both the implicit use of phrenological doctrine and the explicit use of a phrenological medical expert, Andrew Combe. However, absent medical authorities, this appeal to scientific principles could not win out against those medical authorities present—in this case, four physicians who served as witness to the stability of the deceased. The appeals case failed, but phrenological principles were not, here, at issue.

Isaac Ray was also invoked in courtrooms as an expert par excellence on the subject of criminal insanity, cited by both expert witnesses and legal counsel on the subject of insanity in cases throughout the century.[131] Most notably, Ray's *Treatise* appeared in the classic trial of Daniel M'Naghten for the murder of Edward Drummond in England in 1843.[132] The defense counsel in this trial, Alexander Cockburn, made extensive use of Ray's arguments and work in his argument, including lengthy quotations from the *Treatise*.[133] The successful insanity plea in this case was thus supported by Ray's words, as well as the nine physicians called to testify.

The use of Ray, an American, in this British case, moreover, established his work as chief among the corpus of texts on medical jurisprudence, particularly with regard to insanity. A number of defense attorneys in the United States made use of similar tactics, including reading at length from the *Treatise*. For example, in the 1846 trial of William Freeman for murder, the defense attorney relied extensively on Ray's *Treatise*, to the point where he read three sections aloud from the book.[134] The same report of this trial included autopsy findings from Dr. Amariah Brigham, another phrenological enthusiast and associate of the Boston phrenological circle, and phrenological measurements and findings.[135]

In a similar case of the previous year, the trial of Abner Baker Jr. for the murder of his brother-in-law in Louisville, Kentucky, Ray was mentioned along with Beck, Esquirol, Prichard, and Combe on the subject of monomania.[136] Ray's

Treatise, however, was singled out by the presiding judge, Tunstall Quarles, as "an American production of extraordinary ability" on the subject of insanity.[137] Quarles, much like the defense attorney in the M'Naghten and Freeman cases, read long sections of Ray's *Treatise* to the jury, along with passages from Esquirol on monomania.[138] In this case the specter of phrenology was raised, along with mesmerism, as a way to disparage one of the medical experts introduced for the defense. The judge accused the prosecuting attorney of presenting Dr. Richardson, the witness for the defense, as "insane on the subjects of phrenology and mesmerism," although he declared that the same physician "has no faith in mesmerism, and but little in phrenology."[139] Yet Quarles not only persisted in citing Ray but made use of the language of faculties and propensities in so doing.[140] In another case from 1851, the opening remarks made by the defense attorney, George Camp, in the murder trial of John Metcalf Thurston, included a long digression on Gall discussing the "murderous propensity," the evidence for which the counsel cited Ray, before concluding: "I am not stating theories to you . . . I am giving you the detailed facts and history of actual causes observed and reported."[141] Here, the counsel slipped from Gall to Ray, touched on the concept of "murderous propensity" as a part of an extended discussion of monomania, and concluded that these accounts were facts, not theories or mere deductions.

In a case of forgery against Charles B. Huntington in New York in 1856, the defense entered was insanity, and Ray was invoked as a high authority ("he has no superior upon the subject"[142]) on the subject of medical jurisprudence by both the defense and prosecuting attorneys and as a part of the commentary on the trial.[143] Ray was quoted directly by a defense attorney as a part of a witness examination in the trial of Sylvester Breen, alias John Reynolds, for murder later in the century as well, as part of a larger discussion of insanity.[144] However, in the trial of Alvin Worrell for murder in 1857, Ray's theories of intellectual and moral insanity were deemed "too complicated to be of much practical use in the administration of the law" by the counsel for the state, W. V. N. Bay.[145] Yet the definition of monomania that Bay adopted instead was pervaded with the language of propensity: "that form of insanity, in which the mental alienation is partial . . . it may be accompanied with a propensity to homicide, larceny, arson, or any other offence. . . . It may be accompanied with a propensity to murder."[146] The language of propensity was at times a more legible and useful way to describe criminal acts than Ray's articulation of homicidal insanity.

Even if Ray's work was dismissed in this case, his words and his presence were, at other times, of utmost utility. Ray was even called to testify in some cases, such as the 1855 murder trial of Willard Clark, in New Haven, Connecticut, only a few years after Ray published his own guide for medical witnesses on the stand.[147] Ray testified on behalf of the defense, although he had not previously met, conversed with, or examined Clark. His testimony on the mental state of the defendant in this case was cumulative, based on the picture developed by other witnesses as to his actions in the weeks before his crime, and on the medical testimony provided by the two physicians who had been called as witnesses and who had previously examined the defendant. Ray's testimony, including his finding that Clark "was an insane man at the time of the commission of the act," served as a conclusion to the defense's case, and Ray was not cross-examined by the state, unlike the other medical witnesses.[148] The final (albeit lengthy) words of Henry Harrison, the defense attorney, to the jury were a recapitulation of many cases dealing with phrenology, including the Freeman murder trial, Parker's charge to the jury, and quotations from the text of the *Treatise*. Ray's turn as star witness was a coup for the defense: unique to many of these cases, the defendant was found "NOT GUILTY ON THE SOLE GROUND OF INSANITY."[149] Ray's presence had enabled the achievement of a rare reprieve for the morally insane criminal. What phrenology alone, as medical witnessing or medicolegal argument by counsel, could not achieve was seemingly possible, through the use of Ray.

In 1846 in Auburn, New York, Dr. Charles B. Coventry was called to the stand to testify on behalf of Henry Wyatt, a convict at Auburn State Prison, who was then on trial for the murder of a fellow inmate.[150] As a part of his testimony on the nature of criminal insanity, Coventry discussed such medical luminaries as Isaac Ray, Charles Bell, James Cowles Prichard, and Amariah Brigham and commented on both the recent M'Naghten ruling in England and the concept of moral insanity. However, Coventry also included in his testimony other medical authorities: Spurzheim, Gall, and Andrew Combe. He further observed that: "The subject of forensic medicine is treated in connexion with phrenology, because I think they cannot be separated," a revealing statement from a professor of medical jurisprudence and forensic medicine.[151]

Coventry's testimony, with its mix of medical and phrenological experts and attention to the question of moral insanity, was representative of an admixture of these ideas in mid-nineteenth-century America. The particular problems with which medicolegal figures tangled centered upon the state of the field of medical jurisprudence and the question of criminal insanity in particular. In the 1830s and 1840s, when these debates were ongoing, phrenology was yet a viable and valuable option for the making of medicolegal expertise: as Coventry had observed, phrenology and medicolegal knowledge could not (yet) be separated.

Moreover, even after explicit uses of phrenology as medicolegal expertise and phrenologists as expert witnesses were discarded, implicit uses of phrenological language continued to structure medicolegal approaches to problems of criminality, particularly criminal insanity.

Twenty years later, in the 1865 trial of the conspirators in the assassination of Abraham Lincoln, the defense attorney interrogated a medical witness on the stand by asking: "Is or is not a morbid propensity to destroy, proof of insanity?"[152] The counsel—perhaps unknowingly—invoked a lineage of theories of insanity relative to crime, of which phrenological theory was both related and a component, and with which phrenological theories were often combined or confused. Moreover, the use of the phrase "propensity to destroy" suggests the continued utility of phrenological language and theories, whether those using such language were aware of this or not. Indeed, throughout the nineteenth century, commentators on theories of homicidal insanity confirmed this genealogy. As one scholar of medical jurisprudence observed in 1880, writers on the subject of homicidal insanity "have sought assistance from the dead words of the phrenologists. They have found what they call a propensity to destroy or a faculty of destructiveness . . . *i.e.,* a homicidal impulse."[153] While here the author was critiquing both the use of phrenological terminology and the concept of a "propensity to destroy," he simultaneously reinforced the connection between the term and the phrenological lineage from the vantage point of the late nineteenth century. In this way, phrenological language and theories lived on in writings on medical jurisprudence, particularly those focused on insanity, and in popular culture long after phrenology itself had been dismissed by the medical and legal establishments. Phrenology was largely unsuccessful as a component of medicolegal expert witnessing, yet it successfully spread in a more implicit, and often unintentional, fashion.[154]

The continued use of these ideas and this language represents the longevity of what I term a phrenological impulse in courts of law and medicolegal discourse, especially with regard to criminal insanity. While phrenology *qua* phrenology did not become a crucial or central part of medical expert witnessing or medical jurisprudence, phrenological concepts, especially the language of propensities and understandings of criminal insanity, were mediated by figures like Ray, whose gloss on the subject of medical jurisprudence came to influence the development and articulation of medical jurisprudence for much of the nineteenth century. Phrenology thus remained an important foundational and theoretical component that indelibly affected both a broader discourse about criminality and the development of the medical jurisprudence of insanity in the United States.

Chapter 4

The Prison as Laboratory

William Miller was indicted for the robbery and murder of Solomon Hoffman in Williamsport, Pennsylvania, in 1838. Before the trial began, the sheriff and the prosecuting attorney invited Orson Squire Fowler to visit Miller in prison.[1] Fowler was only twenty-nine but was already becoming known as "one of the most distinguished phrenologists in the United States."[2] He examined Miller's head and found that "the sides of the head were bulged out to an extraordinary extent," in the region of the animal propensities, including Destructiveness, which was labeled "very large," as were Acquisitiveness and Secretiveness.[3] Remarking on the size of the animal or "selfish" propensities, Fowler observed that "the immense size of the *whole* of them, acting without the restraints of either the intellect or the moral sentiments . . . would constitute the leading features of character."[4] Any phrenologist, Fowler declared, could predict the results: Miller would be inclined to theft, fraud, and deception, and "Destructiveness 'very large' would add to these, robbery and even murder."[5]

When Miller went to trial, his attorney entered a plea of partial insanity or monomania and introduced Fowler "*without objection on the part of the commonwealth*" as a witness.[6] Fowler repeated his phrenological findings and measurements on the stand, and Judge Ellis Lewis addressed both the plea and Fowler's findings in his charge to the jury. The defense of monomania, or moral insanity, the judge explained, could not be presumed without evidence, as "the science of PHRENOLOGY . . . has not yet been brought to such a state of perfection and certainty as to be received and relied upon in courts of justice."[7] Miller was found guilty and executed two months later. After the case, both

Fowler and Lewis submitted letters detailing these events to the *American Phrenological Journal*, which published them with commentary alongside Miller's confession.

This case was not dissimilar from that of Major Mitchell, which had only occurred a few years earlier. Indeed, the judge's words to the jury echoed those of the judge in the Mitchell case, and these concerns about appropriate evidence and phrenology resonated with the medicolegal community.[8] However, a few details of this case were distinct. First, Fowler, while a remarkable gentleman, was not quite the same sort of phrenologist as the academic members of the Boston Phrenological Society. He and his brother, Lorenzo Niles Fowler, were among the first of a new breed of self-described "practical" phrenologists bringing phrenology to the masses. Second, the phrenologist was invited into the prison setting to examine the suspected murderer by local authorities: the phrenologist was part of the machinery of crime and punishment. Third, the examination of the prisoner served as a demonstration of virtuosity and prediction on the part of the phrenologist. Knowing only the crime committed, this self-professed expert was able to extrapolate Miller's character and crimes. As before, the phrenologist entered the courtroom, with limited success. Here, however, he entered another space, making it useful to phrenology: the prison.

This chapter explores the changing relationship between phrenology and the prison in the nineteenth-century United States, focusing on tensions between discourse and practice. The prison had been a space essential to the application of phrenological theory from its inception, and convicts were used both as research subjects and as exemplars to demonstrate the truth of the science. The Fowlers and their popular, practical phrenology shifted the relationship between penal spaces and phrenological ideology, enhancing a reformist impulse first introduced by George Combe and transforming it into a central tenet of practical phrenology. However, even as a reformist ethos was infused into practical phrenology, phrenologists continued to profit from their association with the penal spaces and practices they critiqued, particularly capital punishment.

Historians, including Roger Cooter and Steven Shapin, have long defined phrenology as a reform science with broad-ranging social and political meanings.[9] More recently, however, John van Wyhe asserted that "reform is inappropriate for a representation of 'phrenology' generally," arguing that instead historians "should associate phrenology with epistemological status and a brash belief in the phrenological practitioner's authority to pronounce on the causes of human behaviour and psychological abilities," rather than reform ethos or efforts.[10] Responding to van Wyhe, Poskett suggested that van Wyhe's use of the term inaccurately represented the broad and often contradictory meanings of "reform," arguing for phrenology as a reform science.[11] I suggest that the personal and public utility of the science often went hand in hand—the uses of phrenology to assert epistemological status and authority were as useful in the service of reformist projects as they were for personal advancement, and sometimes it is difficult to disentangle these seemingly disparate uses and motivations. Early nineteenth-century debates about penal reform, prison discipline, and particularly capital punishment, provide an example of this dynamic: as the Fowlers and others promoted reform movements and mobilized a language of reform, they did so for the sake of both these movements *and* promoting their science (and themselves).

Within the phrenological community, the prison loomed large as a space in which useful bodies were collected and could serve as exemplars of phrenological doctrines. Phrenologists were invited into penal spaces to view convicts and to examine executed criminals, and they came away with knowledge about these bodies, with skulls and busts taken from convicts pre- and post-execution, and with new evidence to support their science. The relationship between phrenology and medical jurisprudence was fraught and uneven throughout this period, but phrenology did find a place within the penal system. If phrenology was efficiently discarded as an elite medicolegal practice, it persisted as a part of the mechanisms of crime and punishment.

Were phrenologists truly "at war with the gallows" and the penal system as they claimed, or were they profiteers hiding behind the language of reform?[12] Did phrenologists enter the prison as would-be liberators, endeavoring to reform minds and bodies and rehabilitate criminals, or did they view such spaces chiefly as laboratories for the development and proof of their science? This chapter explores the tensions inherent to phrenology in the prison, emphasizing in particular the turn to reformist ideology in the science and the simultaneous profit—in terms of material, status, and acclaim—phrenologists experienced from their incursions into these spaces.

Penal Reform, Phrenology, and Criminal Responsibility

The penitentiary was "invented" in the United States at the same time that phrenology was first introduced to medical, legal, and other authorities. As with the case of medical jurisprudence, debates about both prison reform and theories of criminal responsibility emerged as possible sites for the cooperative furthering of both phrenological authority and penology. American phrenological enthusiasts, primed to see the prison as a useful research site by the work of Gall and Spurzheim in Europe, also came to see the ways that phrenology could engage with the shifting politics of penology and criminal reform.

American colonial responses to crime had been primarily corporal in nature—everything from whipping and branding to banishment, to capital punishment, typically by hanging. Jails primarily served as holding sites before physical punishment. Post-Revolution, states began to slowly develop new approaches to punishment: more formal systems of law and an elaborate, tiered system of courts. As the infrastructure of law changed, so too did its punishments: corporal and capital punishment were meted out less frequently and in an increasingly narrow set of circumstances.[13]

In the 1820s, as Frank Morn notes, "two new institutions were invented in America: solitary confinement and silence," which together signaled the creation of the American penitentiary movement.[14] Two competing systems emerged in this period, structuring the building of new penitentiaries and the punishments they embodied: the Pennsylvania system and the Auburn system.[15] The Pennsylvania system or "separate system," exemplified by Eastern State Penitentiary, completed in 1829 in Philadelphia, was focused on near-total silence and solitary confinement, inspired by Quaker ideology. The Pennsylvania system later introduced craft labor and religious study into the system, believing that this would prompt moral reform, though the prisoners remained solitary. The Auburn system or "congregate system," developed in New York at the Auburn Prison in the 1810s, implemented solitary confinement at night, but it also included lockstep marching, uniforms, whipping, and silent, communal work during the day, imposing a factory system of labor in the prison and rendering this a productive—and potentially profitable—space.[16] These institutions and their contingent innovations, though repressive and violent by modern standards and custodial in nature, nevertheless represented a utopian and reformist belief in the potential to rehabilitate criminals, to "cure" the social ailment of crime.[17]

The separate and congregate systems were studied and replicated throughout the United States and in Europe as part of a broader American and cross-continental debate over penal reform.[18] While politicians, philosophers, and penal and state authorities debated the relative dangers and features of these systems, particularly solitary confinement, the goals of these new penal systems were reform, not punishment alone. Solitude, silence, religious study, physical labor, and corporal punishment—these various disciplinary components were evaluated based on their potential to reform, even as reformers became increasingly convinced that some criminals were not salvageable.[19] Christian ideology, inspired by the Second Great Awakening, also influenced reform movements of this era, particularly temperance, directing the shape of the utopian hopes of American penal reform.[20] In the United States, scripture provided one part of the solution; science provided another.

Debates about the nature of punishment and the penal system intersected with scientific debates about criminal responsibility, particularly the question of moral insanity.[21] Phrenologists had much to say on both subjects, and the prisons they entered over the course of the nineteenth century were increasingly modeled on either the separate system or the congregate system.[22] Moreover, the implications of the language of propensity and the organs for understanding crime further complicated questions of both culpability and rehabilitation. Phrenologists emphasized, perhaps paradoxically, that one's organs or faculties indicated deeply fixed aspects of character, but they also averred that "good" faculties could be cultivated and the influence of "bad" faculties could be averted through introspection and self-improvement. Working under these assumptions, a clear benefit to early childhood education emerged, which will be explored in the next chapter: "Our prisons are filled with criminals, who, had they been rightly placed—away from temptations when young and weak—and wisely directed through childhood, would, many of them, subsequently have made useful and honorable citizens."[23]

What was less clear to phrenologists and reformers alike were the benefits of re-education and rehabilitation efforts for people later in life, particularly recidivists. The solution was perhaps indefinite incarceration. As one phrenological author argued, "for those who will not or can not regulate themselves . . . it is the duty of society to restrain, educate, and take care of the weak, the insane, the idiotic, and the intemperate, in some other way besides putting them to death."[24] The reformed penitentiary, to some phrenological writers, came too late to the problem, or remained far too harsh in its methods. They argued that a thorough reform of society and the educational system in particular would obviate the need for the prison altogether, except for those who were incapable of "regulating" themselves.

This emphasis on re-educating and reforming the criminal, which presupposed a changeability of essential characteristics, seems incompatible with a second component of the phrenological reformist ideology with regard to the criminal: the anti–capital punishment position. While for many the idea of capital punishment was barbarous as a concept, as it had been for Combe, practical phrenologists insisted that many criminals, especially recidivists, were "moral imbeciles" who could not be held accountable for their actions.[25] This was especially true for those who were victims of an excess of Destructiveness: "There cannot be the least doubt that many a murderer has forfeited his life on a scaffold, when he should have been confined in a lunatic asylum."[26] The excesses of the animal organs led such unfortunates down a path that terminated in the gallows. Even if such individuals were best placed in asylums and similar institutions, a direct connection was nonetheless made between "bad" organs and "bad" behaviors.

The expectation for the incarceration of offenders was that they could and should be rehabilitated within the prison. But could a "moral idiot" with a "bad head" be made a productive member of society? Were organs—of theft, of murder—immutable and essential to a person's character, or were they changeable and capable of improvement? To argue against capital punishment was to say that such men could not help themselves, yet to argue for better education in prisons was to suggest that such characteristics could be changed, erasing the criminal stain. This tension was never resolved in phrenological texts, which presumed the immutability of a criminal type, linking physical appearance with moral misbehavior. A phrenologist could thus declare at the autopsy table, post-execution, that "judging phrenologically, he had not the slightest doubt" that the murderer was guilty of the crime for which he was executed.[27]

Although this position on crime, initially formulated by Combe and replicated by other phrenologists, has not always been perceived as entirely altruistic, these positions were in line with the most liberal prison reformers of the day.[28] Indeed, American prison reformers were interested in phrenology's explanatory power and its ability to "lead to juster ideas on the subject of crime and its punishment."[29] For penal reformers, phrenology was a useful prop to their arguments regarding the abolition of capital punishment, since it provided proof that criminals could not necessarily be held accountable for their actions. As one reformer argued regarding treatment of the prisoner: "We have him in our power, what then should we do with him? First, we examine his head, (for no philosopher will deny the truth of Phrenology,) and ascertain the state of his organs, and certainly if we find certain propensities largely developed in him, it is wicked to punish him severely for that which he is not so much to blame for."[30] Another reformer of varied interests, Lydia Maria Child, while visiting a penitentiary and a lunatic asylum on Blackwell Island, New York, reflected on the plight of "the morally and the intellectually insane." Phrenology, Child argued, even "with all its absurd quackery on its back, will yet aid mankind in giving the fitting answer."[31]

Some prison reformers took the promise of phrenology to heart and made it the centerpiece of their approach to crime. Most notably, Eliza Farnham, reformer and matron of the women's section of Sing Sing in New York from 1844 to 1848, brought phrenology into the prison.[32] During the beginning of Farnham's tenure at Sing Sing, she edited Marmaduke Sampson's *The Rationale of Crime.*[33] Sampson was an English phrenologist who argued that crime could be attributed to the relative size of different organs of the brain (like Destructiveness) and that such tendencies could be corrected through the stimulation of weaker faculties, through re-education.[34] Farnham's editing work on the volume also included notes and addendums to the text, presaging her reforms to prison life for the inmates under her care.[35] Farnham's reform of the prison, supported by Lorenzo Fowler, included phrenological lectures and education, especially reading to the inmates from Combe's *The Constitution of Man*.[36] However, Farnham's phrenological penal regime was unsuccessful, and much of the criticism from outside observers was devoted to her phrenological tendencies, as phrenology was falling out of fashion among intellectual circles by the 1840s, the period of her tenure.[37] Even if Farnham's application of phrenological theory to prison discipline was short-lived, her attempt suggested the potential for the practical use of phrenology in penal settings.

Phrenologists themselves, at least in the United States, seemed to have been much of the same mind as prison reformers, and their ambitions echoed those of Farnham. When Charles Spear, the editor of *The Prisoner's Friend*, toured New York prisons and attended prison reform and antislavery meetings in May of 1846, he wrote the report of his trip in Fowler's Phrenological Rooms, while the man was in residence: "I have just asked him [Fowler] this question: 'Are phrenologists generally in favor of the abolition of capital punishment?' His reply is, 'Yes.' This is an important fact, for some of the most distinguished men of our time are among the strongest advocates of phrenology."[38]

Prison Reform and the Fowler Brothers

While the editor of *The Prisoner's Friend* might have suggested that "the most distinguished men of our time" were followers of phrenology, by 1848 elite phrenological enthusiasm was in decline. By the end of 1840s, the Boston Phrenological Society was defunct, its large collection of skulls and plaster casts abandoned to an attic, its members dispersed and focusing on other endeavors. Phrenology experienced a sharp decline in elite enthusiasm in this decade, in part due to the critiques of French physiologist Marie-Jean-Pierre Flourens.[39] Flourens's critiques of Gall's theories and the concept of localization more generally had begun in the 1820s, but by the 1840s his position, based on brain lesion experiments on animals, had solidified and triumphed.[40] He and his followers argued against localization through the 1860s, when the new findings of scientists exploring motor centers in the brain collapsed these critiques.[41] As far as American medical elites were concerned in the early part of the century, as France—and especially Paris—went, so too did the cutting edge of medical theory.[42] It was therefore unsurprising that the Boston Phrenological Society, the apotheosis of elite phrenological enthusiasm in America, quietly folded, and that most enthusiasts moved on to other pursuits.[43]

However, already beginning in the mid-1830s, the Fowlers—Orson Squire and Lorenzo Niles—were touring the nation spreading the gospel of phrenology and growing in prominence as practical phrenologists. By the early 1840s, rival lecturers emerged who modeled their practice after that of the Fowler brothers.[44] These practical phrenologists, who gave lectures to popular crowds and examined heads for a small fee, were often lumped in with the professors, physicians, and elite professionals and intellectuals, like Amos Dean and Isaac Ray, who had evinced phrenological enthusiasm in the previous decade, but practical phrenologists were distinct in several ways.[45] The phrenological enthusiasts associated with the Boston Phrenological Society and other early societies, though invested in phrenology, were professionals in other disciplines, including law, medicine, and asylum-keeping. Practical phrenologists, the Fowlers in particular, took phrenology as their profession and primarily addressed not a small, elite set of professionals but an interested public: their goals, training, and audiences were different.

Even as elite enthusiasm faded in the United States, popular, "practical" phrenology flourished. In 1842, Orson Fowler assumed the editorship of the *American Phrenological Journal* (*APJ*), and the brothers set up shop in New York, which shifted the center of phrenology from Boston to New York.[46] Only five years later, the Fowlers' *APJ* claimed twenty thousand subscribers, one of the largest monthly circulations in the United States.[47] The Fowlers were enamored of reform, announcing that the primary work of the *APJ* was to "PHRENOLOGIZE OUR NATION, for thereby it will REFORM THE WORLD."[48] "Reform, *reform*, REFORM," as they argued in the second issue they edited for the *Journal*, "is emphatically the watchword of the age."[49] Reform was also emphatically linked to phrenology, in the Fowlers' eyes: "But the *true* religion, the *best* system of political economy, the *correct* doctrines in regard to banks, the laws of trade, the relations of property, &c., the best system, or rather the only proper method of educating the human mind, together with the only true principles in regard to legislation, civil and criminal jurisprudence, government, matrimony, &c. &c., will each be found to have its counterpart in the doctrines of Phrenology."[50] As this statement suggests, the popularization of phrenology coincided with an increased national emphasis on the possibility of reform.[51] Practical phrenologists, particularly the Fowlers, participated in and discussed a number of reform movements, including crusades for sex education; for fashion reform, especially against tight-lacing; against tobacco and alcohol; health reform, particularly the water cure; abolitionism, especially the Free Kansas movement; women's suffrage; and penal reform and anti–capital punishment.[52]

From the 1840s onward, the *APJ* became a repository for reformist discourse around crime and punishment, among other matters. From its earliest issues and prior to the Fowlers' editorship, like the Boston Phrenological Society's *Annals* and the Edinburgh Phrenological Society's *Transactions*, the *APJ* had long covered issues of crime and punishment. The first issue of the *Transactions*, published in 1824, included among its articles three case studies of noted murderers, an essay on the character of criminals based on studies of the heads of executed murderers, by George Combe, and an essay on Destructiveness and Combativeness, connecting these organs to murder and crime.[53] Likewise, the earliest issues of the *APJ* and the *Annals* similarly reported the cases of famous murderers, thieves, and pirates. However, while crime was discussed in all of these publications, the tenor of the discourse in the *APJ* changed after the Fowlers became the editors. They continued to include profiles of famous murderers in the *APJ*, but they also published reform-minded articles on capital punishment and penitentiaries. The Fowlers politicized the phrenological approach to crime, responding to broader political and cultural debates about crime and punishment.

Capital punishment was a particular object of ire for this new breed of politicized, practical phrenologist. As one writer decried the practice in the *APJ*: "How long must gambling apparatus, brandy-bottles, and the gallows be marks of civilization? When will men learn their true interest, and be prepared for higher joys than mere animal gratification? When will man treat his brother man, who is either unfortunate in his organization, or depraved by an animal education, like a human being, instead of hanging him up like a dog? Not until the rationale of crime and its proper punishment shall be better understood, and law and criminal jurisprudence adapted to the nature of man."[54] This statement highlights the interconnectedness of the various phrenological reform projects of the time, but capital punishment served as the central focus. Similar statements were common accompaniments or epilogues to otherwise typical reports of the execution of criminals. Another author, describing the execution of two men in New York, deplored the "sanguinary spectacle" and concluded that "it is to be hoped that the gallows will not long hold its present conspicuous position among the institutions of the nineteenth century."[55] In another article, on the phrenological character of the murderer John C. Colt, the editors were even more direct, declaring: "Phrenology is directly at war with the gallows."[56]

In other cases, phrenology was presented as the solution for these social problems, a path toward righteousness and reform, as seen in a series of five essays published in the *APJ* in 1845, entitled "The Law of Love a Far More

Effectual Preventative of Crime Than Punitive Measures, Capital Punishment Included." The author of the first essay, J. Kenny, argued against capital punishment and punitive prisons by stressing that the "fatal error" was that men were punished severely after their crime, but nothing was done in advance to prevent crimes by checking the "sinful *propensity itself*."[57] Kenny asked and answered: "But, is there no *substitute* for punishment, as a preventive of crime? There is. *Phrenology* points out a more excellent way. So does the Christian dispensation."[58] Christian doctrine influenced the development of Kenny's thinking and those of other authors in the *APJ*, but it was phrenology that provided the practical mechanism and solution.[59] The four other essays in this series, as well as other essays mobilizing this sentiment and title, elaborated on these themes using examples of unfortunate criminals who ended their lives on the gallows and counterexamples of those whose lives were transformed by love and kindness.[60]

The Fowlers and other writers pursued these arguments in the *APJ* throughout the 1840s and 1850s, emphasizing a dialectic of punishment versus transformative love and kindness. These writers argued that the current system of punishment, including the so-called reformed penitentiary, had been designed "to gratify a spirit of revenge."[61] Prisons were not places of reform, despite the claims of the promoters of the new systems, nor did they deter offenders. If anything, they were schools of crime. Instead, the editors and others argued, society must renounce the principle of vengeance and work toward two goals: protecting society and reforming the offender.[62] These arguments were in line with those of George Combe but modified to fit into American prison reformist discourse, with an added emphasis on Christian doctrine.

Similar arguments were made regarding capital punishment, as writers in the *APJ* argued that the gallows did not deter murderers. Phrenologists turned to the language of propensities to explain their reasoning, as organs like Destructiveness or Acquisitiveness would have led the criminal to his act, and the more circumspect organs—Cautiousness, for example—would be inadequate to respond to the threat of hanging.[63] Further, criminals as a class included those who were insane by virtue of poor or excess development of the organs, or due to an injury to the head, as in the case of Mitchell or Haggerty. Practical phrenologists argued that the deficiencies of the criminal justice system left the criminally insane individual "unprotected against his own perverted nature, to commit the more fearful and life-forfeiting crime of murder."[64] Unfortunately, even when the courts deemed an insane person to be "an unfit subject for the gallows," a hue and cry was raised against "'mistaken leniency'"—proof of the vengeful nature of the penal system.[65]

Practical phrenologists further argued that the spectacle of capital punishment incited others to violence. As one author suggested, "the public condemnation and execution of a human being, by stimulating the faculty of Destructiveness in those who have it already too large, and blunting the Benevolence of those who have too little of it, paves the way to wrangling, fighting mobs, and murder."[66] Thus, the act of witnessing an execution could incite others to violent or criminal behavior, rather than deterring them. The gallows "invariably excited the homicidal organs in the class of minds which they were designed to benefit."[67] While a man with normal or superior development of the organs might have witnessed any number of executions without adverse effect, those most likely to have the propensity to crime would have been encouraged in these inclinations, rather than discouraged. "Murder begets murder," in sum.[68]

In order to eliminate crime, the Fowlers and their fellow reform-minded practical phrenologists argued, several things needed to be accomplished. First, capital punishment must be abolished, as it did not serve as a deterrent to crime, and because it could, in fact, incite a person to commit crime. Second, prisons must be further reformed with an eye to re-education through love and kindness, rather than fear or punishment. Third, criminals could be arrested in their earliest development by educating all children with proper moral instruction. In such a way, even those with overdeveloped animal propensities would fail to turn to crime. Indeed, it was the obligation of society to provide for criminals' restoration to society.[69] For those who considered this to be an impossible task, phrenologists asserted their science as the way forward. Phrenologists argued that criminals should be placed under a "MORAL AND SANATORY regimen, calculated to develop the higher faculties, and remove frenzied excitement from the propensities."[70]

The *APJ*, remade by the Fowlers in the 1840s into an organ of reformist discourse, presented a platform for phrenological reforms to the rehabilitation of criminals and the penal system. The arguments made in the journal elaborated on Combe's writings and drew connections to other reform movements and positions, including post–Second Great Awakening trends in Christian thought and the prison reform movement.[71] Phrenologists did not, however, merely engage with these questions on a theoretical level: they also entered prisons and participated in the system directly. However, it was not as reformers that practical phrenologists entered the prison. Phrenologists in the prison operated primarily in the service of the legitimization of their science, rather than in the spirit of reformist principles.

Phrenologists in the Prison and Postmortem

Despite their critiques of the penal system, phrenologists had a deep-seated relationship with the prison in antebellum America. They were welcomed by wardens, judges, and attorneys into penal settings to examine criminals, which played into the phrenological goals of proving the predictive power of their science. Phrenologists also participated in autopsies or took ownership of the skull or cast of the head of the convict after execution. In these ways, phrenologists made a place for themselves within the penal system.

The phrenological visit to the prison was an early feature of phrenology, following Gall and Spurzheim, as discussed in chapter 1. The prison visit became an important defensive maneuver for practical phrenologists and enthusiasts alike as well as a laboratory for the production of phrenological knowledge. Letters reveal that Spurzheim made a number of prison visits during his brief tour of the United States, including his visit to the Hartford prison, where he identified two murderous co-conspirators for an impressed Amariah Brigham, as discussed in chapter 2. During a similar visit to the Massachusetts State Prison, Spurzheim identified likely recidivists for the warden and explored the causes behind the prisoners' turns to crime.[72]

Other phrenologists made visits to penal spaces for similar demonstrations of virtuosity. George Combe, for example, visited prisons in Dublin as a part of a tour taken in the manner of Spurzheim.[73] In his travels through the United States, Combe visited the Charleston prison, finding that the convicts there had larger animal organs than those of intellect and moral sentiment, though not quite as deficient as the average British criminal.[74] During this trip, he also toured the establishments at Bellevue and on Blackwell Island in New York City, the Auburn Prison in New York, and the Eastern State Penitentiary in Philadelphia, in part to compare the relative merits of the competing systems (he preferred the Auburn system).[75] Combe also corresponded with others interested in prison discipline and penal reform, exchanging letters with writers as far afield as Norfolk Island, in the South Pacific.[76]

Another British phrenologist, James De Ville, examined the heads of 148 convicts on board a prison ship bound for New South Wales, as a phrenological experiment undertaken in 1826. De Ville provided the ship's surgeon, Dr. Thomson, with a "distinct memorandum of the inferred character of each individual convict," with the "desperadoes" clearly noted, especially one, Robert Hughes.[77] The results of this experiment were fruitful for the young science; according to Thomson's notes, a mutiny occurred on board the ship led by Hughes. Thomson's congratulatory report to De Ville ("I will be grateful to De Ville all my life") marked him a convert and suggested a further spread of the doctrine, as "all the authorities here have become Phrenologists."[78] One of Gall's pupils in France, Hubert Lauvergne, made his own phrenological observations at the *bagne* (penal colony) of Toulon, publishing a lengthy volume of his theories on criminality and penology.[79]

Practical phrenologists in the United States replicated similar experiments and examinations in prisons. The Fowlers visited prisons on multiple occasions. In 1834, twenty-three-year-old Lorenzo Fowler, newly out of college, embarked on an extended tour of the United States, beginning in New York and concluding in Mississippi. Fowler's journey through the United States was well documented by a collection of over two hundred phrenological cards and notes from this journey.[80] Lorenzo's clients were varied but fell generally into two types. First, many of these subjects were paying clients, "average" Americans of every age. Lorenzo examined men and women, married and unmarried, old and young, and of many occupations, which he frequently noted along with their name, the location, and the date.

The second type of subjects that Lorenzo examined during this trip were institutionalized populations, particularly convicts in prisons. Clusters of half dozen or more cards taken at the same institution on the same date, or a short range of dates, featured frequently in this collection. Among the roughly two hundred readings Lorenzo performed and recorded in his notes for this trip, at least thirty-five were of convicts within institutions, including jails in Albany, Ithaca, and elsewhere in New York, the Eastern State Penitentiary in Philadelphia, a jail in Louisville, Kentucky, and the Indiana penitentiary. Another fourteen cases were inmates of the Cincinnati Lunatic Asylum. Lorenzo's examinations of convicts and other inmates within these institutions suggests the accessibility of these spaces to practitioners, even early in the days of practical phrenology. His findings, meanwhile, confirmed the phrenological assessment of criminal propensities. Lorenzo summed up one case succinctly: "a very <u>bad head</u> . . . would do any thing to gratify his will."[81] Another, female convict had a "licentious thievish disposition," and yet another, a rapist, was described as having "a bad head—nothing will deter him from his purpose—has not conscientiousness enough to direct his propensities a right."[82]

Despite the Fowler brothers' later embrace of reform positions, at this early moment, when confronted with convicted criminals, Lorenzo saw immutable characteristics, not reformable offenders: these were simply "very <u>bad head</u>[s]," "calculated by nature for the station" they filled.[83] However, these assessments seemed to have been based at times on circumstantial evidence, such as the known crime and sentence. Fowler assessed more than one criminal with lower numerical scores in the animal organs, including Destructiveness, than the "average" clients for whom he had only positive assessments. Despite the importance of organs like Destructiveness for the articulation of criminal theory within phrenology, the science in practice was inflected by the status and identity of its phrenological subjects.

Moreover, while Lorenzo was invested in the commercial gains of phrenology, he simultaneously engaged in an exploratory process involving criminals and mentally ill individuals. Much like Gall's visits to the prison, Lorenzo was entering the same kinds of spaces as he (and his brother) began to develop their own iteration of phrenological practice. Criminals and penal spaces were therefore as much a part of the development of practical phrenology as they were a foundation of classical craniology. Lorenzo Fowler paid attention to two kinds of heads, "good" and "bad," as his notations suggested. This fascination with opposite types would not fade from practical phrenology as it matured; if anything, this relationship would only be continually underlined by the discourse of practical phrenologists, as discussed further in the next chapter.

The Fowlers visited other prisons in the decades after this 1834–1835 trip for the purpose of "testing the truth of their science."[84] To return to the example that opened this book, when Lorenzo visited the Tombs in New York in 1849, for example, he was "invited to the prison and introduced to the several cells by the keeper" to perform "test examinations" on the convicts.[85] During this visit, Fowler examined a series of murderers and proclaimed on the nature of each prisoner in turn. This visit was modeled on similar visits to prisons by Spurzheim and Gall, with examinations of numbers of prisoners in order to demonstrate the "triumphant success of phrenological truth."[86]

The Fowlers were not alone in their visits to American prisons. One writer wrote into the *APJ* reporting on the phrenological characteristics of convicts in a St. Louis jail.[87] Frederick Coombs, a southern phrenologist, visited the New Orleans jail in 1837, and in his subsequent advertising for his lectures, included testimonials from the sheriff and jail keeper on his broadsides.[88] Coombs, in his own words, "found no difficulty in selecting the worst criminal there," and the testimonials noted that his examinations conveyed "exactness and minutiæ of detail that was quite incredible, and has fully convinced us [the sheriff and wardens] of the truth of Phrenology."[89] Phrenologists, including the Fowlers, also examined individual murderers and criminals within prisons, typically in advance of execution, as in the case of William Miller. Articles on the phrenological characteristics of murderers were often based on examinations performed right before execution, with the phrenologist making a personal call, with the warden's permission, to the to-be-executed convict within the jail, or conducted after the execution, on the autopsy table.

Other examinations were conducted as part of an autopsy, with the phrenologist working as part of a group of medical men. William Fahnestock, who testified in the trial of John Haggerty, also participated in a series of experiments conducted on the body of another convict, Henry Cobler Moselman, before and after his execution in 1839.[90] These experiments were conducted by the Medical Faculty of Lancaster with the permission of the sheriff of Lancaster County. Fahnestock's phrenological findings were included in the report of experiments, prefaced with a note that his report was "unanimously adopted, and ordered to be inserted into this part of the general report."[91] The report primarily consisted of caliper, craniometer, and tape measurements of the skull, as he pointedly "refrained from any remarks upon his character."[92] He later published a report on Moselman in the *APJ* reminiscent of a detective story, complete with a reconstruction of Moselman's biography, the events leading to his life of crime and murder, and excerpts from the convict's personal diary, as well as the phrenological report. Unlike the earlier autopsy report, this account included Fahnestock's musings on Moselman's character and tendencies toward certain actions or behaviors.[93] While it was unclear as to whether Fahnestock participated in the trial or how he gained access to Moselman's personal papers, his engagement with this case illustrates the inclusion of phrenological expertise into explorations of the criminal body. Fahnestock was integrated into the medical community of Lancaster and entered the prison as an invited expert, suggesting the potential for a fruitful relationship between the phrenologist and the prison.

In other cases, autopsy reports included phrenological measurements made by medical professionals. After the convicted murderer William Freeman died in his cell at Auburn in New York in 1847, the central question of his case—whether or not he was insane—was put to the test by a panel of medical experts.[94] The postmortem examination was led by two phrenological enthusiasts, Amariah Brigham, the director of the Utica State Asylum, and John McCall, described in the report as "a Phrenologist."[95] As a part of the trial report, an appendix was produced of the findings, including a set of phrenological measurements prepared by Dr. Blanchard Fosgate. Fosgate measured Freeman's cranium twice: first, with the use of a string to measure circumference, and secondly "after the directions laid down in Combe's Phrenology, by callipers."[96] With regard to Freeman's character, he deferred to "Mr. Fowler," quoting directly from an article in Lorenzo Fowler's *Phrenological and Physiological Almanac for 1848*.[97] Fosgate's report was republished in the *American Journal of the Medical Sciences* and in the *American Quarterly Retrospect of American and Foreign Practical Medicine and Surgery*, where the essay was lauded for its "uncommon elegance" and for illustrating "the importance of this science to the welfare of men."[98]

The *APJ* frequently covered pre- and postmortem prison phrenology, dwelling on the findings rather than questions of access. "We saw him during the trial and also after he was executed," the Fowlers noted succinctly on James Stephens, one murderer.[99] Even when the body of the murderer was accessible in the prison, however, readings were often performed on a cast. The murderer Peter Robinson, for example, generously sat for a plaster cast of his head the day before his execution, providing the material basis for a phrenological reading, which was compared to the courtroom confessions.[100] A reading of George Wilson, another murderer, was given "from a cast which was taken by us immediately after his execution."[101] Other accounts made the mechanism of measurement less clear. An article on the murderer and attempted rapist Harris Bell included measurements of the head, but the writer did not discuss how or where the head was accessed.[102] The phrenologist was not always present at the execution or at the postmortem, but nevertheless acquired the skull or bust and presented a postmortem reading. The *APJ* was often vague on the provenance of these objects, which may suggest that some of these skulls or casts were illicitly procured. In the case of Arthur Spring, the editor observed only that "the skull may be seen at our cabinet," but it was unclear as to how the skull of this murderer was acquired.[103]

Articles in the popular press also indicate the frequency with which phrenologists attended or led pre- or postmortem examinations of criminals. In 1835, Dr. W. Byrd Powell, a Professor of Chemistry in the Medical College of Louisiana and a lecturer on phrenology, published a "phrenological exposition" of the noted "land pirate" John A. Murrell, then being held in a Tennessee penitentiary. The governor invited Powell into the prison to examine Murrell, and the organs and characteristics of his head were reported in the press with caliper measurements comparing it to the "usual head." Powell indicated that "Inhabitiveness, Secretiveness, Destructiveness, Acquisitiveness and Constructiveness are large," yet he also noted that, because Benevolence balanced Destructiveness, "he cannot be regarded as possessing a murderous disposition."[104] Orson Fowler also examined Murrell and concurred with Powell, observing that "his notorious rascality does not depend so much upon a bad Phrenological organization, as upon the wrong direction of his mind when young."[105] Murrell's body was disinterred after his death, and his skull became a feature of Southern country fairs in the 1840s, becoming a public spectacle and extending the "career" of this criminal.[106]

In American newspapers, phrenology regularly made its way into discussions of crime and punishment. One account of an execution in 1844 noted that after the hanging of two men for murder in Maryland, the bodies were removed by permission of the sheriff into the courtroom, where "Dr. Worster, the well-known Phrenologist of Philadelphia" examined them and gave "an eloquent lecture" on their characters.[107] Other accounts of executions were more succinct. The entirety of one such notice read: "We understand that the phrenologists, who attentively examined the head of Gibbs, after his execution, found the organ of destructiveness wonderfully developed, and are unanimously of opinion that he was a notorious scoundrel."[108] Here, the execution, the phrenologists' opinion, and the murderous constitution were all linked in a single narrative of the postmortem: the article itself was titled "Organ of Destructiveness." In other short notices, the connection between criminal and phrenologist was implicit but nonetheless clear. For example, a brief mention of the high-profile case of convicted murderer Chastine Cox in 1879 concluded with a simple line: "Prof. Fowler says he has a good head."[109]

Phrenologists were invited into penal spaces more frequently than into courtrooms, and their anatomical expertise was often brought to bear on the heads of criminals. The inclusion of phrenologists in postmortem exams and frequent references to phrenological examination post-execution framed this encounter as the terminal step in the life of a criminal. Some convicted murderers even embraced—or at least acquiesced—to this expectation, leaving their skulls to local phrenologists after their execution. In 1867, one convicted murderer, George Goetz, "bequeathed his head to Professor Koekler, the phrenologist, in consideration of being kept in cigars and whiskey" through the trial and prison stay.[110] In such a way, phrenologist and convict benefited one another. Whether they willingly and knowingly donated their heads or not, many criminals eventually became incorporated into the phrenologist's cabinet of skulls and casts. Prisons were fertile and welcoming spaces for phrenologists throughout the century. How then did practical phrenologists like the Fowlers square their reformist interests with their frequent use of the prison?

The Uses of the Prison

Even though reform-minded, practical phrenologists protested the practice of execution as barbaric, they simultaneously benefited from their access to the bodies of convicted murderers and criminals, making extensive use of the casts and skulls of executed criminals. Even as the Fowlers and their associate Dr. Samuel Wells published jeremiads against capital punishment in their journal, they simultaneously included excited notices regarding the acquisition of new casts taken from the heads of executed murderers for their cabinet.[111] For example, when James Eager, a murderer, was tried and hanged in New York in May of 1845, Dr. Samuel R. Wells, a close associate of the Fowler brothers, cast a bust from the corpse directly after the execution.[112] A Dr. Holmes acquired the body for dissection and delivered the skull to the offices of the *APJ*, which published an account of the phrenological characteristics of Eager. Destructiveness and the other animal propensities achieved predictably high marks, while the moral sentiments were assigned low values. However, the writer averred that Eager was not a murderer by constitution: "he *could* have been made a good citizen."[113] Instead, it was the excitation of alcohol that led him to murder, and as such he deserved "our pity, not the gallows."[114] Indeed, the author concluded, "Society *makes* men bad, and then hangs them."[115]

The anti–capital punishment point of view suggested by these final remarks was reinforced by the next article in the same issue of the *APJ*, "The Law of Love a Far More Effectual Preventative of Crime Than Punitive Measures, Capital Punishment Included," which aimed to introduce a "cool, intellectual view" of the matter of capital punishment, without dwelling on the "horrors of an execution."[116] At first glance, both this essay and the commentary in the account of Eager seem to share the same sentiment against capital punishment and toward penal reform. However, these articles illustrate a curious tension inherent to the phrenological position on crime and punishment. Both essays expressed distaste with the violence of execution from a phrenological vantage point. However, the opening of the account of Eager's execution *also* elucidated the deep relationship between phrenology and the fruits of the gallows and prison. Whatever their political position might have been on the matter, phrenologists benefited from their postmortem examinations and the acquisition of the heads of convicts. Postmortem examinations of criminals were frequently performed at several stages of removal from the corpse, as phrenologists acquired a cast of the head after the execution or examined the bust without ever having been in the presence of the convict, and phrenological cabinets were filled with the skulls and casts of known criminals.[117]

Such skulls and busts were commonly used to test phrenologists. Sometimes these tests were framed as hoaxes and reported in the popular press, with an unidentified skull or bust being presented to a phrenologist, who subsequently interpreted it inaccurately. In 1835, a Professor Sim was tested by a Dr. Kelsey, who "induced some respectable young men to be locked up in jail and submit their head to a Phrenological examination, as convicts."[118] When Sim identified "all sorts of rascally bumps" on the heads of these false criminals, Kelsey got the better of him.[119] More frequently, however, it was the phrenologist who triumphed in these situations. A Mr. Junham was tested by a group of skeptical gentlemen with the heads of an "idiot" and a drummer, and his "wonderful skill in judging of character" turned this test into an advertisement for his services.[120]

These tests of phrenology, whether put to the phrenologist by a skeptic or arranged by him for the purpose of proving the science, were almost exclusively focused on the skulls of criminals. In one example from 1837, Dr. A. C. Dayton procured the skull of a noted murderer, Antoine Le Blanc, and submitted it to three practical phrenologists in turn.[121] First, Orson Fowler and his associate Mr. Brevoort were presented with the skull, which they analyzed in the presence of witnesses. They determined that the individual was male, a thief, and violent, a set of detailed qualities that witnesses agreed were in line with Le Blanc. Lorenzo Fowler was next presented with the skull and produced his own account. The collected readings were judged to be in "almost a perfect agreement, not only in the *general*, but in the *particular* results."[122]

A similar demonstration was performed a few years later, when a skull was presented without details to the Phrenological Society of New York. A committee appointed to examine the skull provided caliper measurements and estimates of the size of the various organs, concluding that the man was of unfortunate organization: "would be quite unfit to be a law unto himself; he would be profligate and corrupt, of a savage, blood-thirsty disposition."[123] Further, "remorse would hardly be felt by him for the most atrocious deeds. He would be pleased with villainy adroitly executed."[124] Following these findings, the man who submitted the skull presented a paper on the life of the man, who was tried for the murder of his wife and child while intoxicated and thereafter executed. As these phrenological readings were in line with the reported events, they were offered as evidence of the truth of phrenology.

These cases were published in the first volume of the *APJ*, when phrenology was still new to American audiences and its proponents were in the process of negotiating for expert status. Such demonstrations were used at this time to promote the expert knowledge of phrenologists. However, many more examples of this kind of demonstration abounded once the *APJ* came under the Fowlers' editorship. For example, Fowler, while giving lectures in Philadelphia, was challenged by Dr. Alfred T. King of the Philadelphia Medical College to examine an anonymous skull before a room of medical students.[125] Fowler found that the individual was "positively deficient in benevolence, humanity, sympathy, kindness, and interest in others . . . in justice, equity, and moral circumspection."[126] King then revealed that the skull was that of Hugh Carrigan, recently convicted and executed for the murder and burning of his wife, along with a host of other crimes. King then "rose and stated that he was astonished, for that he had never before, under such circumstances, heard so correct, so truthful, and so remarkable a delineation of character."[127]

Another phrenologist, D. P. Butler, was interrupted in the middle of a lecture in Boston by a physician in attendance, who presented him with a skull and requested he interpret it. Butler found that the skull suggested a "coarsely organized brain," predisposed to theft, and, due to large Destructiveness, "likely to commit higher crimes, even of robbery or murder."[128] The doctor who presented the skull proclaimed that these findings were "astonishingly correct."[129] The Fowlers also tested themselves. For example, Lorenzo and Orson Fowler each interpreted the same pair of casts of skulls "wholly irrespective of each other, and without either of us knowing what the other had written," in order to produce "the most perfect and thorough test possible of phrenological science."[130] Perhaps unsurprisingly, the two accounts "agree[d] perfectly" such that the "truth of the science is put beyond the reach of doubt or cavil."[131]

Attempts to discredit phrenology and its practitioners were thwarted by the expert phrenologist who perfectly defined the character of the skull, and practical phrenologists embraced these tests as a means of proving the truth of their science, as part of a broader experimental framing of the phrenological encounter.[132] Post-mortem skull readings functioned in a similar way as the prison visits, as a means to test the science and persuade nonbelievers. The use of the criminal bust or skull, specifically, to test this truth speaks to the centrality of the criminal to proving the veracity and utility of the science. By proposing an ability to identify and predict their behaviors, phrenologists asserted criminological expertise and demonstrated their virtuosity.

The skull or bust was a tool, an object that could be used by the phrenologist to prove the truth of his science. The objects of choice for such demonstrations were the skulls and busts of criminals, especially murderers. Phrenologists were not tested, nor did they test themselves, on the heads of "average" or even exemplary men or women. Instead, it was the criminal type that provided proof of the science. Whether the head in question was from a living convict in a prison or taken postmortem, the prison and the gallows served as essential spaces for the production of scientific proof and useful bodies.

Throughout the nineteenth century, tensions pervaded phrenological writing between critiques of execution and the penal system and the utility of the criminal corpse as commodity. Indeed, often the description of the phrenologist's acquisition of the skull or bust was given in the same breath as a condemnation of the violent practices that made this acquisition possible, as in the reform-minded *New York Tribune*: "After the hangman had done his work and judicially strangled John Owen, the latest English victim of a barbarous law, he delivered the body to the phrenologists, who made a cast of the murderer's head. . . . [According to the phrenologists,] the man was morally and physically deformed to such an extent as to be unable to govern his evil propensities unless placed in the most favorable circumstances. To hang such a man is as disgraceful as to hang a confirmed lunatic."[133] The discomfort with capital punishment voiced by this popular paper was in line with the political position of many phrenologists, and yet this group undoubtedly was benefiting from this "barbarous" practice. After all, the assessment of the "deformed" skull that allowed writers to condemn execution could only have been possible through the continued access to the bodies of the condemned.

The frequency of postmortem convict examinations and the use of executed criminals to produce casts or skulls for the cabinet were due at least in part to the ease of access to such bodies in the nineteenth century. A crucial source of bodies for the purposes of medical education and dissection has historically been those of criminals, dating from the Renaissance period, if not earlier.[134] While this changed to an extent in nineteenth-century Britain and the United States, especially due to the passage of the Anatomy Act of 1832 in Britain, which made the bodies of paupers in workhouses a new resource for medical dissection, the association between the criminal and the anatomized body remained.[135] For the readers of popular accounts of crime and punishment, the common coda to the convict's execution, the skull or a cast of the head being taken by a phrenologist, might not have been such a cause for alarm—it may even have been seen as a fitting fate for such villains.

In some cases, this fate could render the phrenologist a potential villain himself. In Indiana in 1880, a young man by the name of Gordon Truesdale "had a desire to procure a collection of human skulls, being an amateur phrenologist."[136] In order to fulfill this desire, Truesdale dug up the corpse of Sarah Platts, a young woman who had died of consumption. He removed her skull, leaving behind the lower jaw and the rest of her body. The disturbance of the grave aroused suspicion about Truesdale, who was well known in the town for his "great hobby" and his "ambition to possess a collection of sculls [*sic*]."[137] Months later, Truesdale became ill and asked a physician whether one "could become poisoned by handling a dead body."[138] His face and head began to swell, becoming "twice their natural size, and lost all semblance to human shape."[139] The physician operated on his face, resulting in masses of offensive matter oozing from each incision. Even so, the prognosis was not good, and Truesdale confessed to the grave robbery just days before his painful, putrid demise, his corpse bursting through the coffin prepared for it and thereafter hastily buried. The tenor of the articles published nationwide about this case demonstrated the extent to which phrenological fortunes had shifted by 1880: phrenology was an amateur hobby, and its practitioner was "lazy and shiftless."[140] The phrenologist here was a literal grave robber, and his death seemed fitting, even karmic: he stole a head, and destroyed his own in the process. The necessity of figuratively (or literally) robbing graves to stock phrenological cabinets was exposed in lurid detail, and the phrenologist, toward the end of the century, was no longer portrayed in a sympathetic light.

Phrenologists were parties to and beneficiaries of capital punishment, their work inextricably connected to the hangman's noose. Phrenologists continued to protest capital punishment and call for reforms to the penal system, but criminal skulls, collected post-execution, and convict heads in prisons continued to be the most useful proofs for their science. Phrenologists were rhetorically "at war with the gallows," but ultimately their discourse, rhetoric, and professional standing were reliant upon its fruits.

While phrenologists themselves never addressed this seeming contradiction, I suggest that prisons and the gallows provided human capital, a laboratory site for the refinement of the science in its early days, and proofs of the science in its latter days, which made this site too valuable to reject. Whether the head in question was from a living convict in a prison or taken postmortem, the prison and gallows served as uniquely useful sites for the production of scientific authority, specimens, and useful bodies. Phrenologists could not reject the prison and the gallows without losing access to both their most valuable research capital and the primary site for demonstrations of the predictive power of their science. This access was especially necessary when the professional and scientific status of phrenology was being challenged, as it was by midcentury. Phrenologists seeking to strengthen their scientific authority and reinforce their professional standing needed the prison, as a space otherwise unclaimed by other scientific disciplines.

The prison not only served the phrenologist; the phrenologist also contributed to the violence and the disciplinary work of the prison. The uses of vision by phrenologists within the prison mirrored and extended its panoptic aspects, contributing to the development of a culture of self-policing. The Foucauldian concept of the panopticon critiques the unequal gaze enshrined in penal architecture and the pervasive nature of observation within the prison, which was designed to produce discipline and which contributed to the unbalanced power dynamic between prisoners, their keepers, and other disciplinary bodies.[141] Moreover, the Benthamite panopticon as described by Foucault was "also a laboratory; it could be used as a machine to carry out experiments, to alter behaviour, to train or correct individuals."[142] It was "a privileged place for experiments on men," enabled by the power of disciplinary vision: a "laboratory of power."[143]

Tom McGlamery has noted that few scholars have considered the self-policing aspects of phrenology and offers his own Foucauldian reading of the practice.[144] While McGlamery mobilizes the concept of the panopticon, he interprets it as a "discursive analogue" to the Benthamite panopticon.[145] "A phrenological America is the ultimate self-policing state," as he states, but the panoptic prison also had a literal and material connection to these practices of self-policing.[146] While the phrenological gaze within the prison was not persistent and constant in the same fashion as the disciplinary gaze within the panoptic prison, the entry of the phrenologist into the prison added to the observational power and unequal gaze imposed upon prisoners, by contributing an aspect of predictive anatomical knowledge and judgment through vision. Phrenologists, including Spurzheim, Gall, the Fowler brothers, and others, gave prison wardens, as well as attorneys and judges, detailed reports on their observations of inmates, sometimes warning wardens of particularly dangerous inmates who might try to escape or behave in a violent manner, and they also acted as expert witnesses on the stand, testifying as to prisoners' potential for future bad behavior, based on the evidence of their skulls, as discussed in previous chapters. This "laboratory of power" and its disciplinary gaze both produced *and* were produced by phrenological vision.

The phrenologist also carried this visual regime out of the prison and translated it into daily life. Practical phrenology, by creating and perpetuating a culture of vision predicated on the identification of "good" and "bad" heads, enabled the production of judgment by appearances in daily life, as we shall see in the next chapter. As Foucault observed regarding the mechanism of the panopticon, "the more numerous those anonymous and temporary observers are, the greater the risk of the inmate of being surprised and the greater his anxious awareness of being observed."[147] As in the prison, so too on the street: power grows more diffuse as more eyes are encouraged and empowered to *look* and *judge*. But beyond the structure of the prison, all people are both *seeing* and *seen*, an inversion of the dynamic of the panoptic prison that does nothing to dilute the disciplinary power of vision. A student of practical phrenology in midcentury America was primed to engage in panoptic practices on the street, seeking "bad heads" and a propensity for crime before its commission. As Foucault has suggested, a panoptic system "was destined to spread throughout the social body; its vocation was to become a generalized function."[148] In mid-nineteenth-century America, phrenology provided the means, Foucault's warning realized: "The gaze is alert everywhere."[149]

Chapter 5

Policing the Self and the Stranger

A young lady, Martha, wrote a short letter to a friend describing an unpleasant trip from Boston to Concord in June of 1839, via a coach that was overly warm, crowded, and dusty. The company was not much better:

> A gentleman opposite stared at me, I put my veil down, & looked out the window, it was really annoying . . . on the whole his gaze was a mystery. When we arrived in Lexington 'twas explained. The stage stopped, some children were playing near, who immediately attracted his observation "What a magnificent head! a splendid head that child has!" & then I perceived that he was a Phrenologist. A lady I knew, whispered to me, that she had minded his staring, & thought it must be embarrassing, & guessed he had been examining my head.[1]

Martha was not alone in serving as the object of an amateur phrenologist's gaze. In the middle decades of the nineteenth century, phrenology became a popular American pastime, promoted by practical phrenologists like the Fowler brothers. Practical phrenologists encouraged individuals to engage in projects of self-improvement while simultaneously turning their attention to the strangers who surrounded them. Phrenology responded to midcentury concerns about an urbanizing nation in transition, providing a tool for managing anxieties about both the self and the stranger.

The nineteenth-century United States was a nation in flux. This period was dominated by large-scale social, cultural, technological, and political shifts that both produced and were produced by urbanization and industrialization as the United States transformed from a primarily agrarian economy to an industrial society. The rapidly expanding city was at the center of these social shifts. In the period from 1830 to 1860, America's urban population grew from roughly 500,000 to 3.8 million: Philadelphia's population grew from 161,000 to over 500,000, Boston grew from 61,000 to 133,000, and New York had the largest population growth, from 200,000 to more than 800,000.[2] By 1860, 101 American cities held more than 10,000 people (up from only twelve in 1820), and eight cities numbered more than 100,000.[3] City growth was fueled, among other factors, by immigration, particularly Irish immigrants driven by economic hardship and political necessity, as well as large numbers of other Europeans, especially Germans.[4] Increasingly, the nation was one of cities, and the cities themselves were a "world of strangers."[5]

As the century progressed, cities were increasingly viewed as "sinister and menacing."[6] Geographic mobility was high amongst the urban population, exacerbated by immigration. The geography of the city itself seemed to produce vice-ridden districts where crime, pauperism, and other illicit behaviors were concentrated. Cities also became sites for mass violence and urban unrest, such as a series of riots and gang wars in the 1830s and 1840s in northern cities. To midcentury commentators, the city appeared to be a breeding ground for vice, crime, disorder, violence, and danger, prompting hostility to the very idea of the city and a desire to exert new forms of discipline and control on this space and its denizens.[7]

Solutions to the city problem were multifaceted. Reform efforts were often allied to or complemented by political and municipal efforts to reorganize the city.[8] In particular, midcentury witnessed the reorganization of policing forces in American cities. Colonial settlements had adopted English policing practices, appointing small numbers of constables and instituting night watches, which were inconsistently recruited and infrequently paid; constables in the north and patrols in the south also policed and surveilled Indigenous and enslaved populations.[9] As the nineteenth century progressed, the growing size and attendant challenges of maintaining order in urbanizing settings necessitated a revision to this system. By the 1830s, as towns were transforming into cities, crises prompted the development of new police forces in American cities, beginning in Boston, New York, and Philadelphia.[10] In New York, the "year of the riots" of 1834–1835 and the unsolved, sensational murder of Mary Roget in 1841 served as catalysts for the 1845 creation of a 200-man "Municipal Police," inspired in part by the Metropolitan Police established in London by Sir Robert Peel in 1829.[11] Boston and Philadelphia also developed their own police forces—Boston was the first, in 1838—and other American cities and towns followed suit in an attempt to control this "plague of strangers."[12] However, these reactive developments did not satisfactorily stem the tide of crime and vice in these cities.[13] Rather than allaying fears and anxieties, policing forces became new sources of concern, with charges of corruption, abuse, ineffectiveness, and illegitimacy leveled against them.[14]

Moral reformist efforts were one attempt to approach the problem of the city; reorganized and expanded police efforts were another. But ultimately the city was the site for a host of cultural anxieties about perceived increasing incidences of crime, violence, vice, and moral decay. These concerns reflected broad-based midcentury anxieties about the place of the individual in a rapidly changing society, joined to fears about strangers in their midst. As Karen Halttunen has argued, in a "fluid social world where no one occupied a fixed social position, the question 'Who am I?' loomed large; and in an urban social world where many of the people who met face-to-face each day were strangers, the question 'Who are you really?' assumed even greater significance."[15] The management of the anxieties invoked by these questions was baked into the cultural products of the midcentury. Self-improvement, as viewed through the conduct manuals and other sources Halttunen analyzes, was one way to manage this expansive set of anxieties. Phrenology and physiognomy were another.

The slippage between physiognomy and phrenology in this period was substantial. Phrenological texts often used the term "physiognomy" and its lessons alongside phrenological concepts. Further, as Sharrona Pearl argues regarding physiognomy in midcentury Britain, "the urban streets became sites of sight, in which all city inhabitants were both observers and the observed."[16] The same was true in the United States with regard to phrenology and physiognomy. The culture of practical phrenology was captivated by the same concerns that motivated urban reformers and municipal police forces: fears of the stranger shaded into fears of the criminal, and practical phrenology reinforced a black-and-white view of human nature in which there were good heads and bad. For the anxious phrenological client, the answer to the question "Who am I?"—hopefully, a good head—was as important as the answer to the question posed to the stranger, "Who are you really?"—potentially, a bad head.

Practical phrenologists in the midcentury United States communicated to an interested public, in Pearl's terms, a "shared subjectivity" predicated on the importance of *looking* in the assessment of character; I argue that, with respect to identifying potential criminals, phrenology possessed sufficient "visual legibility" for it to be useful in this endeavor.[17] If a phrenologist could identify the worst offenders with a rapid eye in the prison, could not a phrenologist (or otherwise well-studied phrenological amateur) identify a bad head—and potential criminal—on the street? In this way the panoptic gaze of the prison, mediated and transformed by phrenological theory, was translated to the midcentury urban street and adapted for daily life and urban concerns.

Phrenology and physiognomy promised to answer these questions and allay these anxieties, providing a means for policing the self and navigating the world of strangers. First, practical phrenology promoted a dichotomy between "good" and "bad" heads and characters. Second, it provided a means for reforming and policing the self and one's close family members, especially children, in the interest of developing a "good" head and character. Third, phrenology mobilized the concept of perfect prediction—a knowledge-producing regime in which one's future potential could be predicted, for better or for worse. Fourth, postbellum political and social change inflected narratives about the criminal potential of racialized others. Phrenologists bridged these ways of knowing and seeing into a single injunction: to look and judge not just oneself, but also those around you, friends and strangers alike. These messages served to promote the utility of practical phrenology (and the fortunes of practical phrenologists), but also provided a set of tools for managing and mobilizing anxieties about the self and the stranger.

Heads, Good and Bad

A recurring motif emerged within midcentury phrenology: good versus evil, the exemplary versus the subpar (or even subhuman). Both phrenological enthusiasts and practical phrenologists wrote extensively on the lives and heads of politicians, statesmen, artists, writers, physicians, phrenologists, and other "great men." These were predominantly *white* and *masculine* models of achievement and greatness: while great women or people of color occasionally figured, they were few and far between. In phrenological cabinets, great men featured prominently, outnumbering any other "type" contained within such collections. In print, biographies and engravings of great men were frequently included, sometimes accompanied by an account of their phrenological characteristics.[18] These great men were culled from history—Cicero, Shakespeare, Milton, Descartes, Newton—as well as from current events.[19]

Great men in phrenological books, cabinets, images, and discourse were compared with their opposite types: "idiots," the "insane," and the criminal. The "idiot" was a common foil, often juxtaposed with great men through illustration, as the visual distinction between the two types of heads underlined phrenological lessons.[20] The text accompanying two such figures explained that the images "are designed to represent the difference between the size and shape of the head of two persons—one possessing a most powerful intellect, and the other being almost entirely deficient in the intellectual faculties."[21] Since the intellectual and reasoning organs were located in the forehead, the angle produced with the lines sketched through the head of the "idiot," the facial angle, illustrated the great difference in the intellectual potential of these two subjects. The facial angle had already been common currency for nearly a century, after its introduction by Petrus Camper in the 1770s, even if it was here applied to intellect, rather than aesthetics.[22]

The comparison between the great man and the criminal offered a different lesson. The dichotomy between the "idiot" and great man illustrated intellectual capability and potential, as the importance of the relative size of the head and brain was one of the first principles of phrenology—essentially, the bigger the brain, the greater the potential mental power.[23] More complex was the task of explaining the significance of the organs, and the contrast between great men and criminals afforded writers the opportunity to make a visible connection between an organ and the expression of that organ as behavior. With criminals and great men, the extremity of the types underlined the significance of the newly defined organs and the animal propensities, not just the broad category of intellect.

Phrenological journals, magazines, and almanacs, from the *Transactions* (Edinburgh) to the *Annals* (Boston) and the *American Phrenological Journal* (*APJ*) and the Fowlers' associated publications, were filled with biographies and accounts of the phrenological characteristics of great men and criminals alike. The juxtaposition of these two types was often implicit rather than explicit. One page of an almanac or a journal might feature the profile of a great man, but on turning the page, the reader would be confronted with the opposite type: a criminal, usually a murderer. *The Phrenological Almanac for 1841*, for example, included profiles of several great men, including Shakespeare, George Washington, and Benjamin Franklin, alongside profiles of three murderers and a thief, as well as an article comparing the effects of small and large Destructiveness.[24]

Sometimes the comparison was explicit. In 1853, the *APJ* published an article entitled "The Good Man and the Murderer. A Contrast," which compared Peter Jeannin, the advisor and financial minister to King Henri IV of France, and "Martin the murderer" (figure 8).[25] While Jeannin's biography took up most of the page and included a high level of detail, little was said about Martin: the reader was not told his first name, the specifics of his crime, his home or nationality, or even the year in which he committed the murder, making "Martin the murderer" difficult to identify as a real historical figure.[26] The portrait of Jeannin was detailed, based on an engraving, whereas Martin's portrait was based on a cast, most likely taken post-execution. The criminal was useful only to the extent to which he served as a comparison and proof of phrenological truth: "Who can look at these portraits and deny the truth of Phrenology? They are

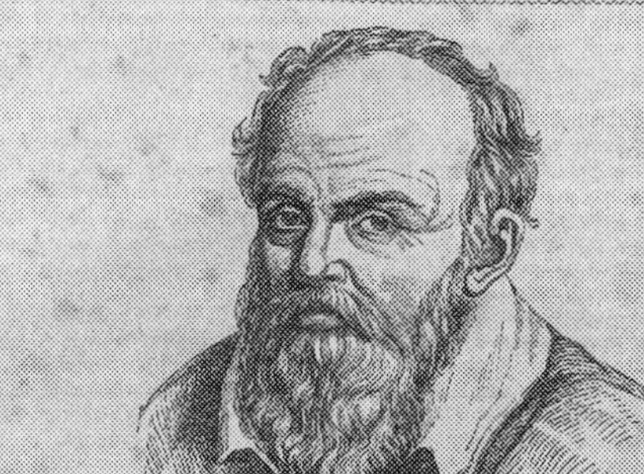

PETER JEANNIN.

THE GOOD MAN AND THE MURDERER.

A CONTRAST.

Such a forehead as this fits a man for the study of every science; it will raise him to eminence in any profession, while the great development of the sincipital region will keep him in the path of righteousness. The whole brain is only compatible with nobleness of mind and elevation of character. All views which emanate from such a head will be extensive, and beyond the reach of common understandings; moreover, they will be ennobled by soundness of judgment and generosity of sentiment.

P. Jeannin, born in 1540, even from infancy displayed great talents; he was brought up to the law, and first appeared in the quality of advocate in the parliament of Burgundy. He soon distinguished himself by his eloquence, and the force of his arguments. He was frank and just. The states of Burgundy appointed him agent for the affairs of the province. It was Jeannin who persuaded the lieutenant-general of Burgundy, De Charny, to postpone the execution of the order for perpetrating, at Dijon, the same horrid massacre of the Protestants on St. Bartholomew's day, which took place at Paris and other cities. He protested that it was impossible the king should persist in such a cruel purpose, and a courier arrived a few days after to revoke the order. This was the more meritorious in Jeannin, as he had been induced, by the zeal which the leaguers affected for religion and the good of the state, to join their party. He was attached to the Duke of Mayenne, and deputed by him to negotiate with Philip II. of Spain, the declared protector of the league.

Jeannin soon discovered that the real design of Philip, in supporting the civil war in France, was to gain possession of some of its best provinces. He, therefore, on his return, exerted his influence to detach the Duke from the Spaniards, and dispose him to acknowledge his lawful sovereign. After Mayenne had returned to his duty, Henry IV. was desirous of engaging Jeannin in his service; and when the latter honestly objected that his majesty should prefer an old leaguer to so many persons of known fidelity, Henry replied that he who had been faithful to a duke, would never be otherwise to a king. This was a true phrenological judgment.

Henry conferred upon Jeannin the office of first president of the parliament of Burgundy, intending that he should dispose of it to another, and devote himself entirely to attendance in the council of state. From this time he became one of Henry's principal advisers and confidants, and was always selected to conduct the more delicate negotiations. He assisted in drawing up the Edict of Nantes. Henry called him *the good man*, communicated to him his most secret thoughts, and consulted him upon his nearest and dearest interests. Having once discovered that a secret of state had been revealed, he complained of it at the council-board, saying at the same time, while he took the president Jeannin by the hand, "I answer for this good man; the rest of you must examine one another."—"Jeannin," said Henry on another occasion, "always thinks well; he never conceals a thought from me, and he never flatters me."

After the death of Henry IV. Jeannin was intrusted by the queen-mother with the management of the most important affairs of the kingdom, especially with the administration of the finances; and in the midst of universal disorder he preserved his integrity of character unsullied. The moderate fortune he left behind him is the best proof of his rectitude. He died at the age of eighty-two, having been minister during twenty-seven years. He possessed a truly elevated mind. On one occasion, when asked by a prince who meant to disconcert him, whose son he was, he replied, "The son of my virtues." His name is illustrious on account of his talents, his virtues, and the services he rendered to his country.

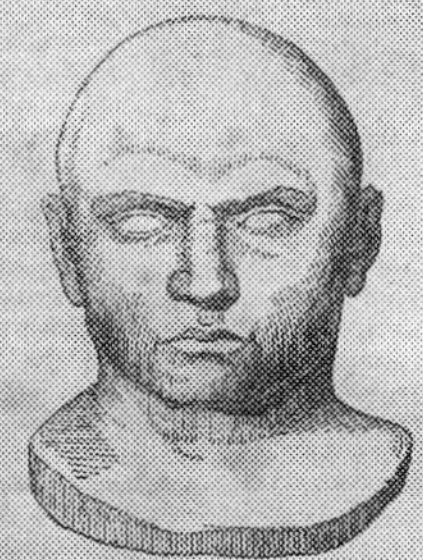

MARTIN, A MURDERER.

In the form of the head of Martin the murderer, we perceive a very marked contrast when compared with that of Peter Jeannin. It is extremely broad at the base, above and about the ears in the region of Destructiveness, Combativeness, Secretiveness, Acquisitiveness and Alimentiveness, while it is contracted in the forehead, and but feebly developed in the top and upper side-head, indicating weak intellectual, moral, and refining qualities of mind. He was the victim of base passion, selfishness, and cruelty, while Jeannin, with a head directly the reverse, was a pattern of intelligence and virtue. Who can look at these portraits and deny the truth of Phrenology? They are extremes of character, it is true, and the developments are also extreme; but if Phrenology be not true, why does it never *happen* that the character of persons with such shaped heads should be just the reverse of what they are? Why is not the character of a Jeannin, a Melancthon, or an Oberlin found in combination with a head like Martin; and why do we never find the character of Martin or Vitellius in connection with a head like Jeannin? Opponents of Phrenology would have found them if such had existed, and nature cannot be bribed to contradict herself to serve the purposes of bigotry and skepticism.

FEMALE SOCIETY.—What makes those men who associate habitually with women superior to others? What makes that woman who is accustomed and at ease in the society of men, superior to her sex in general? Solely because they are in the habit of free, graceful, continual conversation with the other sex. Women in this way lose their frivolity; their faculties awaken; their delicacies and peculiarities unfold all their beauty and captivation in the spirit of intellectual rivalry. And the men lose their pedantic, rude, declamatory, or sullen manner. The coin of the understanding and the heart is changed continually. Their asperities are rubbed off, their better materials polished and brightened, and their richness, like fine gold, is wrought into finer workmanship by the fingers of woman, than it ever could be by those of men. The iron and steel of their character are hidden, like the harness and armor of a giant, in studs and knots of gold and precious stones, when they are not wanted in actual warfare.—*Neal*.

Figure 8. Peter Jeannin and Martin, a murderer, compared, from "The Good Man and the Murderer. A Contrast," *American Phrenological Journal* 17, no. 1 (January 1853): 4. Yale University, Harvey Cushing/John Hay Whitney Medical Library.

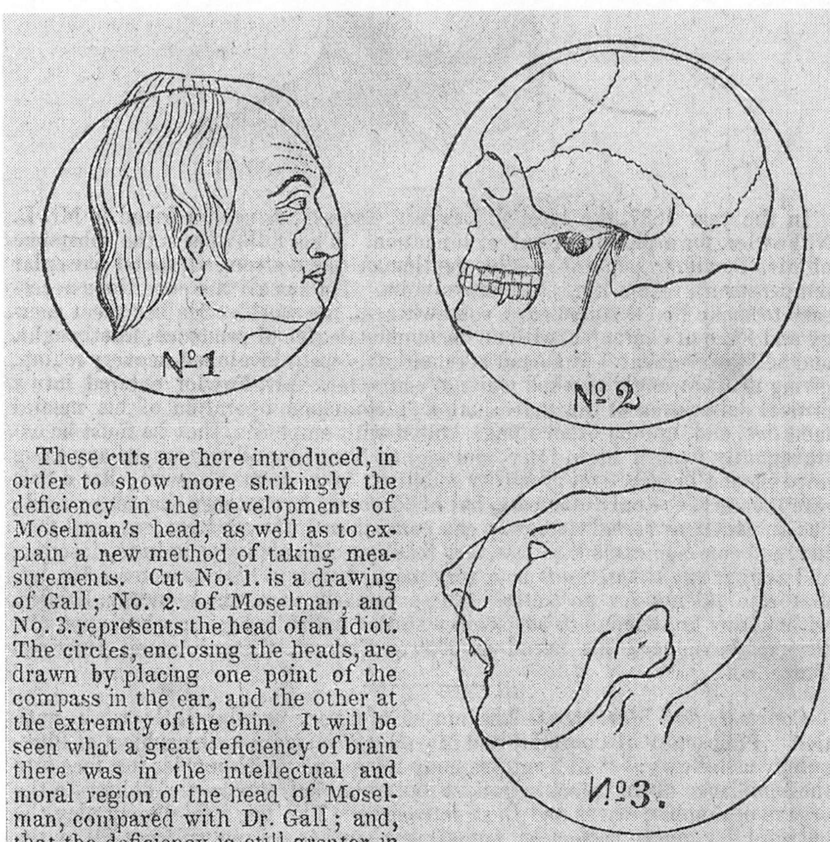

These cuts are here introduced, in order to show more strikingly the deficiency in the developments of Moselman's head, as well as to explain a new method of taking measurements. Cut No. 1. is a drawing of Gall; No. 2. of Moselman, and No. 3. represents the head of an Idiot. The circles, enclosing the heads, are drawn by placing one point of the compass in the ear, and the other at the extremity of the chin. It will be seen what a great deficiency of brain there was in the intellectual and moral region of the head of Moselman, compared with Dr. Gall; and, that the deficiency is still greater in the head of the Idiot, who cannot be considered either as an accountable or a religious being. If this method of measuring the head were applied to animals, it would show, in a most clear and striking manner, what a regular gradation there is from the highest to the lowest of the animal kingdom. This would add much interest to the study of natural history.

Figure 9. Heads of Gall (no. 1), Moselman (no. 2), and an "Idiot" (no. 3), from L. N. Fowler, *Phrenological Almanac for 1842* (New York: 1841): 41. Beinecke Rare Book and Manuscript Library, Yale University.

extremes of character, it is true, and the developments are also extreme; but if Phrenology be not true, why does it never *happen* that the character of persons with such shaped heads should be just the reverse of what they are?"[27]

The most compelling contrast was one which combined all three types. Figure 9, taken from an 1842 phrenological almanac, combined these various comparisons into one image: great man, murderer, and "idiot" together. This image included the profile of Gall, the skull in profile of Henry Cobler Moselman, only recently convicted and executed in Pennsylvania, and a line drawing of an unnamed "idiot" in profile. The three types shown together completed a visual portrait of mental and moral extremes. It was no mistake that the great man presented here was Gall himself, as in figure 3. In the phrenological cosmology, only a phrenologist could stand as the truly eminent great man and example of ideal masculinity and intellectual capacity.[28] By contrasting the founder of the discipline with the most egregious examples of "bad heads," this image aligned the great man with phrenology and simultaneously used the science to define good and bad.

Phrenologists frequently mobilized this dichotomy, contrasting great men with bad heads in lecture halls as well. When William Strathern attended a phrenological lecture in Nottingham, England, on March 14, 1840, he noted in his commonplace book that the heads exhibited to the audience "were known to the world," with such figures as Pitt, Sheridan, Franklin, Sir Walter Scott, Joseph Hume, and George III.[29] However, he also remarked on the heads of various murderers, adding in a footnote that "It struck me as curious that there were 3 heads of 3 Burkes in the Room viz. Burke the Writer, young Burke the Actor and Burke the Murderer."[30] This "curious" combination was in fact a visual trope of the phrenological lecture, intended to convey a message about good and bad heads. One of Strathern's friends, Henry Wild, certainly absorbed this message, declaring that "the index of the face told the secret operations of the mind, and that according as the mind produced good or evil so would the features gradually acquire and incline (to certain extent) a peculiar devellopment that could not be misunderstood to an observant."[31]

Satirical texts also described the phrenological lecture space as highlighting "good" and "bad" heads. As one piece set the scene, among the diagrams displayed at one lecture, "One was a head of Milton, another of Raphael, another of a great murderer, and another exhibited the outlines of an idiot's head."[32] The nineteenth-century adherent to the science would have expected such a scene: large panels and drawings of the great men—and villains—in life, accompanied by their death masks and skulls. Both the specimens and the posters could even be purchased from the Fowler brothers, who outfitted many an itinerant phrenologist and far-flung phrenological society. For twenty-five dollars, one could purchase from the Fowlers "FORTY of our best specimens"—a full cabinet in miniature—which included: busts of John Quincy Adams, George Combe, and Henry Clay; two "idiots" and one "deranged"; three criminals; and several national types.[33]

One set of nineteen posters, produced by Fowler and Wells in the 1850s and 1860s, leaned heavily toward the "great man" representational model, with a number of exceptional women included as well.[34] However, among these great men and women more infamous figures also featured. On the same scroll as George Washington, for example, there was also the depiction of a nameless "Convict," while the poster that depicted Queen Elizabeth and Copernicus also included a generic "Thief" (figure 10). The simplicity of the line drawing of the thief contrasted sharply with the rich detailing of the costumes of the two women just above. The thief and Queen Elizabeth, juxtaposed, suggest the ways that the two types were used rhetorically: great men and women were given the majority of textual and visual detail, whereas the criminal was rendered in simple lines and words, reduced to a type. A hierarchy of attention and individuation emerges from these posters. Great men and women were figures worthy of emulation, but criminals were types rather than individuals, unnamed and unspecific in their infamy.

Accounts of the phrenological developments of great men also suggested to the reader that direct interaction with a skull was not necessary to assess the head or character. If the Fowlers did not need to speak to or examine such figures as Queen Elizabeth or George Washington in order to prepare phrenological assessments, this gave lie to the necessity of manual examination. The writers of these articles did not hide the fact that assessments were based solely on the examination of an image: "The above [illustration] may be considered a correct likeness of WASHINGTON IRVING. . . . The Phrenological indications are in very strict accordance with his fame," began one account.[35] The Fowlers, moreover, offered mail-order services by 1856: one need only send them a daguerreotype and payment to receive a phrenological reading.[36] If judgment by image was sufficient for assessing the head of Irving or a paying client, it would be equally useful for the heads of murderers and thieves. Readers of popular phrenological texts learned that visual examination alone would suffice for assessing criminality, as well as "good" and "bad" heads more generally.

Phrenological lecturers made use of posters as well as busts and skulls, and phrenologists advertised their lectures, readings, and texts with phrenological images. In particular, the phrenological bust, as a material object and as an image, was ubiquitous in nineteenth-century culture and remains a salient shorthand into the present day. The Fowlers' almanacs and journals typically featured an image of the bust on the cover, and phrenological posters, cards, books, journals, and ephemeral materials used the "symbolical head," as it was sometimes called, as a stand-in for the broader science. The way one "read" this head

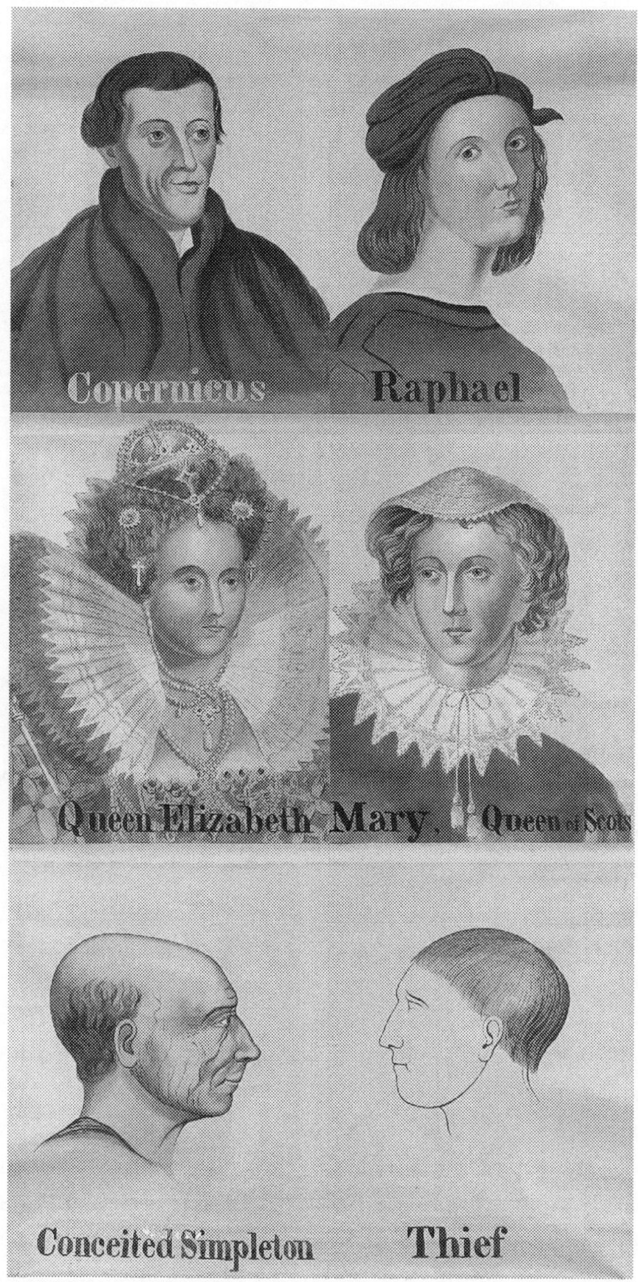

Figure 10. Fowler & Wells portrait posters for Physiognomy Lectures, poster 13. Beinecke Rare Book and Manuscript Library, Yale University.

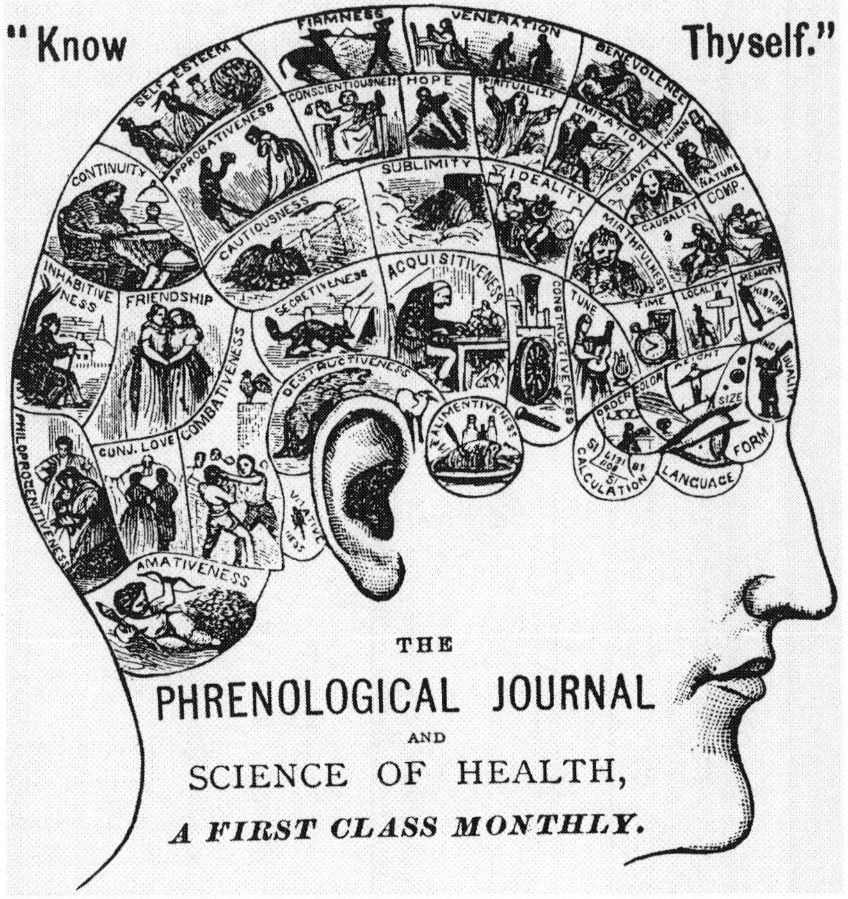

Figure 11. A symbolical head. Credit: Phrenology: Chart. Credit: Wellcome Collection. Attribution 4.0 International (CC BY 4.0).

required visual acuity; while many simply included the name of the organs, others used small cartoons to represent each organ (figure 11). This representational device linked the organ and its location to a behavior, providing a heuristic for remembering phrenological principles. With the ubiquity of the phrenological bust and the broader directive to observe oneself and one's neighbors, a phrenological dilettante had the keys to phrenological visual judgment well in hand.

The visual culture of practical phrenology produced a culture *of* vision. In particular, it promoted the idea that the distinctions that were most apparent and *visible* were those between "good" and "bad" heads. Among those "bad" heads were convicted criminals, but this number might include *potential* criminals. Phrenology advocated a means of empowerment of the individual, the non-elite, to go and *look* and thereafter to judge. The premise of "know thyself" empowered the individual to apply phrenological knowledge to daily life primarily through judgment by sight—whether from images on a page or passersby on the street. After, all, as the Fowlers observed, "a rogue can be detected as well in a church as in a prison."[37]

Know Thyself, Know Thy Child

By the 1840s, practical phrenology became the primary mode of phrenology in America, especially with the influence of the Fowlers. Visiting a phrenologist was a popular pastime, as was purchasing a reading, many of which are available in family archives, copied into letters or diaries. The motives for seeking these readings were not always clear, but there was likely some combination of curiosity and anxiety that led the mid-nineteenth-century American to the phrenologist's office to seek a phrenological reading, which might be received with a mix of "approval and skepticism," and even "consumed . . . as an experiment," as Carla Bittel argues.[38] Practical phrenology can be considered a hybrid practice located between self-help and psychological counseling, between personal and professional forms of self-improvement.[39]

"Know thyself" was a central tenet of practical phrenology, and this dictum often went hand-in-hand with an emphasis on self-education and self-improvement.[40] The goals of this injunction were balanced between individual and community betterment, focusing on eliminating "bad heads" and "bad characters." As the Fowler brothers argued, "SELF-knowledge is . . . both the most useful and promotive of personal and universal happiness and success."[41] As one advertisement in Orson Fowler's *The Practical Phrenologist* proclaimed, "Is not self-knowledge self-POWER? This power a correct phrenological consultation furnishes."[42] If self-knowledge was self-power, the extension of judgment—or surveillance, or policing—from the self to others provided one possible "active, analytical role to users."[43]

But how were these users to learn *how* to use phrenology? The Fowlers explained the principles and theory of their science in great detail, but only vague instruction was provided on how to evaluate and interpret the size of the organs.[44] Even their "how-to" guide, *The Illustrated Self-Instructor in Phrenology and Physiology*, only included a few pages at the end describing the rules for finding the organs by hand.[45] A few other phrenologists included some "hands-on" instructions, with diagrams, for identifying the location and size of organs, or the correct positioning of the hands on the head.[46] Cornelius Donovan, a British phrenologist, stated unequivocally that "the hand is specially adapted to the work of feeling the head," and explained both textually and visually, through a series of plates, how to use the hands to examine the head, seeing as how "most works are silent on this part."[47] However, few phrenological writers explained the method of identifying and assessing the organs by hand or with instruments.

If explicit directions for reading heads by hand were often withheld, implicit lessons on using other tools—particularly vision—were rife in phrenological writing. Indeed, the very key to the dictum of "know thyself" was centered on the promise of vision. Nelson Sizer, one of the Fowlers' collaborators, discussed the ease with which a student of phrenology could estimate by sight: "In the examination of skulls," Sizer wrote, "judgment formed by the eye is quite sufficient."[48] "A cursory glance of the eye will show what portion [of the head] is most developed, and this will indicate the character," explained one article in the *APJ*.[49] Another writer suggested that phrenology revealed, "at the first glance the general drift of the characters of all we may chance to meet."[50] While this knowledge gleaned at first glance required "re-perusal, and much reflection and observation," the phrenological student should be empowered to follow through on this program: "Here are the keys. Unlock and read for yourselves."[51]

Perhaps ironically, the best way to "know thyself" was to pay one of the Fowlers or one of their colleagues (or competitors) for a reading. This may have been a result of simple economics: practical phrenologists made a portion of their living from their examinations of paying clients, which could amount to a tidy sum.[52] In 1835, the Fowlers charged "12 1-2 cents," according to their phrenological cards, but by 1858, Mary Ferguson paid five dollars for a reading and six dollars for a second reading in 1865. Five dollars in 1858 would amount to roughly $159.84 in 2020 currency, and the 12.5 cent examination of 1835 would amount to $3.73 in 2020 currency.[53] This increase in price cannot be attributed to inflation alone, signaling the popularity of phrenological practice by mid-century. Explaining the exact mechanisms of their process of assessing the organs and character could eliminate potential sources of revenue. Yet the self-help principles enshrined within the "know thyself" maxim still operated in the service of practical phrenologists, motivating interested parties to seek out a phrenological reading.

The extant readings of "phrenological developments," disproportionately produced by members of the Fowlers and Wells families and their associates, like Nelson Sizer, were purchased by middle-class Americans and reflected mundane concerns.[54] These accounts were alternately longhand essays reflecting on the character of the individual, or premade charts with subjective numbers, rather than caliper measurements, reflecting the power of the organ.[55] Long-form readings typically provided prescriptive advice alongside an observational character sketch.[56] One reading, for example, of Emily Sawyer by Lorenzo Fowler in 1861, extended for thirteen handwritten pages and included such observations and injunctions as, "You must sleep as much as possible," "You need out-of-door exercise," and "You live too much for others + forget your own interests."[57] Fowler's directions to Sawyer illustrate the extent to which readings provided generalized advice, broadly applicable to the American client.

The foibles and defects of character pointed out in such readings were usually minor.[58] Some readings, for example, noted large Destructiveness but did not suggest that murderous violence would be the outcome. An 1864 reading of Samuel P. Leeds by Nelson Sizer, for example, noted that "Your Destructiveness is rather large. Your feelings are <u>severe</u>, when your temper is excited rather than boisterous—it boils within rather than to boil over."[59] Sizer observed that in a childhood fight, Leeds would have been more likely to take up a weapon than strike out with his fists, yet he did not suggest that Leeds had criminal potential. In another reading given two decades later, Sizer similarly described Mrs. Robert A. Phillips as having "Combativeness and Destructiveness enough to give courage, force, positiveness, and a kind of earnestness which leads you to overdo."[60] Here, a gendered distinction between the interpretation of large Destructiveness was also apparent: Leeds, with his large Destructiveness, prompted an image of boyish fisticuffs, but in Phillips, this organ provided willpower.

While phrenological readings of clients usually focused on the positive, themes of good and bad pervaded. Phrenological readings featured warnings against certain kinds of behaviors, or injunctions to heed particular organs. The reading was never intended to be a portrait of a static character, but instead a guide to better living and behavior. As Fowler wrote in closing to Emily Sawyer: "Cultivate as much as you can the organs marked smallest in your Chart, + properly guide and exercise the stronger ones + thus produce a harmony of mental and physical action."[61] It was not enough to simply "know thyself": one must also work toward constant improvement.

The imperative to educate and improve the self also encompassed the education of the public for social gains, especially the proper education of children—a common theme in phrenological publications. The focus of both phrenologists and their clients on children reflected the changing role of childhood and growing importance of childrearing in America, as the increasingly "interior-focused and emotionally connected family" turned inward, taking personal responsibility for the development of its children, rather than relying on community support.[62] For the midcentury bourgeois family, the lines between education and leisure, between private and public, were permeable.[63] The self-improvement precepts of phrenology fit both goals, to instruct and to amuse, even as it fit into broader cultural interests in popular science, which was by the 1840s well established and even normative in the United States.[64]

Phrenologists argued that early detection of unfavorable tendencies, along with proper education, could change the course of a child's life. Many articles in the *APJ* were focused on the necessity of proper moral education to keep children on the straight and narrow and out of the prisons and gallows. Education was seen as essential to the prevention of crime: "Nearly one half the number of persons convicted of crime in this State, in eight years, had *no education whatever*. . . . Give every human being this [education], and it is our earnest conviction, that it would reduce offenses against our criminal code to an absolute nonentity."[65]

These concerns also provided a path for women to engage with phrenology with the context of the doctrines of "true womanhood" and separate spheres.[66] Mothers were framed in phrenological writing as key to identifying and correcting dangerous traits in their children through phrenology: "'Oh, dear,' sighed a young mother, one pleasant afternoon in early spring, 'what shall I do with little Johnny?' Then she leaned her head upon her hand, and began to meditate upon the evil traits in her little son's character, which were rapidly developing themselves, and which were fast escaping from her control, as she imagined, with the heart-sickening idea that her child might eventually become a reckless youth, and godless man."[67] This anxious mother found her salvation in the phrenological lecture hall and through a phrenological reading, "and she returned to her home rejoicing . . . that she had learned how to deal with their dear little son, so that he should become, in future days, their joy and pride."[68]

The phrenological education of mothers and children was one way to improve both self and society. Lydia Folger Fowler, wife of Lorenzo Niles Fowler and the second woman in America to receive a medical degree, wrote some of her earliest books on the topics of phrenology and physiology for a youth audience, intended as guides to "self-knowledge."[69] Her publications, directed jointly at children and the mothers responsible for educating them, were also excerpted in the *APJ*.[70] Schools might also be sites for phrenological readings, further tying phrenology to childhood education.[71] During a phrenological visit to Louisville, Kentucky in 1835, for example, Lorenzo Fowler visited the "Miss Bliss infant school," where he examined several of the young pupils, either at the behest of the teachers or the parents; on the same trip, he examined children as young as six months old.[72]

Parents brought their children to visit phrenologists as well.[73] While in Louisville, Kentucky, during his cross-country trip in 1835, Lorenzo Fowler performed readings for both Mrs. De Hart and her son, whose measurements were presented as part of the same chart.[74] During this visit, he also examined the entire Wilson family in one sitting: an attorney, his wife, and their daughter.[75] Other parents planned multiple visits to track progress. Mary Ferguson took her nearly three-year-old son, Joseph, to see "Proff Fowler"[76] in Troy, New York, in November of 1858 and paid five dollars for a reading.[77] Ferguson copied the seven-page reading, which she received along with a book with the "bumps marked and what to cultivate," into her diary.[78] She was so pleased with the findings that she returned with a friend to have their heads read as well, the results of which she thought "flattered us a little."[79] Years later, the family visited Fowler when he returned to Troy to receive a reading for their second son, Oakley, for which they paid six dollars.[80] Ferguson reported with satisfaction that the reading "is precisely as he is."[81] Ferguson's diaries suggest that she was not the only concerned parent to take her children to the phrenologist: the first time she attempted to visit, he was engaged with several families and could not fit them in.[82]

A reading was not just a pleasant amusement for an afternoon: it could also suggest "what to cultivate" for even very young children. An 1851 reading of William H. Davis by Orson Fowler was addressed to his parents, interspersed with injunctions as to how to raise and educate the child properly: "One of his largest organs is Destructiveness this renders his anger very severe—be careful not to provoke him. he is therefore a little too sour and hence should always be treated kindly . . . I beg that in his education you would never attempt to use force—because you will just as surely fail as you do."[83] Despite the fact that William had particularly large Destructiveness, Fowler's reading was quite complimentary, noting that he would be "a very superior businessman" and concluding that he had "a good head."[84] The roles of both Mrs. Ferguson and Mrs. Davis in these instances, as the keepers of their children's phrenological readings, were in line with expectations for proper motherhood, particularly their duty to educate their children "*even from the day of birth*."[85] As one phrenologist observed, it was the mother who was the "'*former*' of the infant mind," responsible for "weaving the character and *embroidering the souls*, of her children."[86]

Practical phrenologists argued that "every child born with a sound mind may, by proper mental and physical treatment, *from the day of birth*, be grown up to be a gentle, a benevolent, and a pious adult."[87] Youth was a crucial moment for the development of good character—or bad. Figure 12, an article from the *APJ*, presented the reader with an illustrated account of the "two paths in life" which "lie in possibility enfolded within every infant born into the world."[88] The page contained both hope and a warning: any child could embark on either path, toward dissolution or distinction. The dichotomy between great man and the criminal was here drawn in miniature and related to the life of the average man—or child—with an implied promise that proper education could make all the difference.

Yet the promise of education that phrenologists used to defend their science against claims of materialism—and which supported their reformist position vis-à-vis the prison—was not always upheld. One article in the *APJ*, entitled "Good and Bad Heads," illustrated these extremes using two young boys. While the boy with the "bad" head might have been amenable to transformation, it would take the "best of training" to effect any change at all.[89] A similar account presented the tale of two young boys with an identical religious educational background. One of these boys was pious and moral, whereas the other exhibited a "propensity to steal" from his childhood.[90] The author concluded, "What but Phrenology can explain the reason for this difference between the boys: one a saint from childhood, or rather infancy, and the other, the most extraordinary thief that was ever known?"[91] The lesson from both articles and personal readings by phrenologists was mixed: the child *could* grow to be a good man or a criminal, depending on their education—but only to a point. Some children would inevitably become dangerous adults, due to their "bad" heads. Such morality tales replicated the theme of great man versus criminal, rendering the child's mind the battleground for proper adulthood, or even proper manhood, given that these accounts typically centered on male children.

Phrenological readings of clients occasionally revealed similar findings, presenting advance warning of criminal propensities and behaviors. When performing a phrenological reading on a five-year-old boy, Adam Tailor, in Jeffersonville, Indiana, in 1835, Lorenzo Fowler told his mother that "the most remarkable passion he had was the desire to get," noting his large Acquisitiveness. He asked the mother if the boy had previously taken things that did not belong to him, which she denied. However, she later learned that her son had stolen from her neighbors, validating Fowler's findings.[92] The same day he visited Tailor, Fowler also examined William Buchanan, another young boy who

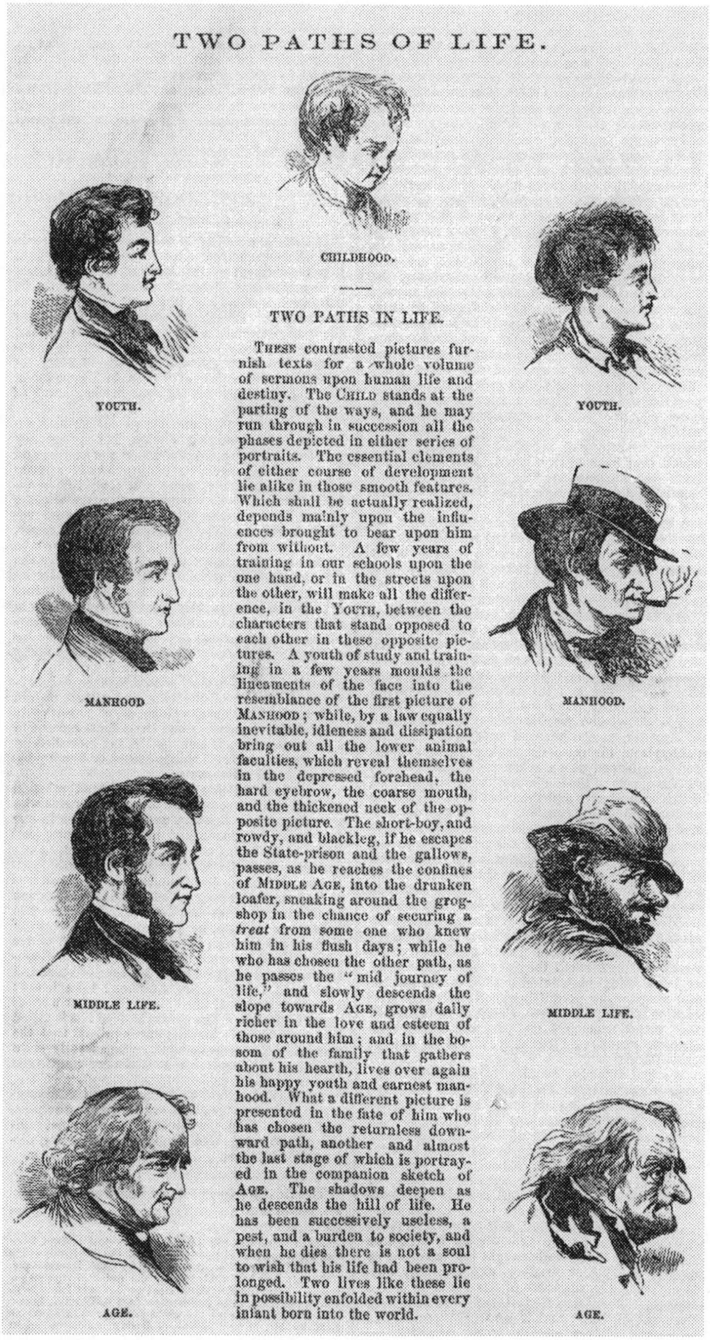

TWO PATHS OF LIFE.

CHILDHOOD.

YOUTH.

YOUTH.

MANHOOD

MANHOOD.

MIDDLE LIFE.

MIDDLE LIFE.

AGE.

AGE.

TWO PATHS IN LIFE.

THESE contrasted pictures furnish texts for a whole volume of sermons upon human life and destiny. The CHILD stands at the parting of the ways, and he may run through in succession all the phases depicted in either series of portraits. The essential elements of either course of development lie alike in those smooth features. Which shall be actually realized, depends mainly upon the influences brought to bear upon him from without. A few years of training in our schools upon the one hand, or in the streets upon the other, will make all the difference, in the YOUTH, between the characters that stand opposed to each other in these opposite pictures. A youth of study and training in a few years moulds the lineaments of the face into the resemblance of the first picture of MANHOOD; while, by a law equally inevitable, idleness and dissipation bring out all the lower animal faculties, which reveal themselves in the depressed forehead, the hard eyebrow, the coarse mouth, and the thickened neck of the opposite picture. The short-boy, and rowdy, and blackleg, if he escapes the State-prison and the gallows, passes, as he reaches the confines of MIDDLE AGE, into the drunken loafer, sneaking around the grog-shop in the chance of securing a *treat* from some one who knew him in his flush days; while he who has chosen the other path, as he passes the "mid journey of life," and slowly descends the slope towards AGE, grows daily richer in the love and esteem of those around him; and in the bosom of the family that gathers about his hearth, lives over again his happy youth and earnest manhood. What a different picture is presented in the fate of him who has chosen the returnless downward path, another and almost the last stage of which is portrayed in the companion sketch of AGE. The shadows deepen as he descends the hill of life. He has been successively useless, a pest, and a burden to society, and when he dies there is not a soul to wish that his life had been prolonged. Two lives like these lie in possibility enfolded within every infant born into the world.

Figure 12. "Two Paths of Life," *American Phrenological Journal* 21, no. 1 (1855): 12. Harvard Medical Library at the Francis A. Countway Library of Medicine.

"had large destructiveness and was the most cruel lad in town," according to Fowler.[93] Similarly, when Miss M. E. Walker was taken by her employer to visit Lorenzo Fowler in Cincinnati in 1835, Fowler noted that "in this case the Propensities rule"; her employer affirmed that Walker "had a bad temper and was difficult to manage."[94] Fowler also claimed that she was "given to falsehood and theft."[95] While the girl denied these accusations, Fowler's notes indicated that only days after his examination, she was convicted for theft and sent to jail. While the crime was committed before the examination, these notes framed Fowler as the one who first identified and brought to light her criminal propensities.

Stories of successes in predicting criminal behaviors could also be passed on secondhand, with phrenologists telling clients about their readings of other heads. When the English author Jane Roberts visited the London phrenologist James De Ville with her friend, Mrs. Phillips, the phrenologist not only provided the two women with their phrenological readings but shared a few stories with them as well. He asserted that evil propensities could be "prevented or cured," yet also conveyed a cautionary tale about warning lords about their servants, who later robbed them—a familiar tale of predictive phrenology.[96] Roberts also recounted a second story, of a gentleman who once brought his young son to De Ville for a reading, only to return years later to inform the phrenologist that the boy was now "lost."[97] De Ville's stories belied his own assertion that evil propensities could be cured, in his discovery of thieves and the failure to reverse the downfall of a young client. These morality tales blended fact and fantasy into stories of the inevitability of crime and punishment. Fictionalized accounts would also play on the same themes of the "two paths of life" and the triumph—or failure—of phrenology to detect evil.

Fantasies of Perfect Prediction

Over the course of the century, fictionalized accounts of the science appeared in newspapers and other periodicals, many of which framed phrenology as an object of mockery or derision. Focusing on the science of "bumpology" and presenting its practitioners as buffoons or even ill-intentioned frauds and fakes, such stories worked to delegitimize the science and frame its believers and practitioners alike as fools. Like attempts to fool or hoax the phrenologist by presenting him with an anonymous skull, these tales sought to undermine the legitimacy and authority of the science. Some of these phrenologists were simply buffoons, with or without their science. One story described a "drunken philosophical, phrenological loafer" who preached a mixed-up version of phrenology while in his cups.[98] Another drunken phrenologist, imprisoned in a local jail for intoxication, protested that the charge was unfair, as "I was intoxicated, drunk, delirious, sir, but it was not with alcohol . . . but it is the effect of those copious libations which I have quaffed at the fountain of science."[99] Sometimes, the humorous anecdote conveyed a grain of phrenological truth: "A PHRENOLOGIST told a man he had combativeness largely developed; 'No,' said the other, 'I have not, and if you say that again I'll knock you down.'"[100]

However, other fictional phrenologists were heroic, deftly able to make sense of human behavior. On the heels of Edgar Allan Poe's invention of Auguste Dupin in "The Murders in the Rue Morgue" (1841) and decades before Sir Arthur Conan Doyle's Sherlock Holmes stories, practical phrenology promoted its own genre of detective story in defense of its claims to legitimacy. Poe has been credited with initiating the genre with "The Murders in the Rue Morgue" and other similar stories.[101] Doyle acknowledged Poe's Dupin stories as a primary inspiration for his own Holmes stories, but literary scholars have recently demonstrated that other writers were also crafting detectives in the early nineteenth century.[102] Poe's own "Murders" included a snide aside to phrenological theory, perhaps anticipating the entry of phrenology into the new genre.[103] Phrenological detective stories were part of an emerging genre responding to social conditions, transformations in the literary market and journalism, and anxieties about law, crime, and human nature in the Anglo-American world. Stories that fit within this genre of writing framed phrenology as a predictive science of criminal behavior; phrenologists could identify wrongdoers, even before the act.[104] While some phrenological detective stories appeared in popular newspapers, most were published in the *APJ* and were likely written by phrenological partisans.

"An Incident in the Travels of a Phrenologist" was widely republished in American newspapers, including the *Daily Evening Traveller* and the *Alexandria Gazette*, as well as the *APJ*, in 1857.[105] The story was told in the first person, from the point of view of a phrenologist who recalled a trip through the Alps in the 1820s, during which time he performed a reading on a "surpassingly beautiful" young woman at the request of her mother.[106] "We were alone; science and nature," he observed, but "hardly had I encircled her head when my heart shuddered;—crime, remorseless, deliberate unfeeling crime—crime unprovoked, unbridled, unhesitating, cold, resolute crime reigned supreme in her head."[107] He concluded that, "never had I witnessed contrast more dreadful: the face and the head."[108] The phrenologist warned his client never to marry, as "there is no affection; you are impelled by violence . . . if your iron will is thwarted, destructiveness will become active."[109] When he spoke the word "destructiveness," the young woman cried out in despair and fled, revealing as she left that she was about to marry a wealthy man. The story ended with a coda: months later, the phrenologist was informed that a recently married young lady had stabbed her husband and absconded with another rich man. Unsurprisingly, this murderess was the same young woman examined by the phrenologist.

This story was unique in that it featured a female villain, as the vast majority of the criminals—real or hypothetical—with which phrenologists were preoccupied were men. The use of a female criminal highlighted the contrast between "face and the head," as the phrenologist observed—between appearances and reality. Destructiveness also featured heavily in this story, as this organ was the crux of the phrenologist's reading, and it was interpreted by his client to be particularly dire. This short story emphasized the relationship between organs and behaviors: the phrenologist did not only identify organs, but criminality itself, concluding that "crime reigned supreme in her head." This article, published in popular newspapers, reinforced a connection between the disposition of the head and criminal behavior, presenting a phrenology as predictive science of criminal behavior.

Other stories circulated, which played on similar themes and replicated this plot: a phrenologist encountered an individual and observed their criminal tendencies via their organs, findings that were confirmed in the revelation of a great crime. The discovery of thieves was a common plot. In one story, "A Thief Discovered," a phrenologist, M. Beraud, attended a dinner party during which he was invited by his host to examine his guests' heads. He stated that the head of one guest had "the organ for *Theft* . . . frightfully large."[110] The accused thief fled the party, as the other members of the party recalled "a series of thievish misdemeanors."[111] The final line of this story suggested that the man "yielded to an instinct which a good education had entirely failed to cure," reinforcing the idea that some heads were simply "bad."[112] In another story, the mayor of New York recounted a tale told to him by an acquaintance in London.[113] According to his story, a gentleman took his twelve-year-old son to visit a phrenologist, who informed him that the boy had large Acquisitiveness. The father scoffed at the idea, but the boy confessed to stealing jewelry from the household and selling it, crimes for which several maids had been accused and dismissed. The writer concluded that this incident "saved the lad from becoming a confirmed thief, if not a robber," a near inversion of the story De Ville told Jane Roberts.[114] In both of these instances, the phrenologist detected the thieving mind, forcing confessions and reinforcing the truth of phrenology.

Murder also figured in these stories. In the widely republished story "The Phrenologist," Professor Leyden was invited to a dinner party hosted by the Baron Hartmann, where he was asked to examine the heads of the guests, echoing the structure of "A Thief Discovered."[115] As Leyden declined to comment on his findings, dinner conversation turned instead to the topic of the recent murder of a young woman. At the same time, a diamond-encrusted snuffbox was passed around the table, only to disappear shortly thereafter. Leyden broke his silence and accused one of the guests of being a "*robber* and a *murderer*!"[116] The accused man was searched, and the snuff box was found in his pocket, which caused him to break down and confess to the murder of the woman as well. The phrenologist was rewarded for his deduction with the "acquisition of the prettiest girl in Germany," his host's daughter.[117] Phrenology triumphed, resulting in the apprehension of an evildoer and the elevation of the science—and a matrimonial reward.

Occasionally, the great men of the phrenological pantheon were made heroic characters in fictional pieces. In "The Phrenologist's Prophecy," set at a ball given by Prince Metternich in Vienna, Gall was asked by his host to judge the guests, especially one of the host's favorites. Gall proclaimed to Metternich that, "your perfect creature, my Prince, is nothing more than a—*perfect villain*!"[118] Years later, a "ghastly, unheard-of crime" (the details of which were not revealed) was committed by this "perfect villain."[119] A second anecdote underlined the point. Gall and Metternich met again years later in Paris where they observed another young man, who Gall proclaimed to be a "cruel Siberian bear."[120] This "bear" was later arrested for conspiracy to regicide and hanged. The fictionalized Gall proved himself twice over, predicting the crimes of horrible villains before the act on the basis of observation alone.

However, most phrenological fiction featured phrenologists as the butt of the joke, rather than the hero of the story, and Gall himself was no exception. In "The King and the Phrenologist," the story seemed at first to replicate the heroic story of "The Phrenologist's Prophecy."[121] Gall, invited by King Frederick of Prussia to dinner, was asked to examine the heads of a few of the guests.[122] After presenting very favorable readings of the two of them, the king revealed that one of the men was a murderer and the other a thief. In this battle of wits between two great men, the skeptical king prevailed instead of the phrenologist—a sign of the decline of phrenology by the last decades of the century.

Short stories in which the phrenologist appeared as a buffoon, rather than as a hero, seem to undermine phrenology's claim to legitimacy. I suggest, however, that both varieties of tales—stories in which phrenologists failed to predict anything of consequence, and those in which phrenologists uncovered the dastardliest of deeds—represented two sides of the same coin. Phrenologists as detectives, successful or not, illustrated the possibility that practical phrenology represented for average Americans. Phrenologists were cast by writers as investigators into the darker side of human behavior: when they read criminality into their subjects, in fiction or in real life, accurately or inaccurately, they were staking a novel claim to be able to scientifically identify good and evil. The potential for phrenologists to be able to correctly identify criminals before the act was both thrilling and unsettling. Phrenology, framed as both arbiter and predictor of good and bad heads, represented a fantasy of perfect prediction that resonated deeply with the readers of midcentury American periodicals, who were living through troubling times.

Race, Crime, and Postbellum Phrenology

In addition to the transformations of American society resulting from urbanization and industrialization, the nation also experienced a major disruption to political and social life and culture in the form of the Civil War.[123] In particular, attitudes toward race, both social and scientific, shifted as a result of Emancipation and the politics of the Reconstruction period. Post–Civil War, attitudes about race and crime also began to form new cultural paradigms and assumptions. While concerns about European immigrants, particularly ethnic groups like the Irish, did not disappear, the relative mobility of the emancipated population and lingering resentment by the Lost Cause–obsessed South prompted a reconfiguration of race and crime. While some European immigrant groups remained objects of suspicion, people of African descent were reframed as dangerous as well. Pre–Civil War, the subjugation of slavery rendered Black bodies abject. Post–Civil War, these bodies were reimagined as potentially violent.

Racial science had long been used in the United States to justify white supremacy and the subjugation of nonwhite peoples.[124] When proslavery advocates and racial scientists wrote about people of African descent before Emancipation, they emphasized the inferiority and low nature of this group, stressing their inability to self-govern, to care for themselves, and to participate in society. Freedom was largely presented as dangerous—to African Americans, more than to whites—as African Americans were considered to be lazy, shiftless, and incapable of caring for themselves. In his infamous essay, "Diseases and Peculiarities of the Negro Race," Samuel Cartwright pathologized behaviors perceived of as unique to Black bodies: first, he coined "Drapetomania," the practice of enslaved peoples running away from their enslavers, reframing this behavior as a mental illness. His second invented mental illness, "dysaesthesia aethiopica," or "rascality," described a condition of laziness which was perceived to be more prevalent among the free Black population than among those enslaved. Cartwright and others writing in the nineteenth century deemed free African Americans to be dangers to themselves: "like children, they require government in every thing."[125]

Racial theory was undergirded in part by phrenology. As Cynthia Hamilton has observed, phrenology was "a contested space that could be colonised by pro- and anti-slavery supporters as well as by those who opposed slavery while affirming the inferiority of African Americans on racial grounds."[126] Phrenology was capacious in meaning and was therefore mobilized by others interested in race, from antislavery activists like Lucretia Mott to proslavery works, including *Types of Mankind* (1854) by George R. Gliddon and Josiah C. Nott.[127] Samuel George Morton's craniology, for example, partially inspired by phrenology, was dismissive of Black intellectual potential and later adapted as a component of scientific racism that supported slavery.[128] George Combe, however, while contributing to the *Crania Americana*, was antislavery, and though reticent on that fact in public lectures and writings, he did communicate his antislavery point of view in private letters, including those exchanged with the proslavery Charles Caldwell.[129] Yet Combe—like many other antislavery advocates—did not believe in intellectual equality between ethnic groups.[130] The *APJ* and other publications by the Fowlers trafficked in mixed messages: abolitionist in nature, but often dismissive of Black intellectual capacity. Many phrenologists, from Gall through Combe and Caldwell, embraced "an essentialist view of humanity in which racial differences were immutable and racial hierarchies were clear."[131] Even when the Fowlers highlighted the "good negro," their framing of these cases as exemplary reinforced racist hierarchies and assumptions.[132] One classic case of the "good negro," Eustache Belin, an enslaved man who saved his enslaver during the Haitian massacres of 1804, not only highlighted his "un-Negro-like behavior" but also his "deferential personality."[133] Eustache, in order to be a "good negro," had to be a perfect servant.

Pre–Civil War and Emancipation, racist assumptions about Black bodies and behaviors resulted in the promotion of an idea of the Black body as abject, inferior, and incapable of higher thought. However, most pre–Civil War writing on the anatomy and character of people of African descent did not include criminality among these negative characteristics. For example, while physician and proslavery advocate John H. Van Evrie, echoing Cartwright, argued that freedom would produce moral defects in the Black population, he also argued that although "the tendencies to petty immoralities are almost universal," "his subordinate nature renders him [the emancipated Black man] less likely to commit great crimes than the superior white man."[134] Moreover, Van Evrie asserted that so-called "negro insurrection[s]" were "nonsensical," as "hybrids and mongrels might perpetuate such monstrous crimes, but the negro—the typical, pure-blooded negro—driven on by his fears and dread of the master race, would only seek its extermination, never the indulgence to *him* of such unnatural propensities."[135] Further: "Nine-tenths of the crime committed by so-called negroes is the work of the mongrel."[136] According to Van Evrie, miscegenation and its products—"mongrels" and "hybrids"—were the true threat, not the "pure-blooded negro," and whites were also more likely to commit "great crimes" than the "pure-blooded negro." The purity of the racial stock was of paramount importance to this writer, but he also expressed doubt as to the ability of the free Black population to commit crime, especially "great" or violent crime.[137]

Van Evrie and others writing on the inferiority of people of African descent in the mid-nineteenth century sometimes mobilized phrenological theory or authors to justify their position. Van Evrie, for example, though largely dismissive of phrenology as a science, nevertheless cited Gall and Spurzheim and used the language of propensity, as did other writers. That neither proslavery nor antislavery advocates, phrenologists or not, did not consider people of African descent to be essentially of a criminal nature is less an expression of charity than it was an assumption of inferiority. Collectively, white scientists and phrenologists writing on race assumed that criminal behavior required a heightened mental ability not possessed by the Black mind.

Post–Civil War, criminality slowly became re-racialized, due to the confluence of Black Code social control, white supremacy, and fears about the movement of the emancipated Black population. The racialization of criminality is largely a story of the twentieth century and therefore beyond the scope of this book, but the shifting tides can be glimpsed nevertheless.[138] While many scholars have located the racialization of crime in the 1960s and 1970s as a national political problem and discourse, recent scholarship has suggested that this process began in the late nineteenth century, resulting in part from increased race-based tensions post Emancipation and increased attempts to surveil, control, and punish African Americans during and after Reconstruction.[139] Estelle Freedman has explored the ways in which sexual violence was racialized in the last decades of the nineteenth century as a means to justify continued violence against African Americans and to enforce white supremacy.[140] Khalil Gibran Muhammad has located a crucial moment of transformation as the 1890 census, which provided statistical data showing that African Americans were overrepresented in the nation's prison population. While this was the result of discriminatory race-based surveillance, laws, and punishments, it was framed as incontrovertible, scientific evidence as to the criminality of African Americans. This racialization of criminality created a recursive justification for further discrimination: "African American criminality became one of the most widely accepted bases for justifying prejudicial thinking, discriminatory treatment, and/or acceptance of racial violence as an instrument of public safety."[141]

Shifting narratives about the racialization of criminality and violence encoded post–Civil War anxieties about the landscape of racial and national identity. By 1915, the physician and ethnographer Robert Wilson Shufeldt summed up a position that by this point was well established in American discourse:

> By nature the negro is, in fact, capable of committing any known crime, in so far as his intelligence will permit him to be the author of it. . . . But lacking in courage, intelligence, forethought, and the necessary staying powers, the criminal negro is perforce restricted to certain of the coarser and grosser crimes in the calendar not requiring these several prerequisites. His murders are clumsy and brutal; his thefts of all kinds are usually paltry and liable to be easily detected . . . in the refinements of criminality in other directions he is fortunately helpless.[142]

Blackness and criminality were by the early twentieth century tightly linked together and overwritten with brutality and incompetence.

Tides were changing with regard to scientific and social attitudes towards racialized, criminal Others, but phrenologists largely missed the boat. Phrenologists continued to write about African Americans postbellum, remarking on their developments, temperament, and skull shape. Race, however, was not a central part of the story phrenologists were telling about crime, even as the public came to embrace an increasingly racialized conception of criminality. Phrenologists were pursuing other ideas about crime, as I shall explore on the next chapter, responding instead to concerns about the slow decline of their science.

Indeed, one sign of the decline of phrenology is the racialization of phrenological practice itself. In the 1820s and through midcentury, most mocking depictions of phrenology focused on white phrenologists, but as the century progressed phrenology was incorporated into racialized media and minstrel shows. As Britt Rusert argues, blackface phrenology "was a clear attempt to delegitimate and mock the field for its inclusivity and for its antislavery leanings," but it also "encoded a cultural anxiety that phrenology might be, or become, a black science."[143] For example, in *Sammy Tubbs, the Boy Doctor, and "Sponsie," the Troublesome Monkey* (1874), the eponymous emancipated student of Dr. Samuel Hubbs was instructed and thereafter presented a lecture on Joseph R. Buchanan's expansion and re-conceptualization of the science.[144] Michael Sappol describes *Sammy Tubbs* as "both minstrel show and anti-minstrel show," noting that minstrel shows frequently mocked both bourgeois scientific performers and the attempts of Black people to comprehend scientific concepts: "The minstrel show thus depicted science as legitimate—a sophisticated, technical body of knowledge that blacks were constitutionally debarred from acquiring—and illegitimate—pretentious bourgeois double-talk."[145]

The legitimacy/illegitimacy of phrenology as science was presented as such in other examples of nineteenth-century minstrelsy, conveyed by fictional Black "lecturers" portrayed less sympathetically than Tubbs, and perhaps referencing real Black phrenologists on the lecture circuit.[146] One collection of midcentury minstrel songs, jokes, and similar materials ended with a "Grand Burlesque Lecture on Phrenology," accompanied by an illustration of one Black man phrenologizing another seated Black man.[147] The heavy dialect of the stump speech aside, this "burlesque lecture" nevertheless incorporated real phrenological organs, like Locality, Adhesiveness, and the moral sentiments, alongside other scientific jargon, mocking the tenets of phrenology through the farce it made of the Black lecturer.[148] A contemporaneous magic lantern slide (figure 13), similarly portrays an elegantly dressed Black phrenologist giving a phrenological lecture, with phrenological busts as props, to a Black audience.

The Darkey Phrenologist, a one-act minstrel play, exemplifies the twin absurdities of both phrenology and the Black "professor."[149] In this play, Professor Mephistopheles Faust and his assistant, Orlando, engaged in a rapid-fire exchange explaining the basic dictums of phrenology, including the organ of Destructiveness and its impact on criminal potential, before being interrupted by the Professor's mother-in-law, Dinah Crow:[150]

PROF. De perdigious prominence at de back ob de object am where de animal bumps lies. Yer can see from de furdest part ob de room de two bumps protrudin' from behind de enormous ears, which, dough dey am much larger dan dose ob any udder animal ob de same asinine nature, am not near capacious enuff to cubber de two enormous bumps, which, bein' as big as turkey eggs, am visible 'bout half a mile away. Dese, my friends, am de organs ob destruction, an', by deir size, probe wivout a doubt dat de subjec' now

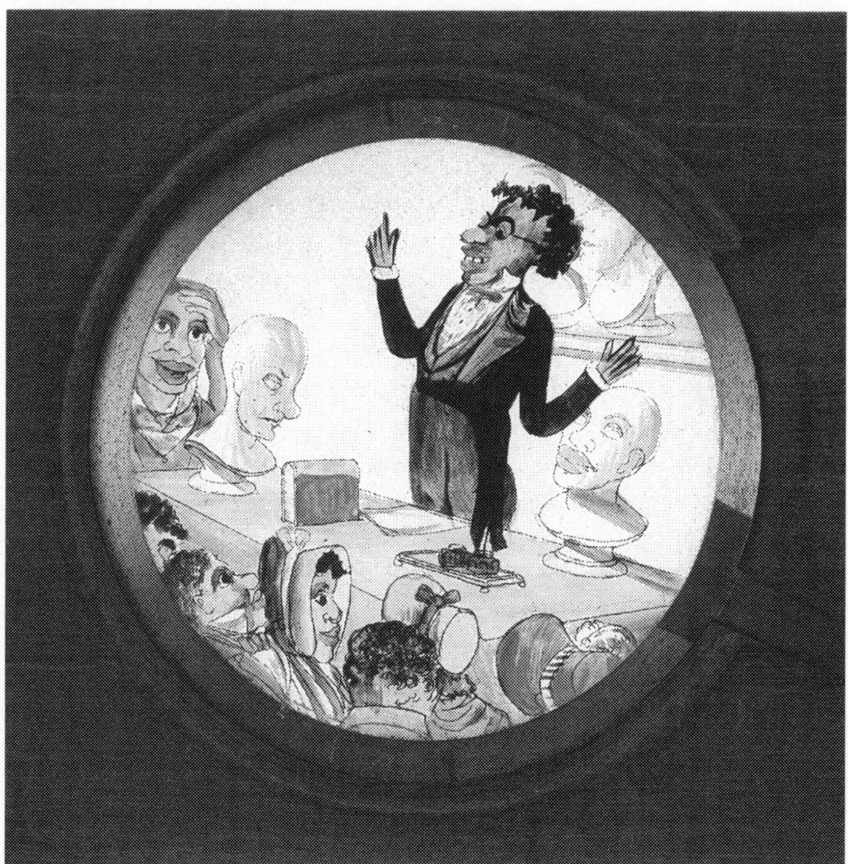

Figure 13. Single-lever magic lantern slide with moving figure, c. 1850s. Louise M. Darling Biomedical Library History and Special Collections for the Sciences, University of California, Los Angeles.

under manipulation couldn't help kermittin' a murder, eben if he tried eber so much to avoid doing' so.

ORL. I feels bery much inclined dat way just now.

PROF. What's dat yer say?

ORL. Oh, nuffin. Only if anyfing bery serious should happen to you, yet must blame de bumps for it, yer know, an' not me.

PROF. Yer can hear, my friends, de nature ob de vile subjec' before yer assertin' itself, which probes dat my estimate ob his character am quite right. We can derefore only pity him. De unfortunately doomed criminal can't eben help himself. He am chock full ob craft an' deceit, an' his interlect am like a brick wall—[151]

In this play, the depiction of phrenology, particularly the operation of Destructiveness and its mitigation of criminal responsibility, was presented as farcical. Phrenological tenets and theories of criminality, by the turn of the century, were fit only for a risible explication in the context of a minstrel show.

Minstrel shows continued to use phrenology, albeit as an object of mockery. Other commentators, including racial theorists, found less utility in phrenological theory as the century progressed. As Nott and Gliddon, leaders in proslavery racial science in the nineteenth century, argued in 1857, while "little doubt can be entertained of the general adaptation of the skull to its contents . . . in the 'mapping-out details,' to which the followers of Gall and Spurzheim have so unwarrantably resorted, Phrenology is no longer a science."[152] The last statement—"Phrenology is no longer a science"—would have been profoundly troubling to phrenologists. Indeed, phrenologists in the last decades of the nineteenth century were much more preoccupied with the internal politics of their profession than with external political concerns or racial discourse. Practical phrenologists were invested in the Civil War, yet even as the war progressed, the *APJ* continued to focus more attention on matters of perennial interest to the phrenological community, including criminality.[153] Post–Civil War, phrenologists expressed more concern with their profession than continuing national tensions. American phrenologists were entering into their own struggle for a place in the medical and scientific pantheon within a scientific landscape that had been happy to leave these theories in the past.

It is hard to identify the extent to which real individuals engaged in practices of surveillance in daily life, yet the discourse of "bad" heads and visual identification was both pervasive and long-lasting. A century after the first introduction of craniology, Destructiveness in particular was still being framed as the organ that led directly to crime. As figure 14, published in *Vaught's Practical Character Reader* (1902), suggests, Destructiveness was considered to be the root of all evil—and most criminal acts—even in the dawn of the new century, a hundred years after Gall engaged in his penal research program in Germany, and decades after the introduction of Cesare Lombroso's theories of criminal anthropology.[154]

Aside from the reinforcement of the association between the organ of Destructiveness and a host of bad and criminal behaviors, the text also made continual judgments about head shapes as well. The *Reader* relied heavily on visual evidence to demonstrate correspondences between heads and characters, including "dangerous" head shapes. Figure 15 connected Destructiveness

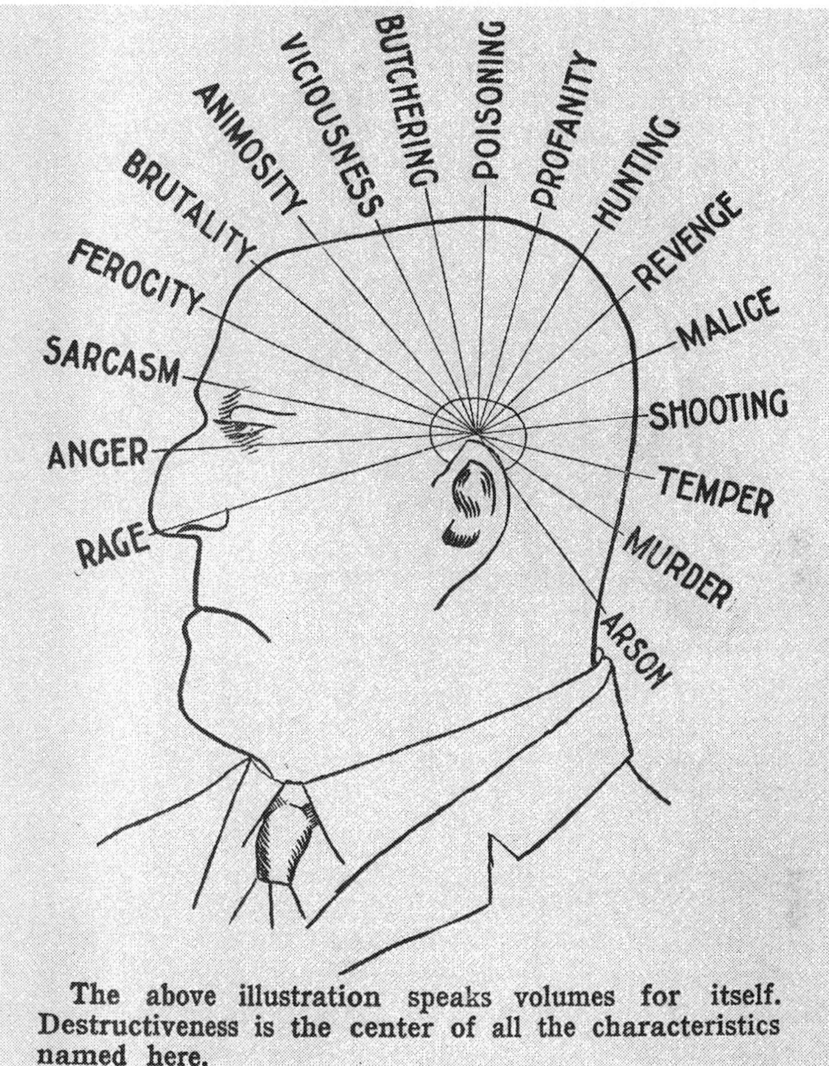

Figure 14. Destructiveness as the center of negative characteristics, from L. A. Vaught, *Vaught's Practical Character Reader* (Chicago: L. A. Vaught, Publisher, 1902), 39. Harvard Medical Library at the Francis A. Countway Library of Medicine.

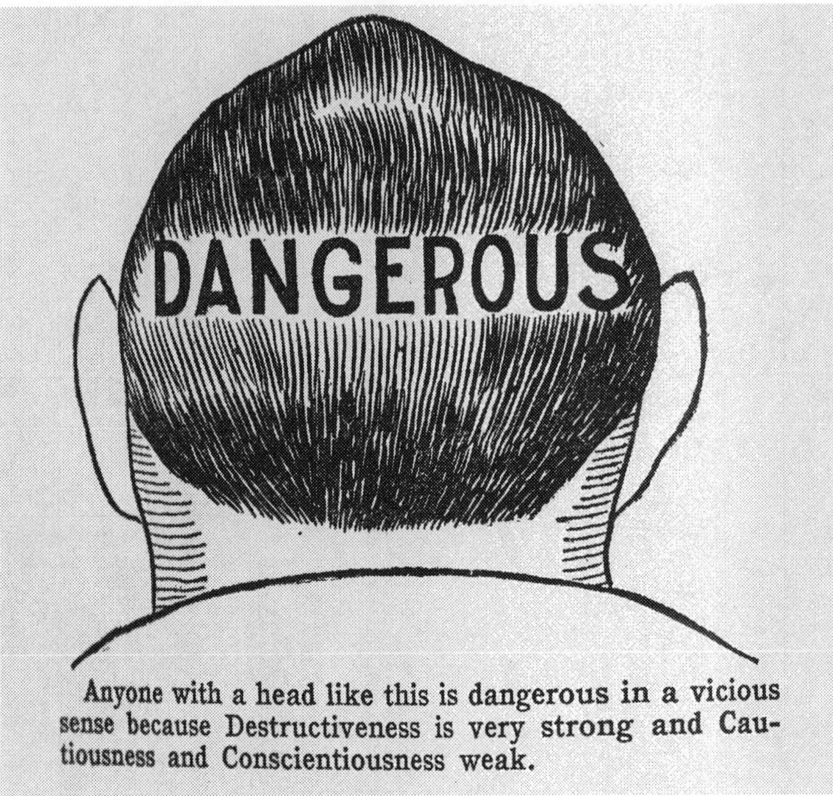

Figure 15. A dangerous head, from L. A. Vaught, *Vaught's Practical Character Reader* (Chicago: L. A. Vaught, Publisher, 1902), 38. Harvard Medical Library at the Francis A. Countway Library of Medicine.

directly to the formation of a head shape that signaled danger, similar to the head shape and assessment of midcentury phrenologists as depicted in figure 2. Figure 16 illustrated a second type of "bad" head for a "selfish, tricky and deceitful" character, instructing "all men, women and children" to "make use of every opportunity you have of looking at heads from a back view."[155] Vaught's *Reader* reproduced phrenological ideas about "good" and "bad" heads, reinforced the association between Destructiveness and danger, and instructed readers to use visual clues to pass judgment based on appearances in daily life.

In the last decades of the nineteenth century, other criminal sciences emerged to take up the mantle of perfect prediction that practical phrenologists had attempted to claim for their science. In the last third of the nineteenth century, Cesare Lombroso's positivist criminology in Italy, Francis Galton's efforts toward fingerprinting in Great Britain, and Alphonse Bertillon's anthropometric

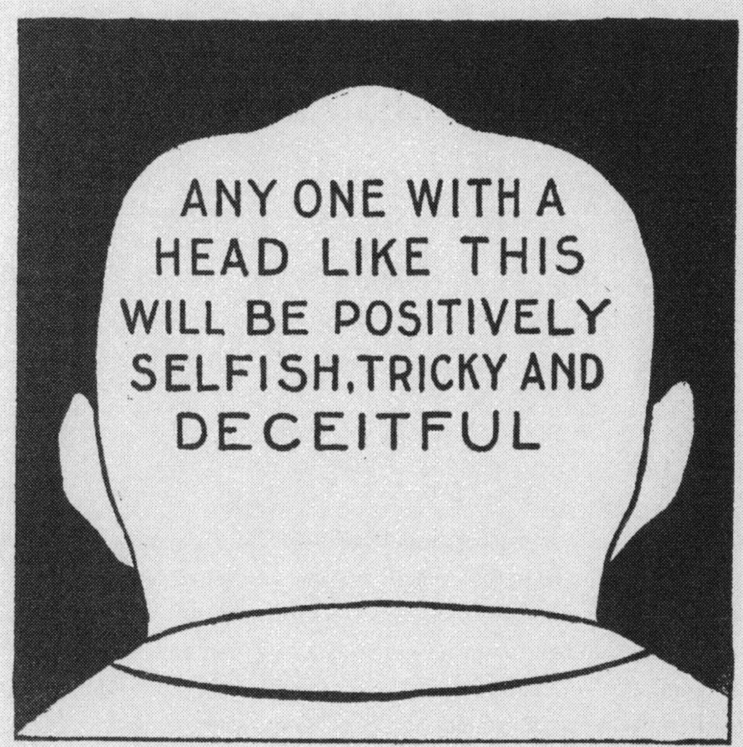

Figure 16. A selfish, tricky, and deceitful head, from L. A. Vaught, *Vaught's Practical Character Reader* (Chicago: L. A. Vaught, Publisher, 1902), 11. Harvard Medical Library at the Francis A. Countway Library of Medicine.

systems of identification in France were all introduced as new, scientific forms of predictive policing. While phrenological science would persist in popular culture and usage throughout the century, the leaders of science had moved on. Phrenology would continue to be a popular diversion as well as a serious enterprise for some, even as new forms of criminal science were developed in the final third of the century which offered new ways of thinking about crime, supplanting this vernacular criminal science.

Chapter 6

A Victory for Phrenology?

Dr. Samuel R. Wells, an associate of the Fowler brothers, served as an expert witness for the defense in the case of Lawrence Sullivan, on trial for the murder of John O'Brien in New York in 1870. On the stand, Wells identified himself as "an expert in regard to what caused insanity, temporary or otherwise, by the delineation of the character or by the organization as a whole," and his testimony repeated similar themes and arguments as those used in the cases of Major Mitchell and John Haggerty.[1] He argued that the defendant was an "imbecile" rather than an insane man, yet "a very slight provocation would quite unbalance him, as he is but an unfortunately or illy developed person; he is A CHILD WITH A MAN'S BODY."[2] The jury returned a guilty verdict on the charge of murder in the first degree, sentencing Sullivan to execution. However, some concerned parties petitioned the governor to appoint a commission to assess Sullivan's mental condition. This petition was granted, and Sullivan was examined by a group of physicians including Jacob S. Mosher, the state's Surgeon General. The committee declared the convict to be "hopelessly insane, with no probability of his recovery," and he was committed to the Auburn Lunatic Asylum, in lieu of execution.[3]

At first glance, this might have looked like a "victory for phrenology," as the case was described in *The Phrenological Journal and Life Illustrated*, for which Wells served as an editor alongside the Fowlers.[4] Wells argued that Sullivan was mentally incompetent, which was the eventual determination made by the state. As this article argued: "Phrenology positively declared what Sullivan's mental condition was, and in December, 1871, that declaration was fully sustained and confirmed by the highest medical authority and by the

Executive of the State . . . had Phrenology not intervened in this case, nothing could have saved Lawrence Sullivan from the gallows."[5] However, this account neglected an essential fact of the case: Wells's testimony was excluded by the judge.[6] When the case came to the New York Supreme Court, the exclusion of this testimony was the foundation for its appeal, but the exclusion stood and the appeal failed.[7] While the eventual commitment of Sullivan to Auburn as insane was presented as proof of the truth of phrenology, Wells's phrenological testimony was not considered to be admissible evidence.[8]

Was this indeed a victory for phrenology? An anonymous writer in *The Phrenological Journal* wrote optimistically, "let us hope that this sad case has opened a new era in the administration of criminal jurisprudence," presumably one with a permanent place for phrenology in the courtroom.[9] However, if anything, this case represented the converse: this was one of the last times that phrenology made its way into the courtroom.[10] While in the early decades of the century the expert nature of phrenology was still being debated in courtrooms, as in the Major Mitchell trial, four decades later phrenology's star was falling.

A decade later, in the fall of 1881, when Charles Guiteau was tried for assassinating President James Garfield, a series of medical experts testified as to whether or not the infamous murderer was in fact mentally ill.[11] During cross-examination, one of the star expert witnesses for the state, Dr. Edward Charles Spitzka, was asked how his examination of Guiteau was conducted while the defendant was in prison. Spitzka responded simply: "I represented myself as a professor of phrenology, in order that he should not suspect that I was a medical expert."[12] Spitzka drew a sharp line around medical expertise, excluding phrenological knowledge from its bounds. When asked to clarify the nature of his "phrenological dodge," he stated that "Phrenology is not a science; it is charlatanism; and all procedures of a charlatan are dodges."[13] By the last decades of the nineteenth century, other medical and scientific models for understanding the criminal mind were emerging as more attractive alternatives. The prediction of a "new era in the administration of criminal jurisprudence" may have come to fruition, but a very different set of scientific practices would benefit. Phrenology was left to the wayside by both the mainstream scientific community and popular sentiment.

Studies of the brain and mind transformed over the course of the nineteenth century, displacing phrenology from the neurological pantheon. The retreat from phrenology among American physicians and scientists was prompted in particular by the interventions of Marie-Jean-Pierre Flourens, who in the 1840s conducted experiments discrediting cerebral localization as represented by phrenology.[14] While elite intellectuals largely abandoned phrenology, they retained an interest in cerebral localization. In the 1860s, the work of Pierre Paul Broca in France and Carl Wernicke in Germany on different forms of aphasia served as proof positive of the possibility of localizing brain functions, spurring the development of the field of neurology.[15] As with the brain, so too the mind. Psychiatry also developed over the course of the nineteenth century, with one-time asylum superintendents becoming professionalized and medicalized, the asylum itself completing its reconfiguration into a therapeutic space—if one with only limited curative success.[16]

And then there was criminology itself. Criminal science was "invented" in the last decades of the nineteenth century, with the emergence of theorists like Cesare Lombroso and practices like Bertillonage, as this chapter will explore. While physicians were looking to Europe, preoccupied with lessons of laboratory science and the "new" scientific medicine, phrenologists also looked to new European innovations.[17] Yet whereas American physicians considered the potential for reinvention and reform of their profession through European models, phrenologists were largely considering problems of memory and positioning. Phrenologists were less invested in adapting their theory in pace with new intellectual and technological developments than they were with asserting their primacy in a scientific lineage or claiming that new sciences were "really" phrenology.

This chapter examines the scientific approaches to criminal minds and bodies that emerged in the last third of the nineteenth century, focusing on the ways in which late nineteenth-century phrenologists incorporated these new sciences and their practitioners into their self-conception of their project. I analyze not only the phrenological impulse within various sciences, but also the desire of partisans to identify phrenology in other sciences—and the desire of nonphrenologists to distance their scientific developments from phrenology. In the face of the new sciences of criminal anthropology and criminal identification, and the broader collection of studies of cerebral localization, practical phrenologists maintained that they belonged in the lineage of these practices, to diminishing returns. Phrenologists' insistence that these scientific developments were in fact continuations of older phrenological practice resounded within the echo chamber of phrenological literature, yet this connection was also drawn by nonphrenologists as a way to critique these new practices.

This chapter explores processes of remembering and forgetting within the phrenological and criminological communities. Latter-day practical phrenologists attempted to reframe phrenology as the origin point for neurology and criminology, producing their own genealogies that located their science in relation to these newer, respectable bodies of scientific knowledge. At the same time, criminologists and neurologists working on cerebral localization worked hard to distance their projects from that of phrenology. Discourses around "old" and "new" phrenologies, phrenological responses to criminal sciences, and critiques of criminology together reveal the concerns of phrenologists and nonphrenologists alike with regard to self-construction and positioning practices within these fields of inquiry.

Old and New Phrenology

Over the course of the nineteenth century, both phrenologists and nonphrenologists frequently commented on the existence of a "new" phrenology (or phrenologies) as a way of framing the development of new scientific approaches toward the brain. As Tabea Cornel has explained, "the designation *new phrenology* was (and remains to be) a flexible instrument for 'boundary-work' from within and outside the mind and brain sciences," used to position disparate practices and disciplines "inside or outside the borders of 'good science.'"[18] Throughout the nineteenth and twentieth centuries, innovators within the brain sciences and critics of these disciplines used "new phrenology" both positively and negatively to frame such developments. My interest here is with how phrenologists made use of or responded to this discourse of "new" phrenology, as well as how phrenologists specifically framed criminological developments as examples of such new phrenologies.

The juxtaposition of new versus old was itself not new. Phrenology itself had often been compared to an older science, physiognomy. When it was first introduced at the turn of the nineteenth century, phrenology was often explained or framed as the "new physiognomy."[19] By comparing the two, phrenologists were borrowing some of the authority of a well-known science that had roots in antiquity. At the same time, this well-known practice could help interested parties understand the stakes and import of the new science. This comparison highlighted the ways in which phrenology was both different and *improved*. Phrenology was framed as a new, more scientific way of answering the questions that physiognomy had long been thought to solve. Phrenologists stressed not only the novelty of the approach, but also the improvements to its practices through the advancement of scientific principles.

Phrenology was still a new science in the United States when it began a process of reinvention by its practitioners. James Stanley Grimes, a practical phrenologist, proffered a "new phrenology" as early as 1839. His *New System of Phrenology*, however, was not very different in content or argument to the works of Gall and Spurzheim or the works of contemporaries like Caldwell.[20]

Similarly, the Fowler brothers' brand of practical phrenology, popularized in the 1840s, could also be considered to be a "new" phrenology, distinct in some ways from the academic and anatomically focused Continental phrenology of the earlier part of the century. By focusing on an interested public and positioning themselves as interpreters of the "normal" skulls of paying clients, practical phrenologists participated in a vernacularization process that transformed both the practice and perception of phrenology. This new phrenology popularized by the Fowler brothers was intended to "render it highly *practical*, and to adapt to the *million*"[21]—science at the service of an interested public, rather than the preserve of an educated and cloistered elite. Other contemporaneous scientific practices, like Joseph R. Buchanan's psychometry, also purported to present a "new phrenology."[22]

Through the late nineteenth century, phrenologists used "new phrenology" primarily to frame developments *within* phrenology, not external to it, a rhetorical survival strategy of a science in decline.[23] After the 1870s, much of the discussion around a "new phrenology" focused on the contributions of neurologists to the localization of the mental organs and the explication of human behavior.[24] Comparisons drawn between localization and phrenology linked these practices and theories rhetorically, if teleologically. Writers for popular publications, not just phrenological periodicals, explained the discoveries of Broca and others as the "new phrenology" to suggest the significance of these findings, and it proved difficult at times to separate these new and old practices. Disputes and ambiguities between localizationism and diffusionism were marked by the uses of "new phrenology" to differentiate partisans for or against localization.[25] Debates about localization mobilized the language of the "new phrenology" not to make points about phrenology itself, but instead to make claims about the scientific merits—or lack thereof—of these new fields of study.[26]

At the same time, for phrenologists, this boundary-work was largely beside the point: phrenological partisans considered these new sciences to be validations of their theories. They argued that these "new" phrenologies were in fact continuations of the same ideas and practices. This identification of various "new phrenologies" could even be reduced to a farce. As one joke announced: "A new phrenology is out which tells character by the way you shut a door."[27] As far as many commentators outside phrenology were concerned, phrenology was a risible practice that had been effectively disproven by Flourens in the 1840s.[28] The decline of academic enthusiasm for phrenology was no doubt connected to this high-profile critique and associated attempts to distance studies of the brain from phrenology, though it did not materially affect the development of popular practical phrenology. If phrenologists declined to give credence to Flourens's perspective, they were not loath to embrace later localization projects.

Late nineteenth-century practical phrenologists paid particular attention to studies of aphasia, which were central to localization theory. Pierre Paul Broca's identification of anatomical proof for the localization of functions in the brain, using aphasia as an object of inquiry in the 1860s, was presented by phrenologists as a continuation or confirmation of phrenology.[29] Phrenologists viewed Broca's anatomical study as nearly identical to the foundations of phrenology: "In France an eminent savan [*sic*], M. Broca, has also been at work in experiments and observations relating to the brain and nervous system, and has also obtained results which are testimonials to the accuracy and fidelity of the great fathers of Phrenology, Gall and Spurzheim."[30]

Practical phrenologists often incorporated these scientists into their self-presentation of the lineage of their science, such that Broca and others became the heirs to Gall and Spurzheim within the pages of phrenological periodicals and texts. Even if one "new phrenology" existed in the guise of practical phrenology, this other "new phrenology"—cerebral localization—promised a return to and revival of the oldest traditions and theories of the field. This relationship was underlined frequently by phrenologists, who deemed Broca and his colleagues to be part of their phrenological project: "The 'New Phrenologists,' as the experimenters and theorists in motor localization are called."[31]

However, phrenological commentators also took umbrage with the credit received by Broca and others for the findings of Gall and Spurzheim. As one phrenologist writing in the British *Phrenological Magazine* observed, the seat of the faculty of speech was "discovered by Broca, though foreshadowed by Gall."[32] This author argued that Gall's suggestion of a speech center "has been fully established by later anatomists, and then complacently concluding that there are no foundations in fact for the assumptions of the phrenologists."[33] This irritating fact was "a specimen of the kind of treatment phrenology gets at the hands of these pseudo-scientists," who failed to accord appropriate respect to phrenology.[34] Moreover, these same "pseudo-scientists," protested that "'this is the new phrenology—not the old,'" with the old being their "*bête noir* [*sic*]."[35] As another British commentator asked rhetorically, "You would now, very probably, ask your phrenological friend *why* the name of Broca appeared in your text-book and not that of Gall—Broca's investigations having merely confirmed, and in some ways modified and elaborated the original discovery of Gall."[36] According to this author, this injustice was due to ignorance and prejudice, as "the fact is that the modern investigator of the functions of the nervous system, with his scalpel, electrodes, and dissecting knives, is toiling up a height climbed long ago."[37] Phrenological partisans argued that the contributions of their science were intentionally erased by the promoters of cerebral localization, rather than remembered as an essential step toward these discoveries.

Similar points were made within American phrenological publications. In the American *Phrenological Journal and Life Illustrated*, for example, the editors remarked upon Broca's known antipathy to phrenological theory. And yet, they observed with amusement, "for seventy-five years facts of a similar nature, stated as the result of fifty times more experiment and examination than the above paragraph indicates, have been constantly spread before the public and explained on scientific principles," although the scientific community remained aloof and newspapers had ridiculed phrenologists.[38] Broca's findings, they argued, were not much different in substance than those of Gall and Spurzheim. Indeed, they insisted that the recently published *Cerebral Convolutions of Man* (1873), by anatomist Alexander Ecker, was not an improvement on an 1820 paper of Spurzheim, published as part of his *Anatomy of the Brain* (1835). Perhaps "if the words 'phrenology' and 'Spurzheim,' however, could be eliminated from it, and some jaw-cracking French name applied to it, it would, probably, at once secure *caste* and respect among some of our celebrated scientists and professors."[39] Phrenological theory, American and British phrenologists argued, was not dissimilar and was in some ways superior to the cutting edge of anatomical localization theory. They asserted that prejudice against phrenology and the intentional erasure of phrenological origins in cerebral localization prevented scientific appreciation for the theories of Gall and Spurzheim, which were finally finding validation in the new discoveries of cerebral localization.

From the phrenological point of view, the development of these new sciences was unequivocally a victory for phrenology, even if the frequent dismissal or erasure of phrenology rankled. Much phrenological writing during the period from 1870 to 1900 made use of the new language of cerebral localization, images of the brain, and the findings of Broca and others without directly discussing the antipathy of these anatomists and physiologists for phrenology.[40] Phrenologists were quick to embrace cerebral localization as part of their project, but were highly sensitive to critiques of their science from outside of phrenological circles. They were perfectly content to assess bodies of scientific knowledge as "old" and "new" phrenologies, but only in order to argue for continuity, assuring the place of phrenologists in the scientific pantheon. Commentators who presented the "old" phrenology as outdated or unscientific and used it as a foil to the new sciences of cerebral localization were seen as unfairly prejudiced and worthy of attack.

This dynamic is perhaps best seen through the response to an article, "The Old and New Phrenology," published in *Popular Science Monthly* in 1889 by Dr. Moses Allen Starr.[41] A neurologist who had studied with Jean-Martin Charcot and Sigmund Freud, Starr became the chair of nervous disease at the College of Physicians & Surgeons of Columbia University the year before this essay was published, replacing Edward Seguin.[42] Starr, whose perspective might be interpreted as representative of mainstream medical thought, provided in this essay a largely dismissive reading of phrenology as a means to present more recent advances in the field of neurology. He began with a simple observation—"ALMOST every one has at some time wondered whether there is any truth in phrenology"—but quickly answered his own question: "It is pretty well agreed among scientists, at present, that the old system of phrenology has no actual basis of fact."[43]

Starr generously credited phrenology with spurring the study of the brain, stating that "to this old system of Gall modern science really owes a great deal; for, like every false idea, it had within it a little kernel of truth, and the interest excited by the claims of its supporters awakened a discussion which has led to a discovery of the greatest importance in the saving of human life."[44] He traced the history of studies of the brain after Gall, beginning with Flourens and German experiments before focusing on more recent research as steps towards a "new phrenology," by which he meant the physiology of the brain, especially the localization of motor areas.[45] Starr concluded that the "old phrenology" was "wrong in its theory, wrong in its facts, wrong in its interpretation of mental processes," whereas the "new phrenology" was "scientific in its methods, in its observations, and in its analysis."[46] In this article, the "old" and "new" phrenologies were set up in direct opposition to one another, with a clear contrast drawn between an old, wrong science, and a new, modern, and correct scientific theory.

A month after Starr's publication appeared, *The Phrenological Journal and Science of Health* (*PJSH*) responded with a defense of the science. The author, R., was concerned that the Starr article, written by a professor of a well-known scientific institution, "may have a prejudicial effect upon the uninformed and delay the general acceptance of the true physiology of the brain and philosophy of mind."[47] The author noted that he had similarly responded to and critiqued an article on the same subject published ten years earlier by the *Popular Science Monthly*, also on the subject of "The Old Phrenology and the New," making this a new salvo in what was perceived to be—for phrenologists at least—a continuing battle for the status of their science and its place in the history of studies of the brain.[48]

The author observed that if Starr had only connected phrenological theory of the faculties and motor functions, his article would be useful. But instead Starr attempted to disprove the "'Old Phrenology,'" displaying his ignorance: "We can assure Dr. Starr that there are many scientists, doctors and others, who openly express their belief in the truth of the 'Old Phrenology'; and many others who, in spite of a contemptuous sneer when it is mentioned in public, yet instinctively heed its dictates."[49] Moreover, the opponents of phrenology, Starr included, were "ready enough to admit its truth when it goes to support their own hypotheses."[50] R.'s impassioned defense of the maligned "'Old Phrenology,'" particularly his emphasis on the similarities between the practice, theories, and findings of these sciences, was characteristic of the defensive phrenological stance, as was the slightly hysterical tone of the essay.

In this case, "'Old Phrenology'" was taken as an affront, but phrenologists also mobilized this phrase to make rhetorical points in defense of phrenology and its place in the genealogy of the brain sciences. Phrenologists were also doing boundary-work, but this time in the history of their field and its teleology. This connection between old and new was drawn most frequently by the late nineteenth-century practical phrenologist and physician, Henry Shipman Drayton. Drayton wrote prolifically on phrenology and other topics, like mesmerism, frequently making arguments connecting neurology and physiology with phrenology. While he played with the dichotomy between old and new, this was primarily used to disavow any such distinction: for Drayton, as with other latter-day phrenologists, modern practices of anatomical localization were simply continuations of phrenological theory.

For example, in an article published in the *PJSH* in 1892 entitled "Old and New Phrenology," Drayton mused sardonically on rhetorical comparisons between old and new: "it is one of the fashions or fads of the day to draw contrasts between the past and the present . . . for the purpose of showing the superiority of our era, and how much our forefathers were behind in everything."[51] He sketched a retrospective of studies of the functions of the brain, remarking on the enthusiasm with which Gall and Spurzheim's "epoch-making truths" were greeted at the turn of the century.[52] Decades later, however, Broca and others, though "building on the foundation of G. and S. and developing a center in the brain for Language about where Gall had said it was located," were received even more warmly, displacing the work of phrenology's founders:

> What excitement, then! The world of physiology and psychology rang with their names. Hurrah! new light on brain function; hurrah! now it is

> demonstrated that the brain is divided into areas having special duty and service in the economy of life. Hats are thrown up; great enthusiasm reigns in the societies and academies of the learned.
>
> But now we venture to ask "What of the old Phrenology, with its gracious, helpful tenets regarding the mind and character of men?" "Oh," one of the muscular disciples replies, "that is *passé*, exploded, relegated to the limbo of chimeras and fallacies. Our system of muscle action is the new and true Phrenology. The world has no longer any use for the old."[53]

What then, Drayton asked, of the many anatomists and theorists of the brain of the past century, a long list of "good and useful men" who expressed interest in phrenology—including Bell, Pinel, Dickens, and Emerson, along with the Fowlers, Wells, and Sizer—who must therefore have been "victims of a sheer delusion"?[54] Surely, Drayton concluded, "our stalwart champions of a new and muscular Phrenology" were unaware of the tenets of the older system, for the work of recent contemporaries sounded suspiciously similar to those of the "old Phrenology."[55]

Drayton also wrote letters to newspapers to protest misleading coverage of phrenology. In an 1892 letter to the editor of *The Sunday Inter Ocean* responding to a dismissive account of phrenology in the same paper, Drayton argued that "physiologists who busy themselves with experiments upon motor centers of the brain are approaching closer and closer to the position of Gall and Spurzheim," and moreover, that "Broca's discovery of the center for spoken language is nothing more than a confirmation of Gall's center."[56] Drayton ended this letter on an optimistic note: "Phrenological science is advancing; it has a growing constituency among people of education and scientific acquirements."[57] This optimism may seem unwarranted, especially with the benefit of hindsight, as phrenology was certainly in decline by the 1890s.

Drayton's writings encapsulate a common point of view among late nineteenth-century American phrenologists: *all* advances in studies of the mind and brain were viewed as extensions of phrenology. Phrenologists connected their science with every advance in the study of brains, skulls, and mental disorders, framing themselves—or, at least, Gall and Spurzheim—as the originators of a great and widespread field of science. If they sometimes positioned themselves as the ignored Cassandras, proclaimers of a great truth dismissed due to the prejudice and indifference of the scientific community, they simultaneously gloated over any perceived correlation between traditional phrenological theories and new scientific discoveries.

Within this cosmology, *all* scientists working on the broadly defined study of the skull or brain became phrenologists:

> If we look over the arena of mental, psychological, physiological science today, in the spirit of candor we can not but note how the genius of Gall and Spurzheim has stamped its modes of action and development. . . . It is mind and brain or brain and mind that interests each and all, yet their departments are respectively distinct.
>
> In Germany, Benedikt, Hitzig, Schiff, Nothnagel, Munk; in France, Charcot, Manouvrier, Tarde, Luys, Dupuy, Delauney, Richet; in Italy, Lombroso, Garofalo, Mantogazza; in England, Ferrier, Gowers, Galton; in America, Hughes, Buttolph, Hall, Sanford, Schurman, and then that large class of men in all these countries, who stand prominent in their field of advanced Phrenology.[58]

To latter-day phrenologists, it mattered less that such individuals might have considered themselves to be part of their cohort: "their affirmation or denial of premises advanced by psychologists is of little real importance. . . . They can not help being phrenologists."[59] Even though these scientists were "unwilling to declare themselves disciples of Gall and Spurzheim," they appropriated these teachings and named them "new," forgetting or erasing phrenological origins.[60] Thus, "most of them are, so far as belief in the nature of the brain is concerned, phrenologists, although they might not accept the name."[61]

For phrenologists, it did not matter if a scientist accepted, cited, or rejected phrenology as such; by virtue of approaching topics of mind and brain, he declared himself to be a phrenologist. In this way, *all* scientists could be made into phrenologists, providing much-needed borrowed authority to a science in decline. This strategy further allowed for the continuation of phrenology, if only as a "new" phrenology, and this framing of the mind sciences as broadly and historically inclusive of both "new" and "old" phrenologies also charted a path for a phrenological future. Among these anointed "new" phrenologists were not only anatomists like Broca, however. This cohort included scientists devoted in particular to scientific studies of crime as well, especially Cesare Lombroso.

Positivist Criminology

According to Cesare Lombroso, his theories came to him in a "literal flash of light" while he was conducting an autopsy on a criminal in 1871, which led him to make connections between the skull of the convict and those of lower animals and "inferior races."[62] Lombroso was an Italian psychiatrist who in the

1870s, while a professor of psychiatry at the University of Pavia, conducted research on convicts and inmates of prisons and asylums that led to his articulation of a biological criminology focused on the elucidation of the type of the "born criminal," thus founding criminal anthropology.[63] Lombroso was strongly influenced by contemporaneous intellectual currents in Continental thought, including French positivism, German scientific materialism, and British evolutionism, as well as his own training as a psychiatrist.[64] The associations between evolutionary theory and Lombroso's theories of born criminals are perhaps best known, in part due to the strong hereditary thrust of his theories, as well as his focus on degeneration.[65] Despite the fact that Lombroso's published works were not translated into English for years or decades, if at all, these theories became influential for a brief period throughout Europe and in the United States.[66] Indeed, they would have a more lasting legacy in the United States than in Europe, where they were more quickly disputed and discarded.[67]

Lombroso and his school of positivist criminology or criminal anthropology have been closely tied to the "birth" of criminal science. The term "criminology" itself was not in use before Lombroso, nor did his predecessors refer to themselves as "criminologists."[68] Nicole Hahn Rafter has argued that scholars and scientists who speculated on the causes of crime prior to Lombroso's 1870s innovations "did not think of themselves as specialists in the production of scientific information about crime."[69] If this was the case for phrenologists, it was only because they made sweeping claims to expert knowledge in so many fields that they therefore did not claim to specialize in theories of crime. Moreover, as Daniel Patrick Thurs notes, "antebellum science talk reflected the fuzziness of science as a category . . . Americans talked about the 'sciences' rather than 'science.'"[70]

Specialization in science, particularly medicine, was largely a piecemeal and gradual trend in the nineteenth century, and medical and scientific practitioners, their patients, and the public often viewed specialization with suspicion.[71] Yet despite their self-presentation as general experts on many aspects of the human mind and society, phrenologists might be considered to be criminologists *avant la lettre*. They considered their field of knowledge to constitute specialized, explanatory knowledge relevant to crime, especially in retrospect, when confronted with the growing success of the field of criminology. Lombroso, like so many other late nineteenth-century scientists, was yet another "new phrenologist"—a pretender to the throne who garnered acclaim for unattributed phrenological ideas.

When phrenologists prepared genealogies of the history of criminology at the end of the century, they asserted their place within this history, positioning the founders of phrenology as founders of criminology as well. For example, in an essay published on "The Science of Crime" in the *PJSH* in 1899, the author, Burton Peter Thom, asserted Gall as the true founder of scientific criminology: "while his work extended far beyond the borders of what we should now call criminology, he devoted much attention to the problems of the criminal organization and its varieties, many of his observations according well with the results of recent investigation."[72] Thom described Lombroso as "the distinguished Italian savant who has done more than any other man to establish the extent of its application," but he presented Gall as the founder of this scientific approach to crime, with Lombroso responsible for extending and popularizing the science.[73] Thom was uninterested in narrowing the focus of phrenology to the problem of crime alone, no matter how respected the field of criminology had become. Instead, he positioned phrenology as expert knowledge in many fields, one of which was criminology. In this retelling of the history of criminology, phrenology became the origin point for this "scientific system of ever-widening scope."[74]

While Lombroso connected his insights to theories of atavism, he was also replicating connections familiar to phrenology. Gall had studied animal skulls in relation to human skulls in order to identify particular organs, and connections between animal and human skulls were drawn by phrenologists throughout the century, especially with attention to the organ of Destructiveness, along with different ethnic types.[75] The explanatory framework may have been quite different in these two approaches to the criminal, but the conclusions were similar.

During the development of phrenological theory in the early part of the century, the prison was similarly used as a laboratory for the examination and measurement of the skulls of criminals. Phrenologists were invited into prisons to examine both living and dead convicts, included in autopsies, and provided with the skulls (or casts of heads) of criminals, as this book has explored. Similarly, Mary Gibson has observed that for Lombroso, "the prison was a laboratory in which he used a variety of odd machines to measure and experiment on the physical body," and further that Lombroso conducted autopsies on the bodies of dead convicts.[76] While phrenologists did not apply a systematic or classificatory system to criminals, as did Lombroso, these two areas of scientific inquiry shared a set of methods, assumptions, sites, and thematic interests. Lombroso himself had further replicated a familiar theme of phrenological writing, as his focus was not only on criminal types, but also on great men, as in his 1888 *L'uomo di genio in rapporto alla psichiatria* (translated into English as *The Man of Genius*). Lombroso also combined these two themes in his work on "criminals of genius."[77]

Lombroso's contemporaries often made comparisons between phrenology and criminal anthropology as a means to critique Lombroso. Phrenologists made similar connections, but cast them in a positive light. A review of the English translation of *La donna delinquente* (*The Female Offender*) in the British magazine *The Speaker*, for example, found Lombroso's connection between physical and psychological characteristics among criminals to be less than convincing: "The lesson taught by phrenology ought always to be remembered when anatomical are considered as associated with psychological peculiarities . . . the study of the offender, whether male or female, is best approached from the social and not from the anatomical side."[78] Unsurprisingly, phrenologists found this aspect of Lombroso's argument to be worthy of praise rather than censure. A review of the same work, which appeared in the *PJSH*, observed with approval that Lombroso "proceeds upon the strictly phrenological principle that mental processes are closely related to physical conditions."[79] Further, the editors remarked that "Prof. Lombroso's work contains a great deal of information of practical advantage to phrenologists, although many of his ideas are already familiar to our profession."[80] Even when praising the work of Lombroso, phrenologists could not resist asserting the primacy of phrenological theory.

Lombroso's criminological peers drew similar connections. At the Second International Congress of Criminal Anthropology, held in Paris in 1889, Lombroso opened the conference with a paper on "The Latest Discoveries in Criminal Anthropology." Léonce Manouvrier, a French anthropologist, delivered the second paper, which attacked Lombroso's theories, especially the concept of the "born criminal." Manouvrier "pronounced the theory of his opponents to be but a recitation of the exploded science of phrenology," arguing that the anatomical differences Lombroso identified "belonged as much to honest men as to criminals."[81] This conference marked a schism in the criminological community, as well as the beginning of the decline of Lombroso's primacy, at least in the European context, although he continued to draw disciples in Italy, who closed ranks after this meeting.[82] Coverage of this conference within the *PJSH* omitted these negative references to phrenology and this attack on Lombroso.[83] Instead, it was used as further evidence "confirmatory of the 'old' phrenological centers of ideation."[84] The conference presenters were described as "new" phrenologists for whom "every certain step . . . but brings them nearer to the 'old' phrenologists."[85] "Palman [*sic*] qui meruit ferat," the article concluded—give credit where credit is due, to the "old" phrenologists.[86]

However, phrenologists were not in perfect accord with Lombroso. While they were quick to identify elements of his work relating to phrenology, they still objected to the pessimism of his approach. Late nineteenth-century phrenology had not outgrown the utopian outlook imposed upon it by the reformist impulses of the Fowler brothers at midcentury. Positivist criminologists, according to phrenologists, "treat the inveterate offender against law, social and civil, as one defective constitutionally, and akin to the insane or idiotic."[87] This was unpalatable to late-century phrenologists, who maintained that all men were "amenable to training and improvement, whatever may be the degree of moral degeneration or perversion."[88] It was on this point that phrenologists most frequently and stridently voiced their disapproval of positivist ideology, setting their approach apart from the mainstream of criminology.

Even though phrenologists did not always approve of the implications of Lombroso's theory of born criminals, they reinforced this connection in the service of supporting their claims to the longevity and influence of phrenology. This rhetorical strategy frequently intersected with the insistence on connections to the broader articulation of the "new phrenologists." For example, Bernard Hollander, a physician and leader of British phrenology, presented a paper at the Anthropological Institute in London in February 1889 in which he made an impassioned case for the correspondences between the findings of phrenology and physiology.[89] Sir George Ferrier, a British neurologist, responded to Hollander's paper arguing that, while "a scientific phrenology might one day become possible," at the present time Hollander had not provided sufficient evidence.[90] Hollander countered this critique with specific evidence: "He [Gall] noticed the resemblance between the skulls of murderers and the skulls of carnivorous animals; the predominance of the temporal lobe struck him, and both Prof. Benedict [*sic*] and Lombroso—the authorities on criminal anthropology—testify as to its correctness. . . . He reasoned that there must be in the case of murderers an organ giving an impulse to destroy or kill ('destructiveness')."[91] Hollander focused on the contributions of criminal anthropology to legitimize Gall's contributions. Perhaps his recourse to Lombroso was ill-chosen, as 1889 was also the year of the Second International Congress of Criminal Anthropology, which signaled the decline of Lombroso's status and the rise of different schools of thought in criminal science.[92]

Lombroso's reputation did not decline quite so quickly in the United States, and American phrenologists continued to cite him to reinforce the status of their science. As late as 1909, the *PJSH* included a special Christmas message for its subscribers in its December issue: "we are gratified to be able to announce that he [Lombroso] was a firm believer in Dr. Gall's theory of

Craniology."[93] A decade earlier, the editors of the journal had written to Lombroso to ask his opinions on Gall and cerebral localization, to which he replied that while "The system of Dr. Gall may not be considered by all correct on every point" it was "nevertheless the result of an immense and diligent series of studies in the nerve centres, which makes it the precursor of Criminal Anthropology."[94] Lombroso and criminal anthropology, even in the new century, continued to be an important touchstone for the self-fashioning of phrenology and its genealogy.

Explanatory systems for crime only held so much promise. At the end of the century, new schemes were also developed to identify both convicts and recidivists, with a renewed focus on identifying and tracking criminals after the act, rather than predicting their movements before a crime. These identification systems were similarly prefigured with phrenological techniques and technologies.

Measuring Skulls

Gall and Spurzheim had initially proposed only visual and manual examinations of skulls when they introduced phrenology in the first two decades of the nineteenth century. However, in the 1820s, George Combe introduced and advocated for the use of calipers and a new instrument he called a craniometer for the production of phrenological measurements.[95] By 1841, Combe had decided that the craniometer "ha[d] not been found to be practically useful," and advocated for the exclusive use of the calipers.[96] These instruments were also adopted by Samuel George Morton as he developed his *Crania Americana*.[97] While many measurements were conducted of the criminal skull by phrenologists, especially in the earlier decades of the century, these measurements were never conducted systematically, collated or compared, or analyzed in the aggregate. Individual phrenologists wrote prolifically on the criminal type and behaviors, but their conclusions were not systematized, aside from a general agreement regarding the significance of certain propensities. However, tape measures, craniometers, and especially calipers remained valuable tools, which came to be associated with the practical phrenologist.

By the last decades of the nineteenth century, new explanatory and measurement systems had emerged to take up the problem of the criminal, including the practical system of anthropometry, developed by Alphonse Bertillon in 1880s Paris.[98] Bertillon was a police officer who developed a scientific approach to managing criminals, especially recidivists. His father, Louis-Adolphe Bertillon, and older brother, Jacques Bertillon, were well-known statisticians; Louis-Adolphe was also an anthropologist, and Jacques originally trained as a physician. The scientific and statistical training of his family members may have influenced his own measurement-based approach to crime. Alphonse and his brother were raised in a house that held anthropometric measurement tools, including the calipers, due to their father's anthropological work and association with the theories of Adolphe Quetelet.[99] While he would also contribute to the standardization of the mug shot, and worked on fingerprinting and handwriting analysis, it was his system of anthropometry, later known as Bertillonage or the Bertillon system, for which he was best known.

Bertillonage required the measurement of various parts of the human body, from the height of the body and length of the feet down to more unusual measurements, such as the length of the forearms, the distance from shoulder to shoulder, and so forth. Central to these measurements was a series of measurements of the head and facial features. All of these numbers would be inscribed on a card, often with a criminal's mug shot, collected centrally in an innovative and complex filing system. In this system, the measurements of the body allowed for the identification of criminals—specific, quantifiable, and measurable data, rather than subjective or descriptive data alone. The system was, claimed the *New York Times*, "better than photographs," for identifying criminal offenders.[100]

Bertillonage was also initially more popular than fingerprint identification, a process developed in British colonial India in the 1850s, though usually associated with Francis Galton's work with fingerprints and his fingerprint classification system developed in the 1880s.[101] Galton himself advocated for the use of the Bertillon system and did not believe that fingerprinting would be useful outside of the colonial context.[102] Even though both fingerprinting and anthropometric identification schemes were developed in the same period, Bertillonage was greatly preferred and expediently implemented by both scientists and state authorities, dominating discussions of criminal identification through the first decades of the twentieth century.

The system was introduced and tested in Paris in the early 1880s before spreading through France.[103] The early successes of Bertillonage, especially its use in identifying recidivists, led it to catch on quickly throughout the Western world. It was adopted in Britain, Germany, and in the British colonies (especially India) in the same decade, and various municipalities and states in the United States introduced the system in the 1890s.[104] These laws and the use of this system would last in the United States into the 1920s or 1930s, in some cases.[105] Unlike phrenology, which was frequently framed by enthusiasts and practical phrenologists as an expert practice with few techniques explained in detail to the public, the Bertillon system was described and explained in great detail, both textually and pictorially, and it was received positively in the

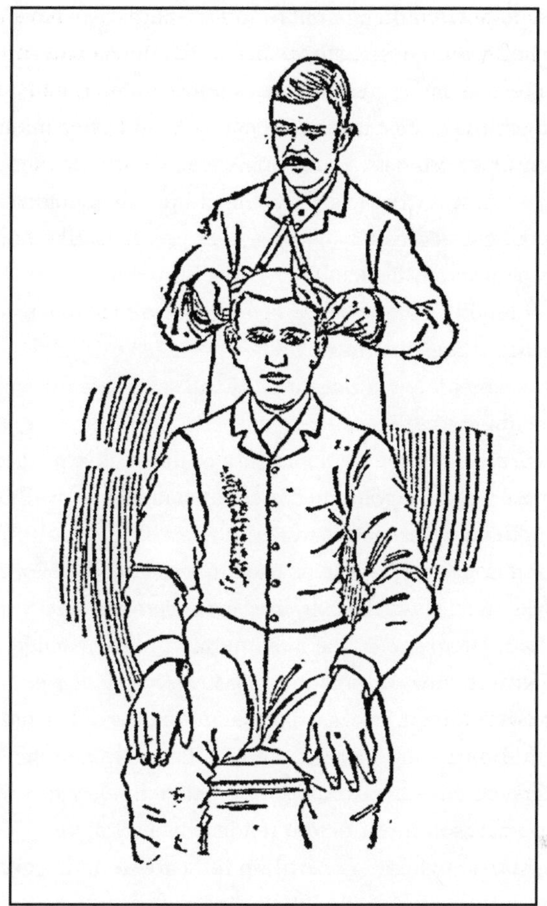

Figure 17. A police officer measuring the head of a convict with calipers, from "Adroit Criminals. How They Are Identified in the Bertillon System of Measurement . . ." *The Sunday Inter-Ocean* (Chicago, IL), November 17, 1889. Credit: from NewsBank, Inc. and the American Antiquarian Society. All Rights Reserved.

United States. Not of least importance was the ease of use of Bertillonage; a police officer only needed to read a short manual or attend a few days of practical demonstration to be able to put it into practice.[106] In images, its instruments dominated, with a familiar feature: the calipers, wielded by a police offer to measure the head of a prisoner (figure 17).

While these measurements of the body were taken initially in millimeters, for the sake of organization these numbers were reduced to descriptive data, with each number transforming into "short," "medium," or "long" for filing purposes. Once a card was inscribed, the relative sizes of different body parts, beginning with height, would be used to sort the cards into smaller and smaller categories—height would designate the first of the divisions, which would continue down along the list of measurements into smaller sorted groups. An officer could use his filing system to look up newly arrested or convicted offenders, in order to identify recidivists or criminals who crossed state or national borders. Despite the complexity of this system and its filing practices, it was used and preferred in some cases for decades over practices like fingerprinting or the mug shot. "The scientific accuracy of the Bertillon system," the *Scientific American* concluded in 1904, "is now beyond question," dismissing the potential of other technologies, including fingerprinting.[107]

Head measurements were only part of the set of measurements, but they were detailed and given pride of place on Bertillon cards. As explained by the *Scientific American*: "The length and width of the skull are taken by means of a caliper compass having a graduated arc scale reading to millimeters. . . . The measurement of the width is obtained with somewhat greater difficulty, because there are no fixed points which can be used in every subject. For this reason the extremities of the two legs of the caliper compass are placed on each side of the head, and shifted slightly until the maximum width is reached."[108] This span was identical with the measurement for Destructiveness in phrenological discourse. While Bertillon had stressed the significance of the hand and ear for identification, as Bertillonage spread, commentators framed the head measurements instead as the most significant: "in practice the length and width of the head are in most cases quite sufficient to identify a criminal."[109]

Phrenologists, though giving Bertillon little attention in comparison to figures like Broca and Lombroso, included him in their pantheon of "new phrenologists" as part of their continual project of self-fashioning.[110] For example, in two essays on "rogues" published in *The Phrenological Journal and Life Illustrated* in 1888 and 1898, the author's reports of phrenological and physiognomic observations of criminal types were paired with discussions of Bertillonage.[111] In the 1898 essay "In a Gallery of Rogues," Henry Drayton described the system of Bertillonage measurement before reflecting on the value of phrenology and physiognomy: "But really, on close inspection, with the assistance of some knowledge of physiognomy and Phrenology, it is not difficult to differentiate the good from the bad in human nature."[112] Drayton suggested that even though Bertillonage "work[ed] exceedingly well," a skilled phrenologist could identify offenders even before the act.[113]

Phrenologists, at least as represented by the *PJSH*, were mostly accepting, if somewhat dismissive, of the possibilities of Bertillonage. It "appears to work fairly well," one writer observed, "but for the most part the method is regarded as involving too much detail for general introduction."[114] Instead, phrenologists proposed a superior plan: "an examination of the size and contour of the head, which, if made by an experienced hand and eye, will furnish in brief a positive clue to the character of an individual."[115] They advocated for the use of phrenological examinations to supplant Bertillonage and also suggested the casting of the head in plaster as a record, reimagining the police station as a phrenological cabinet. "The addition of an officer versed in phrenological methods to the police organization has often been urged," as they suggested, but instruction provided by a practical phrenologist could "render a person of average intelligence sufficiently skilful" to make this phrenological knowledge of service to the police.[116] In lieu of Bertillon's system they proposed a phrenological police.

Both the proposed phrenologically trained police officer and the police officer trained in Bertillonage had the same toolkit: the tape measure and calipers. However, unlike the phrenologists, the practitioners of Bertillonage were not presenting an explanatory system, with an aim to predict or explain the actions of criminals as individuals or in the aggregate. No discussion was conducted of the significance of these various measurements, nor were statistical studies done comparing them. Instead, the Bertillon system had a goal of identification alone, and criminals were measured and their cards filed post-arrest or post-conviction. The aim was to identify recidivists, especially given the frequent use of aliases and the movement of criminal offenders, not to theorize about criminal types. Bertillonage was about controlling a deviant and problematic population through the use of detailed measurement and recordkeeping, rather than identifying criminals before the act. Bertillonage attempted to reduce an aggregate into individuals; phrenology, along with positivist criminology and other fields of anthropology, collected individuals into aggregate types.[117]

Despite the very different effects of these practices, however, Bertillonage and phrenology shared techniques, technologies, and assumptions regarding the practice of measuring bodies in general and of measuring criminals in particular. The image of the phrenologist with his calipers and that of the police officer with his instrument were nearly identical, as were the instruments themselves. While more measurements were taken within Bertillonage of the prisoner's body, the method of measuring the head in both instances was the same, even if the underlying assumptions and ensuing interpretations were largely different: both sciences did assume that the shape of both the skull and skeletal system was immutable. The term "craniometry" itself, an alternate name used as a shorthand for both systems, is suggestive. This perception of similarity is shared by more recent commentators: at least one scholar has referred to Bertillonage as "Bertillon's phrenology."[118]

The differences between the two systems are as suggestive as the similarities. Phrenology was a science founded by a set of medical experts and largely promulgated by physicians and scientific men, at least in its early days. While Bertillon's father and brother were both well-respected scientists and statisticians, he himself had little scientific training, working as a clerk in in the Paris Préfecture de Police.[119] In spite of the these origins, phrenology was controversial within the scientific community; while it became a popular vernacular science and remained so into the twentieth century, it was never wholly accepted in scientific circles, and never successfully incorporated into the penal or justice systems, despite efforts by phrenologists throughout the century. Bertillonage, on the contrary, was adopted widely and accepted with a great measure of faith by scientists and penal experts, becoming for a time an essential step on the criminal's journey through the penal system. While Bertillonage was applied to thousands of criminals in the United States, France, and other countries, the system was never used to try to explain the criminal or to construct a type—it was solely used for identification.

Why did these two anthropometric sciences of crime have such different fates? The eighteenth and nineteenth centuries witnessed an increase in numeracy among lay observers, accompanied by an increased trust in the measurements and measurement systems of scientists as they entered the public sphere.[120] Over the course of the nineteenth century, such faith became more pronounced, and tools of measurement also became more common and accessible for nonexperts. Phrenology, which often hid and obscured its measurement techniques, or presented obscure numbers and measurements without explanation, was unable to muster trust in its system. Even though phrenologists continued to discuss measurement practices and technologies, phrenology was associated primarily with the subjective practices of "bumpology"—feeling the head with the hands. An attempt to present their science as a specialized system, to keep it somewhat inscrutable in order to preserve their place as experts, paradoxically rendered phrenology less trustworthy as a science to the public. Conversely, Bertillonage made its practices and instrumentation visible, legible, and simple to understand—a transparent system with clear methods and goals. The prominent use of technology inspired faith in Bertillonage: the objectification of the criminal, explicitly and specifically, did not cause great concern for the public.

Moreover, underlying sentiments motivating these two approaches also affected their reception. Phrenological criminological thought conveyed optimism that criminals could be re-educated or that criminal types could be identified and helped before the fact. However, late nineteenth-century criminology inspired pessimism, particularly Lombroso's articulation of the criminal type as immutable. Criminals were *born*, rather than *made* by education and circumstance, according to Lombroso: they could not be fixed, but they could be identified, corralled, and controlled. Bertillonage was based on similar pessimism—namely, that identification was the only worthy goal within the penal system, and that recidivists in particular were the most important to identify and place in jail.

The increased faith and visibility in measurement practices and scientific instrumentation, coupled with an increased pessimism regarding the ability to reform criminal minds, together account for the perceived success of Bertillonage, as compared to phrenological criminal science. While the Bertillon system of the late nineteenth century shared tools and techniques with phrenology, it acquired a status of popularity and trust that phrenology was unable to achieve. The utility of caliper measurements to assess the criminal body, while introduced by phrenologists in the early part of the century, found its fullest expression in the measurement practices of Bertillonage. The ubiquity of the calipers and other tools of measurement applied to the criminal body served to undergird the authority of the science, even conducted as it was by lay practitioners.

In 1906, Jessie Fowler, who took on the family business after the deaths of her father and uncle, attempted to reinforce the message that it was "Not Bumps, But Calipers" that were essential to phrenological theory.[121] A long interview published in the *Charleston News and Courier* was accompanied by an illustration of her performing a phrenological examination on a stoic gentleman in her phrenological cabinet (figure 18). In this illustration, Fowler stood above a seated gentleman, calipers poised to measure his skull from temple to temple. If not for the phrenological accoutrements and the gender of the examiner, this image might have easily passed for the measurement of the criminal skull by a police officer trained in the Bertillon system (figure 17). As her phrenological peers might have argued, it was only a trick of fate that it was a police officer, rather than a Fowler scion, who found a place in the system of criminal identification and control, just as such phrenological partisans argued it was an unfair result of prejudice that privileged the "new phrenology" over the old, erasing its contributions.

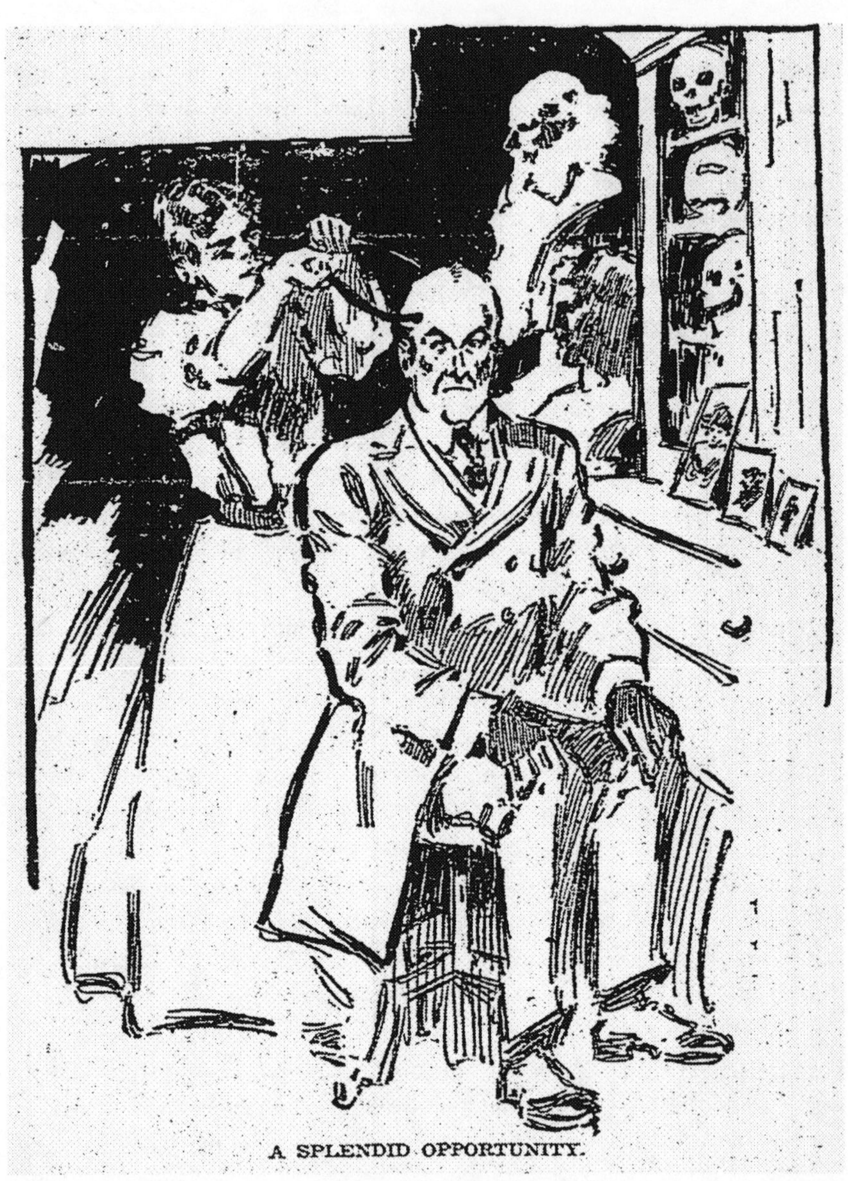

Figure 18. Jessie Fowler measuring the head of a client with calipers, from "Not Bumps, but Calipers. Miss Fowler Talks about Skulls and Upsets a Popular Notion about Phrenology," *Charleston News and Courier*, published as *The Sunday News* (Charleston, SC), January 21, 1906. Credit: from NewsBank, Inc. and the American Antiquarian Society. All Rights Reserved.

If the modern sciences of brain and crime were content to forget or erase their similarities to phrenological practices and discourse, practical phrenologists continued to insist on the role of their science in the development of these fields, staking their claim to interpret criminal minds well into the twentieth century. In so doing, they participated in a continuing project of self-fashioning and remembering to the point of diminishing returns, interpreting erasures of phrenology as "victories" instead.

Phrenologists were not alone in seeing clear connections between phrenology and the mind sciences, and studies of cerebral localization in particular. It is a commonplace for historians of science and medicine to tie phrenology to the neuro disciplines, focusing on the interventions of Gall in particular.[122] Historians have embraced phrenology as a component of the history of the mind sciences and more generally of the history of science. A phrenologist transported to the present might be pleased to find that the place of phrenology has been secured within the historical record, perhaps reading this as the ultimate victory for phrenology.

Epilogue

Phrenological Futures

A dispatch from the future appeared in *The Phrenological Journal and Science of Health* in 1892, imagining a world in which phrenology had truly triumphed. Among other achievements, the author predicted that by the 1940s, phrenologists would serve as chairs of phrenology in illustrious universities, which would require students to sit for phrenological examinations before enrollment. Further,

> Then there is the work of the courts. What abominable work they used to make of criminal trials! A mere farce, often. But how is it now? Police judges are selected and elected because they are supposed to be competent phrenologists. Jurors are sworn in when they have correctly answered certain phrenological questions.
>
> An experienced and reliable phrenological examiner is always called in to examine the accused and the witnesses phrenologically, telling the court what mental conditions he finds and how the jury should receive the testimony of each and all.[1]

This "Dream of Fifty Years Forward" recalls the phrenological promises of the farcical Sir Thomas of chapter 1's *The Phrenologist*, who desired that "every judge, magistrate, police officer, constable, and all persons concerned in the preservation of his Majesty's peace shall be Phrenologists."[2] Nearly seventy years after the publication of the play, which poked fun at the pretensions of phrenologists, American phrenologists were still earnestly imagining a world in which Sir Thomas's proposal and these latter-day phrenological dreams might become a reality, with the reform of the courts, prisons, and police at the center of these ambitions. But it was not to be. Within the span of these imagined fifty years, phrenology faded from sight. The last issue of *The Phrenological Journal and Science of Health* itself was published less than a decade later, in 1911. The disappearance of this journal signaled the end of a phrenological era in the United States.

Phrenology by the early twentieth century was increasingly perceived as a relic of an "almost forgotten medical theory."[3] Writing in the 1920s, a century after the introduction of phrenology in America, John Collins Warren Jr. reflected on the cabinet of the Boston Phrenological Society, which had been donated in the 1850s to his grandfather, John Collins Warren Sr., to form the newly created Warren Anatomical Museum at the Harvard Medical School.[4] Warren Jr. observed that these theories "have long since been set aside in the advance of our knowledge of anatomy and physiology."[5] Warren's fond memories of visiting his grandfather's collection included a familiar juxtaposition: great men "cheek by jowl" with celebrated criminals: "The formidable array of plaster casts of the heads of all sorts and conditions of men which decorated the railing surrounding the gallery of the Anatomical Museum is one of my earliest recollections of the Harvard Medical School. . . . The busts of the intellectual Cicero and Caesar and the death mask of the great Napoleon stood literally cheek by jowl with those of degenerates and celebrated criminals."[6] Yet while these busts—some of them, at least—remained within the Warren Anatomical Museum, they no longer appeared in its public displays. Phrenology had been dismissed from the halls of science, banished to dusty backrooms—real and metaphorical—as "memorials of an interesting episode" in the history of science and medicine.[7]

Yet in the same decade that John Collins Warren Jr. produced his eulogy for the departed science, phrenology was still, paradoxically, making headlines. In August of 1928, nearly a year to the date after the murder of a merchant by the name of Coleman Osborne, two men and one woman were due to be executed by the state of Georgia for the crime.[8] The convicted parties were Clifford and Eula Mae Thompson, a young, white married couple, and James Hugh Moss, an African American professional baseball player. According to the reporting, Clifford Thompson and Moss had shot and robbed Osborne at his store in Chatsworth, Georgia. All three were convicted of murder and sentenced to the electric chair, but Eula Mae issued a last-minute confession alleging that her previously unknown lover had been the man to pull the trigger, not her husband or Moss. This confession resulted in an attempt by the defense attorneys to seek clemency for their clients, necessitating the governor's attention.[9]

The governor of Georgia at this time was Lamartine G. Hardman, a Georgia native who followed his father's footsteps into the medical profession, graduating from Georgia Medical College in 1876, before completing further study at the University of Pennsylvania, the New York Polyclinic, and Guy's Hospital in London.[10] Aside from his medical practice and experiments in anesthesiology, he was a leader in the agricultural industry and eventually entered politics, with his first position in 1902 as an elected member of the Georgia House of Representatives.[11] By the time he became governor in 1926, he was a wealthy member of Georgia society and a prominent political figure with a known medical background.

Hardman commuted the death penalty to life in prison for Eula Mae, but declined to allow clemency for Thompson and Moss, who were electrocuted on August 3, 1928, after a stay of several hours while he considered the case.[12] Hardman's decisions, according to multiple news outlets and his own statement to the press, were based on phrenology.[13] As one newspaper observed, the outcome of this case "will depend upon the faith in phrenology of Governor Hardman."[14] As Hardman justified his decision, "believing that the verdict is just and that the parties are guilty . . . and reading as best I can their physiognomy and phrenology, I feel that the court rendered a righteous verdict."[15] Moreover, his decision to commute Eula Mae's sentence was based on his feeling "the bumps on her head—and decid[ing] that she could be redeemed."[16] Later the same month, Hardman was asked by counsel to repeat the same process by the defense attorney for George Fickling, an African American man convicted of murdering his brother-in-law, whose execution was also originally scheduled for August 3, 1928.[17] The attorneys reportedly asked Hardman to "study a picture of the defendant and apply thereto the governor's knowledge of phrenology with a view to determine whether or not Fickling has the features or characteristics of a degenerate or a criminal."[18] Hardman's assessment is unknown, but the case was eventually transferred on appeal to the Supreme Court of Georgia, and Fickling's sentence of execution was affirmed by the Supreme Court the following year.[19]

Except in the case of Eula Mae Thompson, latter-day appeals to phrenology were less than successful, not unlike those attempts to use phrenology in courtrooms a century earlier. The three men condemned to the chair ended their lives there, and Eula Mae's reprieve could be attributed to discomfort with sentencing the first woman to the electric chair in the state of Georgia, rather than to phrenology. It does not seem that any other enterprising defense attorneys in this state attempted a recourse to phrenology after this point, even if Governor Hardman was an open adherent. These events appeared to be the last gasp of phrenology in the medicolegal or criminological realm; phrenology would never again make its way into legal proceedings. Twentieth-century approaches to crime and criminals, in courts and out, had left behind the science. The phrenologists' dream was dead.

The history of science and crime in the twentieth century has focused primarily on developments within forensic science: the ever-enlarging and ever more precise practices of analyzing crime scenes and evidence, including DNA testing, in order to determine perpetrators and the events of a crime.[20] The increasing focus on the "stuff" of crime—trace evidence, fingerprints, DNA leavings, weapons, and the scene of the crime—has drawn attention away from the criminal perpetrator him or herself. The focus on the aftermath, the effect of crime, seems to suggest a turn away from the criminal. Yet the promise of predictive criminology has not fallen entirely by the wayside. The twentieth and twenty-first centuries have seen the increased prominence of offender profiling; for example, the practice of interpreting the criminal act in order to identify personal or psychological traits of the criminal, and thus identify the perpetrator.

Attention has also turned to predictive sciences, with attempts by biologists to identify a "criminal gene"—a return to the hereditary positivism of Lombroso, albeit with a decidedly science-fiction cast. For example, in 2015, a cohort of genetic researchers based in Finland published a study in *Molecular Psychiatry*, entitled "The Genetic Background of Extreme Violent Behavior," which presented findings based on the genetic study of 900 Finnish prisoners. The researchers identified two genetic factors associated with violent behavior: specifically, a monoamine oxidase A low-activity genotype and a CDH13 gene, positing "both low monoamine metabolism and neuronal membrane dysfunction as plausible factors in the etiology of extreme criminal violent behavior," a factor in at least 5 to 10 percent of all violent crime in Finland.[21]

Various media reported on this research when it first became available as an advance article in 2014, including the BBC, the *Los Angeles Times*, and *Bloomberg*, as well as a number of popular science and medical blogs. The coverage of this study was sensational in nature, flattening the detail of its results and extrapolating out to discuss a "criminal gene."[22] While some of the coverage was circumspect—*Bloomberg*'s headline was "Extreme Violent Crimes Tied to Gene in Study of Criminals"[23]—others took the study's conclusions to the extreme: "Are Criminals Born with a MURDER GENE?" asked the British tabloid *Daily Mail Online*.[24] Some essays warned about drawing unnecessary conclusions—"This Isn't Minority Report," claimed *Medical Daily*[25]—while others made more polemical connections, as in an essay in the conservative online magazine *The New Observer*: "Scientists Find that Nazis were Correct about Heredity and Criminality."[26]

This Finnish study was hardly the first to identify a "criminal gene"; similar studies and popular responses to these studies can be identified going back at least the past two decades. This conversation regarding the possibility of a criminal gene has also often been revived when major crimes hit the national and international media circuit, as in the case of the 2012 Newtown shooting, which prompted discussion of searching perpetrator Adam Lanza's genes for explanations.[27] The promise of an explanation for violent crime—even if in only 10 percent of criminal actions, as the Finnish study suggested—is compelling to modern commentators and audiences alike. This fascination with the criminal gene at first glance appears to be a complete repudiation of any sort of phrenological influence in the study of crime. After all, the scientific study of genes—the submicroscopic, molecular building blocks of life—is about the furthest one can get from subjective studies of the shape of a skull or head. Bypassing psychological and sociological studies, genetic study of criminal behavior seems to elude any connection to phrenology and studies of the mind. Instead, genetic research promises a completely objective, measurable, and hence materialistic solution to the problem of criminal prediction.

However, these genetic studies, which might be considered postmodern manifestations of Lombrosan hereditary ideology, have a counterpart in other recent studies of crime, in which one might detect a much more phrenological bent. Researchers in the field of neurology, for example, have been producing in recent years PET (positron emission tomography) and fMRI (functional magnetic resonance imaging) studies of the brains of criminals.[28] The connection between these modern efforts to map the mind and phrenology remains suggestive to observers. As one reporter, writing on the work of self-described neurocriminologist Adrian Raine, has observed, the discipline of neurocriminology "remains tarnished, for some, by association with 19th-century phrenology, the belief that criminal behaviour stemmed from defective brain organisation."[29] Indeed, studies that promise to localize tendencies to certain behaviors, such as violent acts, suggest to observers the same assumptions as phrenology. Even if organs like Destructiveness have been discarded, the identification of areas of the brain with increased metabolic activity in criminal offenders does not seem dissimilar from the articulation of the phrenological organs.

But perhaps the organs themselves have not been entirely forgotten. Studies by psychologists, anthropologists, and sociologists have also suggested intriguing connections between facial shape and characteristics such as trustworthiness, aggression, and selfishness. Social scientists have published a series of articles in recent years exploring the relationship between facial width-to-height ratios (fWHR) and the behavior of businessmen, finding that men with wider faces were more likely to lie, cheat, and engage in other unethical behavior,[30] and that wide faces incite selfish behavior in others, a self-fulfilling prophecy that also elicits selfish behavior in individuals with wider faces.[31] These studies, intended to explain certain factors in business practices and trends, seem to have little import for the science of crime, but related studies on fWHR push these findings into the realm of the criminal, particularly through the focus on aggression. Various studies in the past decade have pointed to the relationship between a high fWHR and high levels of aggression towards others,[32] as well as a gendered cue of potential threat behavior.[33] This recent focus on fWHR has pointed toward a peculiar, though contested,[34] finding: that a high fWHR, which is to say, a broad or wide face and head, suggests to the viewer traits of aggression, lying, cheating, and untrustworthiness, characteristics that are both positively associated with wider heads and the expectation of which produces social pressure to behave in this way, known as facial stereotyping.

The images included in these studies depict wide faces and heads compared to narrow faces and heads, either with pictures of real heads or more cartoonish illustrations, as with one press image that juxtaposed an angry, wide, red face next to a serene, narrow, blue face.[35] Such illustrations and the message they contain—that wide faces signal aggression and are dangerous and untrustworthy, whereas narrow faces are safe and worthy of trust—seem to replicate the image and lesson of small and large Destructiveness common to nineteenth-century phrenology, as seen in figure 2. These recent psychological studies, which similarly suggest an association between wide heads and "bad" behaviors, seem to reproduce phrenological findings of nearly two centuries ago. Either phrenologists were ahead of the curve, or they were responding to the same set of assumptions or intuitions about facial shape that psychological researchers have recently identified. One of these studies of fWHR, moreover, not only replicated familiar phrenological findings and images; it also focused, as the abstract makes clear, on identifying a "propensity for aggression."[36] Knowingly or not, these researchers, through their return to the language of the propensities and the visual language of the criminal mind, are participating in and perpetuating a phrenological framework.[37]

There is also a subtler link between phrenological criminology of the nineteenth century and contemporary discussions about crime and punishment: an underlying desire for prediction motivated by fantasies of futurity, much like the "Dream of Fifty Years Forward." By this, I mean to suggest a generalized embrace of and faith in technological or scientific solutions to human problems. What was a phrenological chart but the promise of one's brain, mind, and potential made manifest and portable, on paper—a record of one's inner self and future potential, for good or ill? Phrenological writings on crime were particularly suggestive of these fantastical futures: phrenologists posited a world in which one's criminal potential could be identified in childhood, redirected, identified before the act, and reformed. This was the promise of perfect prediction before the act, to reform the nation and make a better world for tomorrow: it would not be out of place in a Philip K. Dick novella or a *Black Mirror* episode.

Recent attempts to identify a criminal gene or to use neuroimaging to identify a criminal brain are not so different, at their heart, from phrenological efforts to identify criminal types based on skull shapes. All of these scientific projects are driven by a matrix of anxiety about strangers, about risk and danger, and about the future—about uncertainty in an ever-changing world. These are attempts to use scientific theory and objective, identifiable markers—whether skulls, genes, or brain scans—to alleviate these anxieties through the promise of alternately identifying, disciplining, or reforming the criminal, either before or after the act. Phrenology was discarded in the past for various reasons, not least because of its failure to solve the problems it purported to solve. Yet scientists and an interested public in the present remain transfixed by the possibility of a similar solution—finally identifying a biological, "natural" sign, written on the body or brain or genetic code, that could render the criminal a problem of the unenlightened past. There is a lingering cultural desire to consign the criminal as type, like phrenology itself, to the waste bin of history, for the sake of a better, safer tomorrow.

As I was completing this book, an article from online news magazine *The Outline* popped up on social media, shared with me by friends and colleagues familiar with my work, entitled "People Keep Trying to Bring Back Phrenology." The author, Tom Whyman, was responding to recent news coverage regarding Unilever's plans to use facial recognition technology in job interviews, which prompted widespread commentary in the Twittersphere relating this innovation to phrenology. As Whyman states: "the truth is that phrenology has never really been discredited . . . its *foundational assumptions* did not simply go away. Rather, they were dispersed across other disciplines." Further: "The logic of phrenology works to encode the past into the present—to make old injustices impossible to overcome."[38]

The problem is not that people keep trying to "bring back" phrenology, but that phrenology has never really left us; or, rather, that we have never truly abandoned phrenology. Its lessons, language, assumptions, and images have been thoroughly dispersed throughout and incorporated into American science, medicine, law, culture, and society. Dismissing phrenology as "dead science" only strengthens its cultural valence and its ability to proliferate: choosing to believe that phrenology has been left in the unenlightened past, fully discarded, paradoxically provides a pathway for the spread and re-legitimization of phrenological thinking. Modern-day cultural assumptions and narratives were created within this epistemology, and the strand of phrenological thinking that spreads, morphing into "new"—though still recognizable—forms is not the utopian promise of phrenology as self-improvement, but dystopian claims about "bad heads" and minds requiring reform at any cost, if not wholesale elimination.

Theories of criminal minds and behaviors have been and continue to be a chief area where the lingering effects of phrenological thinking can be glimpsed and that expose the most troubling features of the seductive nature of this epistemology. This book has explored the origins of phrenological theory and the extent to which concerns with criminality directed the shape of the science. I have discussed the centrality of the criminal to early debates about phrenological truth and how criminals as exemplars came to anchor phrenological cabinets, discourse, and representation. I have explored how courtrooms and prisons, and the language used to frame criminality within these spaces, were shaped by phrenological thinking, even as phrenological language and images also directed how the public imagined the dangerous Other in midcentury America. I have also discussed the extent to which phrenological criminology predated and shared assumptions, language, and techniques with more traditionally accepted origin points for criminal science. In so doing, I have aimed not only to demonstrate the ways in which the criminal shaped phrenology, but how phrenology shaped American science, medicine, law, and society in turn through its construction of the criminal mind.

A phrenological impulse infused the work of significant medical and legal figures of early nineteenth-century America and led to the continuing influence of phrenological theory over the course of the nineteenth century. Even if phrenology itself was discarded by elite intellectuals by midcentury, with phrenology becoming increasingly vernacular, its language and images, its assumptions and its promises, continued to inflect the discourse of criminal science and medical jurisprudence throughout the nineteenth century. Though often hidden from view or reframed as something different or "new," this phrenological impulse lives on in American culture, a dark mirror reflecting and shaping ever-evolving phrenological futures.

Acknowledgments

As much as a monograph tends to be a portrait of the historian, it is also a portrait of the broader academic network that produced the scholar. This book would not have been possible without the support, advice, suggestions, and critiques of colleagues, mentors, peers, friends, and others along the way.

This book began as a dissertation project in the Program in the History of Science and Medicine at Yale University, under the direction of John Harley Warner, with Paola Bertucci and Frank Snowden serving on the committee. John was an invaluable resource throughout the dissertation process and long after. He helped me to identify the language of propensity that is a key concept in this text, and he also guided me through the process of revising the dissertation into a book. Frank asked me some of the most crucial questions during the research process, helping me to identify the stakes in this story. Paola's incisive critiques molded this book into something sharper, and her mentorship has been significant for my career. Other members of the Yale faculty were also generous with their time—including Joanna Radin, Bill Rankin, and Henry Cowles. I am also grateful to Naomi Rogers, my advisor during my first years at Yale, who encouraged me to pursue my ever-changing research interests and provided me with more than one push in the right direction. My path started even earlier, at Harvard, and to Anne Harrington I owe a special debt: as an undergraduate, she inspired me first to change my concentration and then to pursue graduate study in the history of science and medicine. At Harvard, Phil Loring advised my senior thesis, guiding me in my first major research project.

At Yale, I was supported by a community of scholars who provided feedback on my work in progress. My peers were key sources of support along this path—particularly Mary Brazelton, Deborah Doroshow, Jenna Healey, Kate Irving, Heidi Knoblauch, Kelly O'Donnell, Joy Lisi Rankin, Rachel Rothschild, Robin Scheffler, Ying Jia Tan, and Marita von Weissenberg. To Jenna and Kelly I owe special thanks: aside from my partner and my peer reviewers, no one has read and provided feedback on as much of the manuscript as the two of them, and I know that my work is better because of their thoughtful critiques.

This research was supported by a number of grants and fellowships, in addition to funding and internal grants from Yale, including the Audrey and William H. Helfand Fellowship in the History of Medicine and Public Health at the New York Academy of Medicine; the James and Sylvia Thayer Short-Term Research Fellowship for UCLA Library Special Collections; the History of Medicine Travel Grant for the David M. Rubenstein Rare Book and Manuscript Library of Duke University; and the Larry J. Hackman Research Residency for the New York State Archives. Funding for early stages of this project was provided from Yale through the Beinecke Rare Book & Manuscript Library, the MacMillan Center, and the Center for Language Study. The revision process was supported by funding from the Department of History at Mississippi State University.

This work similarly could not have been completed without the assistance of archivists and librarians at various institutions, particularly: Nickoal Eichmann-Kalwara, Digital Scholarship Librarian of the University Libraries at the University of Colorado–Boulder, formerly of Mississippi State University; James D. Folts, Head of Researcher Services, New York State Archives; Melissa Grafe, the John R. Bumstead Librarian for Medical History at the Cushing/Whitney Medical Library at Yale University; Dominic Hall, Curator of the Warren Anatomical Museum at Francis A. Countway Library of Medicine; Rachel Ingold, Curator of the History of Medicine Collections at the David M. Rubenstein Rare Book & Manuscript Library at Duke University; Russell Johnson, Curator, History & Special Collections for the Sciences, Louise M. Darling Biomedical Library, UCLA; Scott Podolsky, Director of the Center for the History of Medicine in the Francis A. Countway Library of Medicine; and Arlene Shaner, Historical Collections Librarian, the New York Academy of Medicine.

I have benefited from the generosity of many members of my professional societies, particularly the History of Science Society, the American Association for the History of Medicine, and Cheiron, who provided feedback on this work in progress. I appreciate the kindness of James C. Mohr, who provided thoughtful critiques which shaped the third chapter of this book. I greatly benefited from Carla Bittel's expertise and mentorship; she has read and provided feedback on several chapters and portions of this book over the years. Tabea Cornel provided suggestions on the sixth chapter of this book, helping me to clarify my argument. I appreciate the commentary, feedback, and mentorship provided by many other colleagues over the years, including: Susanna Blumenthal, Thomas Broman, Janet Browne, Ellen Dwyer, Cathy Faye, Mary Fissell, Delia Gavrus, Christopher Green, Andrew Hogan, Rana Hogarth, Sherrie Lyons, Scott Phelps, Sarah Richardson, David K. Robinson, Julia Rodriguez, Laura Stark, Fenneke Sysling, Harry Whitaker, and Debbie Weinstein, among many others. I also appreciate the community of similarly minded scholars who met in summer 2015 in Potsdam, New York, at the "Phrenology, Anthropometry, and Craniology: Historical and Global Perspectives" conference, which I organized with Stephen T. Casper and Julia Rodriguez. The group of scholars at this meeting helped me to find my path toward the final shape of this book.

As I revised this book at Mississippi State, I've benefited from the support and mentorship of many of my colleagues here, especially Arialle Crabtree, Alexandra Finley, Margaret Hagerman, Carolyn Holmes, Alexandra Hui, Andrew Lang, Matthew Lavine, Shane Miller, Davide Orsini, Julia Osman, Judy Ridner, Morgan Robinson, Megan Smith, Tara Sutton, and Eric Vivier. My department head, Alan Marcus, has been very encouraging of this endeavor, and I appreciate his support.

In the development of this book, I am grateful to my editor, Peter Mickulas, whose patience and guidance have been invaluable. I appreciate the thoughtful feedback of my two peer reviewers, Susan Branson and Stephen T. Casper. I met Susan at a Newberry Seminar while I was in early stages of this project, and she provided encouragement then and valuable suggestions as a reviewer. Stephen has been a long-term mentor of mine. In addition to his incisive critiques as a reviewer, his advice and encouragement has profoundly shaped my career.

A version of chapter 3, with some material from chapter 1, appeared as "A Propensity to Murder: Phrenology in Antebellum Medico-Legal Theory and Practice," *Journal of the History of Medicine and Allied Sciences* 74, no. 4 (October 2019): 416–439, DOI: 10.1093/jhmas/jrz055, published by Oxford University Press. I thank the journal and the press for permission to include this material.

I have relied throughout this process on the love and support of friends and family, near and far. My mother, Sharon Sportack Thompson, and her partner, William Huneke, have been sources of unwavering encouragement and optimism.

This book would not have been possible without the support of Scott DiGiulio, my partner, copilot, and most constant editor. This book is dedicated to him.

Notes

Introduction

1. N. Sizer, "Article LXVII: L. N. Fowler's Visit to the Tombs," *American Phrenological Journal* 11, no. 9 (October 1849): 316–317.
2. On phrenology, see Mary A. Armstrong, "Reading a Head: *Jane Eyre*, Phrenology, and the Homoerotics of Legibility," *Victorian Literature and Culture* 33, no. 1 (2005): 107–132; David Bakan, "The Influence of Phrenology on American Psychology," *Journal of the History of the Behavioral Sciences* 2, no. 3 (1966): 200–220; Christopher J. Beshara, "Moral Hospitals, Addled Brains and Cranial Conundrums: Rationalizations of the Criminal Mind in Antebellum America," *Australasian Journal of American Studies* 29, no. 1 (2010): 36–60; Carla Bittel, "Testing the Truth of Phrenology: Knowledge Experiments in Antebellum American Cultures of Science and Health," *Medical History* 63, no. 3 (2019): 352–374; Carla Bittel, "Woman, Know Thyself: Producing and Using Phrenological Knowledge in Nineteenth-Century America," *Centaurus* 55, no. 2 (2013): 104–130; Rhonda Boshears and Harry Whitaker, "Phrenology and Physiognomy in Victorian Literature," in *Literature, Neurology, and Neuroscience: Historical and Literary Connections*, ed. Anne Stiles, Stanley Finger, and François Boller (Amsterdam: Elsevier, 2013), 87–112; Susan Branson, "Phrenology and the Science of Race in Antebellum America," *Early American Studies* 15, no. 1 (2017): 164–193; Jason W. Brown and Karen L. Chobar, "Phrenological Studies of Aphasia before Broca: Broca's Aphasia or Gall's Aphasia?," *Brain and Language* 43, no. 3 (1992): 475–486; G. N. Cantor, "A Critique of Shapin's Social Interpretation of the Edinburgh Phrenology Debate," *Annals of Science* 32, no. 3 (1975): 245–256; G. N. Cantor, "The Edinburgh Phrenology Debate: 1803–1828," *Annals of Science* 32, no. 3 (1975): 195–218; Shalyn Claggett, "Putting Character First: The Narrative Construction of Innate Identity in Phrenological Texts," *VIJ: Victorians Institute Journal* 38 (2010): 103–126; Charles Colbert, *A Measure of Perfection: Phrenology and the Fine Arts in America* (Chapel Hill: University of North Carolina Press, 1997); Roger Cooter, *The Cultural Meaning of Popular Science: Phrenology and the Organization of Consent in Nineteenth-Century Britain* (Cambridge: Cambridge University Press, 1984); Roger Cooter, "Phrenology and British Alienists, c. 1825–1845. Part I: Converts to a Doctrine," *Medical History* 20, no. 1 (1976): 1–21; Roger Cooter, "Phrenology and British Alienists, c. 1825–1845. Part II: Doctrine and Practice," *Medical History* 20, no. 2 (1976): 135–151; Roger Cooter, *Phrenology in the British Isles: An Annotated Historical Biobibliography and Index* (Metuchen, NJ: Scarecrow Press, 1989); R. J. Cooter, "Phrenology: The Provocation of Progress," *History of Science* 14, no. 4 (1976): 211–234; Tabea Cornel, "Something Old, Something New, Something Pseudo, Something True: Pejorative and Deferential References to Phrenology since 1840," *Proceedings of the American Philosophical Society* 161, no. 4 (2017): 299–332; Macdonald Critchley, "Neurology's Debt to F. J. Gall (1758–1828)," *British Medical Journal* 2, no. 5465 (1965): 775–781; Nicholas Dames, "The Clinical Novel: Phrenology and *Villette*," *NOVEL: A Forum on Fiction* 29, no. 3 (1996): 367–390; John D. Davies, *Phrenology: Fad and Science; A 19th-Century American Crusade* (Hamden, CT: Archon Books,

1971 [1955]); David de Giustino, *Conquest of Mind: Phrenology and Victorian Social Thought* (London: Routledge, 2016 [1975]); Paul Eling and Stanley Finger, eds., "Gall and Phrenology: New Perspectives," special issue, *Journal of the History of the Neurosciences* 29, no. 1 (2020); Stanley Finger and Paul Eling, *Franz Joseph Gall: Naturalist of the Mind, Visionary of the Brain* (New York: New York University Press, 2019); Samuel H. Greenblatt, "Phrenology in the Science and Culture of the 19th Century," *Neurosurgery* 37, no. 4 (1995): 790–805; Jason Y. Hall, "Gall's Phrenology: A Romantic Psychology," *Studies in Romanticism* 16, no. 3 (1977): 305–317; Cynthia S. Hamilton, "'Am I Not a Man and a Brother?' Phrenology and Anti-slavery," *Slavery and Abolition* 29, no. 2 (2008): 173–187; Victor L. Hilts, "Obeying the Laws of Hereditary Descent: Phrenological Views on Inheritance and Eugenics," *Journal of the History of the Behavioral Sciences* 18, no. 1 (1982): 62–77; Edward Hungerford, "Poe and Phrenology," *American Literature* 2, no. 3 (1930): 209–231; Bill Jenkins, "Phrenology, Heredity and Progress in George Combe's *Constitution of Man*," *British Journal for the History of Science* 48, no. 3 (2015): 455–473; Enda Leaney, "Phrenology in Nineteenth-Century Ireland," *New Hibernia Review* 10, no. 3 (2006): 24–42; Sherrie Lynne Lyons, *Species, Serpents, Spirits, and Skulls: Science at the Margins in the Victorian Age* (Albany: State University of New York Press, 2009); Angus McLaren, "Phrenology: Medium and Message," *Journal of Modern History* 46, no. 1 (1974): 86–97; Angus McLaren, "A Prehistory of the Social Sciences: Phrenology in France," *Comparative Studies in Society and History* 23, no. 1 (1981): 3–22; Patricia S. Noel and Eric T. Carlson, "Origins of the Word 'Phrenology,'" *American Journal of Psychiatry* 127, no. 5 (1970): 694–697; T. M. Parssinen, "Popular Science and Society: The Phrenology Movement in Early Victorian Britain," *Journal of Social History* 8, no. 1 (1974): 1–20; James Poskett, *Materials of the Mind: Phrenology, Race, and the Global History of Science, 1815–1920* (Chicago: University of Chicago Press, 2019); James Poskett, "Phrenology, Correspondence, and the Global Politics of Reform, 1815–1848," *The Historical Journal* 60, no. 2 (2017): 409–442; Marc Renneville, *Le langage des crânes: Une histoire de la phrénologie* (Paris: Institut d'Édition, Sanofi-Synthélabo, 2000); Robert E. Riegel, "The Introduction of Phrenology to the United States," *American Historical Review* 39, no. 1 (1933): 73–78; Cynthia Eagle Russett, "How to Tell the Girls from the Boys," in *Sexual Science: The Victorian Construction of Womanhood* (Cambridge, MA: Harvard University Press, 1989), 16–48; Steven Shapin, "Phrenological Knowledge and the Social Structure of Early Nineteenth-Century Edinburgh," *Annals of Science* 32, no. 3 (1975): 219–243; Steven Shapin, "The Politics of Observation: Cerebral Anatomy and Social Interests in the Edinburgh Phrenology Disputes," special issue, *Sociological Review* 27 (May 1979): 139–178; Sally Shuttleworth, "Reading the Mind: Physiognomy and Phrenology," in *Charlotte Brontë and Victorian Psychology* (Cambridge: Cambridge University Press, 1996), 57–70; Donald Simpson, "Phrenology and the Neurosciences: Contributions of F. J. Gall and J. G. Spurzheim," *ANZ Journal of Surgery* 75, no. 6 (2005): 475–482; Michael M. Sokal, "Practical Phrenology as Psychological Counseling in the 19th-Century United States," in *The Transformation of Psychology: Influences of 19th-Century Philosophy, Technology, and Natural Science*, ed. Christopher D. Green, Marlene Shore, and Thomas Teo (Washington, DC: American Psychological Association, 2001), 21–44; David Stack, *Queen Victoria's Skull: George Combe and the Mid-Victorian Mind* (London: Hambledon Continuum, 2008); Martin Staum, "Physiognomy and Phrenology at the Paris Athénée," *Journal of the History of Ideas* 56, no. 3 (1995): 443–462; Madeleine B.

Stern, "Emerson and Phrenology," *Studies in the American Renaissance* (1984): 213–228; Madeleine B. Stern, *Heads & Headlines: The Phrenological Fowlers* (Norman: University of Oklahoma Press, 1971); Madeleine B. Stern, "Mark Twain Had His Head Examined," *American Literature* 41, no. 2 (1969): 207–218; Madeleine B. Stern, "Poe: 'The Mental Temperament' for Phrenologists," *American Literature* 40, no. 2 (1968): 155–163; Fenneke Sysling, "Science and Self-Assessment: Phrenological Charts 1840–1940," *British Journal for the History of Science* 51, no. 2 (2018): 261–280; Owsei Temkin, "Gall and the Phrenological Movement," *Bulletin of the History of Medicine* 21, no. 3 (1947): 275–321; Daniel Patrick Thurs, "Phrenology: A Science for Everyone," in *Science Talk: Changing Notions of Science in American Popular Culture* (New Brunswick, NJ: Rutgers University Press, 2007), 22–52; Stephen Tomlinson, *Head Masters: Phrenology, Secular Education, and Nineteenth-Century Social Thought* (Tuscaloosa: University of Alabama Press, 2005); Richard Twine, "Physiognomy, Phrenology and the Temporality of the Body," *Body & Society* 8, no. 1 (2002): 67–88; Pieter Verstraete, "The Taming of Disability: Phrenology and Bio-power on the Road to the Destruction of Otherness in France (1800–60)," *Journal of the History of Education Society* 34, no. 2 (2005): 119–134; Anthony A. Walsh, "The American Tour of Dr. Spurzheim," *Journal of the History of Medicine and Allied Sciences* 27, no. 2 (1972): 187–205; Anthony A. Walsh, "Phrenology and the Boston Medical Community in the 1830s," *Bulletin of the History of Medicine* 50, no. 2 (1976): 261–273; Kenneth J. Weiss, "Isaac Ray's Affair with Phrenology," *Journal of Psychiatry & Law* 34, no. 4 (2006): 455–459; Kenneth J. Weiss, "Isaac Ray at 200: Phrenology and Expert Testimony," *Journal of the American Academy of Psychiatry and Law* 35, no. 3 (2007): 339–345; Christopher G. White, "Minds Intensely Unsettled: Phrenology, Experience, and the American Pursuit of Spiritual Assurance, 1830–1880," *Religion and American Culture* 16, no. 2 (2006): 227–261; John B. Wilson, "Phrenology and the Transcendentalists," *American Literature* 28, no. 2 (1956): 220–225; John van Wyhe, "The Authority of Human Nature: The *Schädellehre* of Franz Joseph Gall," *British Journal for the History of Science* 35, no. 1 (2002): 17–42; John van Wyhe, *Phrenology and the Origins of Victorian Scientific Naturalism* (Aldershot, UK: Ashgate, 2004); John van Wyhe, "Was Phrenology a Reform Science? Towards a New Generalization for Phrenology," *History of Science* 42, no. 3 (2004): 313–331; Arthur Wrobel, "Orthodoxy and Respectability in Nineteenth-Century Phrenology," *Journal of Popular Culture* 9, no. 1 (1975): 38–50; Robert M. Young, "Gall and Phrenology: Speculation *versus* Observation *versus* Experiment," in *Mind, Brain, and Adaptation in the Nineteenth Century: Cerebral Localization and Its Biological Context from Gall to Ferrier* (New York: Oxford University Press, 1990 [1970]), 9–53; S. Zola-Morgan, "Localization of Brain Function: The Legacy of Franz Joseph Gall (1758–1828)," *Annual Review of Neuroscience* 18, no. 1 (1995): 359–383.

3. Riegel, "The Introduction of Phrenology to the United States," 73.
4. Phrenology operated alongside other approaches to visual judgment on the basis of appearance in the nineteenth century, especially physiognomy. See Karen Halttunen, *Confidence Men and Painted Women: A Study of Middle-Class Culture in America, 1830–1870* (New Haven, CT: Yale University Press, 1982); Lucy Hartley, *Physiognomy and the Meaning of Expression in Nineteenth-Century Culture* (Cambridge: Cambridge University Press, 2001); Christopher J. Lukasik, *Discerning Characters: The Culture of Appearance in Early America* (Philadelphia: University of Pennsylvania Press, 2011); Sharrona Pearl, *About Faces: Physiognomy in*

Nineteenth-Century Britain (Cambridge, MA: Harvard University Press, 2010); Melissa Percival, *The Appearance of Character: Physiognomy and Facial Expression in Eighteenth-Century France* (London: W. S. Maney & Son, 1999); Ellis Shookman, ed., *The Faces of Physiognomy: Interdisciplinary Approaches to Johann Caspar Lavater* (Columbia, SC: Camden House, 1993).

5. Walsh referred to this cohort as "scientific phrenologists" and notes that there was a broader group of educated men, particularly in Boston, who studied phrenology as a leisure activity. Walsh, "Phrenology and the Boston Medical Community," 271, 273.
6. On phrenology and crime or criminology, see Michael Dow Burkhead, *The Search for the Causes of Crime: A History of Theory in Criminology* (Jefferson, NC: McFarland & Company, 2006), 67–72; Beshara, "Moral Hospitals, Addled Brains and Cranial Conundrums"; Finger and Eling, *Franz Joseph Gall*, 382–390; Arthur E. Fink, *Causes of Crime: Biological Theories in the United States, 1800–1915* (Philadelphia: University of Pennsylvania Press, 1938), 1–19; Nicole Hahn Rafter, "The Murderous Dutch Fiddler: Criminology, History, and the Problem of Phrenology," *Theoretical Criminology* 9, no. 1 (2005): 65–96; Stern also discusses the Fowler brothers' attention to penal reform in her work, and Davies includes a chapter on penology in his (Stern, *Heads & Headlines*, 39–41; Davies, "Phrenology and Penology," in *Phrenology*, 98–105).
7. On medical jurisprudence, see John Starrett Hughes, *In the Law's Darkness: Isaac Ray and the Medical Jurisprudence of Insanity in Nineteenth-Century America* (New York: Oceana Publications, 1986); R. Gregory Lande, *Abraham Man: Madness, Malingering and the Development of Medical Testimony* (New York: Algora Publishing, 2012); James C. Mohr, *Doctors and the Law: Medical Jurisprudence in Nineteenth-Century America* (Baltimore, MD: Johns Hopkins University Press, 1996 [1993]); Daniel N. Robinson, *Wild Beasts & Idle Humours: The Insanity Defense from Antiquity to the Present* (Cambridge, MA: Harvard University Press, 1996); Charles E. Rosenberg, *The Trial of the Assassin Guiteau: Psychiatry and the Law in the Gilded Age* (Chicago: University of Chicago Press, 1976 [1968]).
8. For example, David A. Jones's *History of Criminology* devotes a mere two pages to phrenology in a book of more than two hundred pages and focuses exclusively on the work of Gall and Spurzheim and the European context. David A. Jones, *History of Criminology: A Philosophical Perspective* (Westport, CT: Greenwood Press, 1986), 136–137. Arthur Fink and Nicole Hahn Rafter have more to say about the role of phrenology in the history of criminology. See Fink, *Causes of Crime*, 1–19; Rafter, *Creating Born Criminals* (Urbana: University of Illinois Press, 1997), 75–79, 94; Nicole Rafter, "Phrenology: The Abnormal Brain," in *The Criminal Brain: Understanding Biological Theories of Crime* (New York: New York University Press, 2008), 40–64; Rafter, "The Murderous Dutch Fiddler."
9. On the history of criminology, see Piers Beirne, *Inventing Criminology: Essays on the Rise of* Homo Criminalis (Albany: State University of New York Press, 1993); Burkhead, *The Search for the Causes of Crime*; Simon A. Cole, *Suspect Identities: A History of Fingerprinting and Criminal Identification* (Cambridge, MA: Harvard University Press, 2001); Fink, *Causes of Crime*; Jonathan Finn, *Capturing the Criminal Image: From Mug Shot to Surveillance Society* (Minneapolis: University of Minnesota Press, 2009); Mary Gibson, *Born to Crime: Cesare Lombroso and the Origins of Biological Criminology* (Westport, CT: Praeger, 2002); David G. Horn, *The Criminal Body: Lombroso and the Anatomy of Deviance* (New York: Routledge, 2003); Jones, *History of Criminology*; Rafter, *Creating Born Criminals*; Ysabel Rennie, *The Search*

for Criminal Man: A Conceptual History of the Dangerous Offender (Lexington, MA: Lexington Books, 1978).

1. Origins and Organs

1. R. T. Webb, *The Phrenologist; A Farce, in Two Acts: Containing a Popular Summary of that Pseudo, or Real Science* (London: Printed for the author, by C. Slater, 1824), 8.
2. Webb, *The Phrenologist*, 21.
3. Webb, *The Phrenologist*, 25.
4. Webb, *The Phrenologist*, 26.
5. Webb, *The Phrenologist*, 30.
6. Webb, *The Phrenologist*, 30.
7. John van Wyhe, "The Authority of Human Nature: The *Schädellehre* of Franz Joseph Gall," *British Journal for the History of Science* 35, no. 1 (2002): 22. Gall's middle name has been alternately been given as Joseph or Josef; I use the former, following scholars including van Wyhe, as well as others like Stanley Finger and Paul Eling. Stanley Finger and Paul Eling, *Franz Joseph Gall: Naturalist of the Mind, Visionary of the Brain* (New York: New York University Press, 2019).
8. van Wyhe, "The Authority of Human Nature," 18. On Gall and his theories, see also Jason W. Brown and Karen L. Chobar, "Phrenological Studies of Aphasia before Broca: Broca's Aphasia or Gall's Aphasia?," *Brain and Language* 43, no. 3 (1992): 475–486; Macdonald Critchley, "Neurology's Debt to F. J. Gall (1758–1828)," *British Medical Journal* 2, no. 5465 (1965): 775–781; Finger and Eling, *Franz Joseph Gall*; Jason Y. Hall, "Gall's Phrenology: A Romantic Psychology," *Studies in Romanticism* 16, no. 3 (1977): 305–317; Donald Simpson, "Phrenology and the Neurosciences: Contributions of F. J. Gall and J. G. Spurzheim," *ANZ Journal of Surgery* 75, no. 6 (2005): 475–482; Owsei Temkin, "Gall and the Phrenological Movement," *Bulletin of the History of Medicine* 21, no. 3 (1947): 275–321; Robert M. Young, "Gall and Phrenology: Speculation *versus* Observation *versus* Experiment," in *Mind, Brain, and Adaptation in the Nineteenth Century: Cerebral Localization and Its Biological Context from Gall to Ferrier* (New York: Oxford University Press, 1990 [1970]), 9–53; S. Zola-Morgan, "Localization of Brain Function: The Legacy of Franz Joseph Gall (1758–1828)," *Annual Review of Neuroscience* 18, no. 1 (1995): 359–383.
9. van Wyhe, "The Authority of Human Nature," 18–19.
10. van Wyhe, "The Authority of Human Nature," 19–21.
11. van Wyhe, "The Authority of Human Nature," 25–26; John D. Davies, *Phrenology: Fad and Science; A 19th-Century American Crusade* (Hamden, CT: Archon Books, 1971 [1955]), 7; Roger Cooter, *The Cultural Meaning of Popular Science: Phrenology and the Organization of Consent in Nineteenth-Century Britain* (Cambridge: Cambridge University Press, 1984), 39–40.
12. van Wyhe, "The Authority of Human Nature," 26–29. On this tour, see Finger and Eling, *Franz Joseph Gall*, 224–273; John van Wyhe, *Phrenology and the Origins of Victorian Scientific Naturalism* (Aldershot, UK: Ashgate, 2004), 209–211.
13. Franz Joseph Gall and [Johann] G. Spurzheim, *Anatomie et physiologie du système nerveux en général, et du cerveau en particulier, avec des observations sur la possibilité de reconnoître plusieurs dispositions intellectuelles et morales de l'homme et des animaux, par la configuration de leurs têtes*, vol. 1 (Paris: F. Schoell, 1810).
14. Franz Joseph Gall, *Sur les fonctions du cerveau et sur celles de chacune de ses parties, avec des observations sur la possibilité de reconnaitre les instincts, les penchans, les talens, ou les dispositions morales et intellectuelles des hommes et*

des animaux, par la configuration de leur cerveau et de leur tête, 6 vols. (Paris: J.-B. Ballière, 1825).

15. van Wyhe, "The Authority of Human Nature," 26–27, 30.
16. Cooter, *The Cultural Meaning of Popular Science*, 3; John van Wyhe, "Was Phrenology a Reform Science? Towards a New Generalization for Phrenology," *History of Science* 42, no. 3 (2004): 314.
17. Cooter, *The Cultural Meaning of Popular Science*, 3.
18. Cooter, *The Cultural Meaning of Popular Science*, 3–4. Gall's works exclusively addressed manual examinations; instruments, like the calipers, were introduced and promoted by later phrenologists, particularly George Combe. François Joseph Gall, *On the Functions of the Brain and of Each of Its Parts*, vol. 3, trans. Winslow Lewis Jr. (Boston: Marsh, Capen & Lyon, 1835), 139–140; Lucile E. Hoyme, "Physical Anthropology and Its Instruments: An Historical Study," *Southwestern Journal of Anthropology* 9, no. 4 (1953): 413–414.
19. Cooter, *The Cultural Meaning of Popular Science*, 3–4.
20. Cooter, *The Cultural Meaning of Popular Science*, 4.
21. According to Gall, reports of this trip were originally published in May 1805 in *Freymüthige*, and also in Demangeon's 1806 *Physiologie Intellectuelle*, with later accounts appearing in other periodicals. François Joseph Gall, *On the Functions of the Brain and Each of Its Parts*, vol. 6, trans. Winslow Lewis Jr. (Boston: Marsh, Capen & Lyon, 1835), 295; "Article I [Review of works of Gall and Spurzheim]," *Foreign Quarterly Review* 2, no. 3 (London: C. Roworth, 1828): 14–15; "Article XIII: Dr. Gall's Visit to the Prisons of Berlin and Spandau," *The Phrenological Journal and Miscellany* 3, no. 10 (Edinburgh, 1826): 297–306; "Phrenology. Visit of Dr. Gall to the prison at Berlin, and Fortress of Spandau, with his phrenological observations on the prisoners," *Atkinson's Casket or Gems of Literature, Wit and Sentiment* no. 5 (May 1835): 287.
22. "Article XIII: Dr. Gall's Visit to the Prisons of Berlin and Spandau," 305.
23. "For the Emerald: Some account of Doctor Gall's system of Craniology, condensed from the Monthly Magazine," *The Emerald, or Miscellany of Literature* 1, no. 8 (June 1806): 89.
24. "For the Emerald," 90–91.
25. [Gall; craniology], *Middlebury Mercury* (Middlebury, VT), February 4, 1807.
26. "Craniology," *Commercial Advertiser* (New York), February 2, 1806.
27. "Phrenology. Visit of Dr. Gall to the prison at Berlin," 287.
28. Thomas Sewall, *An Examination of Phrenology; in Two Lectures* (London: James S. Hodson, 1838), 4.
29. van Wyhe notes that the minister of police in Vienna, Earl Saurau, helped Gall acquire criminal skulls. van Wyhe, "The Authority of Human Nature," 22.
30. Gall, *Sur les fonctions du cerveau*, 1:350, 393–400, 428, 430, 455.
31. Johann Gaspar Spurzheim to Honorine (Perier) Pothier Spurzheim, October 21, 1815, Box 1, Folder 4, Papers of Johann Gaspar Spurzheim, 1813–1835, B Ms c22, Harvard Medical Library, Francis A. Countway Library of Medicine, Boston, MA (hereafter cited as Spurzheim Letters); Johann Gaspar Spurzheim to Honorine (Perier) Pothier Spurzheim, April 17, 1816, Box 1, Folder 6, Spurzheim Letters.
32. J. L. Levison, "Dr. Spurzheim's Visit to Hull," *The Phrenological Journal and Miscellany* 5, no. 17 (1829): 82–87, at 85–86. See also "Phrenology. Visit of Dr. Gall to the prison at Berlin," 287–288.
33. The term "phrenology" was coined by American physician Benjamin Rush, though not originally intended to indicate this field of study. On the origin of "phrenology,"

see Anthony A. Walsh, "Phrenology and the Boston Medical Community in the 1830s," *Bulletin of the History of Medicine* 50, no. 2 (1976): 261; Patricia S. Noel and Eric T. Carlson, "Origins of the Word 'Phrenology,'" *American Journal of Psychiatry* 127, no. 5 (1970): 694–697. For a detailed account of precursor sciences of the self or soul, see Fernando Vidal, *The Sciences of the Soul: The Early Modern Sciences of Psychology*, trans. Saskia Brown (Chicago: University of Chicago Press, 2011).

34. Spurzheim's original English text, for example, was entitled *The Physiognomical System of Drs. Gall and Spurzheim*. J. G. Spurzheim, *The Physiognomical System of Drs. Gall and Spurzheim* (London: Baldwin, Cradock, and Joy, 1815); Sharrona Pearl, *About Faces: Physiognomy in Nineteenth-Century Britain* (Cambridge, MA: Harvard University Press, 2010), 186, 189–191.
35. Cooter, *The Cultural Meaning of Popular Science*, 4; Christopher J. Lukasik, *Discerning Characters: The Culture of Appearance in Early America* (Philadelphia: University of Pennsylvania Press, 2011), 27–29.
36. See for example: Marin Cureau de La Chambre, *L'art de connoistre les hommes* (Paris: Chez Iacques d'Allin, 1667); *The True Fortune-Teller, or, Guide to Knowledge: Discovering the Whole Art of Chiromancy, Physiognomy, Metoposcopy, and Astrology* (London: E. Tracy, 1698).
37. Ellis Shookman, "Pseudo-Science, Social Fad, Literary Wonder: Johann Caspar Lavater and the Art of Physiognomy," in *The Faces of Physiognomy: Interdisciplinary Approaches to Johann Caspar Lavater*, ed. Ellis Shookman (Columbia, SC: Camden House, 1993), 2–4.
38. Shookman, "Pseudo-Science, Social Fad, Literary Wonder," 4–7. Cooter notes that Lavater was also a student of medicine who incorporated attention to the skull to his system of physiognomy. Cooter, *The Cultural Meaning of Popular Science*, 4–5.
39. Cooter, *The Cultural Meaning of Popular Science*, 40.
40. Davies, *Phrenology*, 8–9; Victor L. Hilts, "Obeying the Laws of Hereditary Descent: Phrenological Views on Inheritance and Eugenics," *Journal of the History of the Behavioral Sciences* 18, no. 1 (1982): 63.
41. Davies, *Phrenology*, 8–9; Hilts, "Obeying the Laws of Hereditary Descent," 63–65; Stephen Tomlinson, *Head Masters: Phrenology, Secular Education, and Nineteenth-Century Social Thought* (Tuscaloosa: University of Alabama Press, 2005), 62–63.
42. Davies, *Phrenology*, 8–9.
43. van Wyhe, "Was Phrenology a Reform Science?," 322.
44. Johann Gaspar Spurzheim to Honorine (Perier) Pothier Spurzheim, October 21, 1815, Box 1, Folder 4, Spurzheim Letters; Johann Gaspar Spurzheim to Honorine (Perier) Pothier Spurzheim, April 17, 1816, Box 1, Folder 6, Spurzheim Letters.
45. Cooter, *The Cultural Meaning of Popular Science*, 7.
46. Davies, *Phrenology*, 9–10. While Cantor dates the beginning of the Edinburgh phrenology debate to 1803, he suggests that it did not take off in earnest until the 1815 review of Spurzheim's text by John Gordon in the *Edinburgh Review*. G. N. Cantor, "The Edinburgh Phrenology Debate: 1803–1828," *Annals of Science* 32, no. 3 (1975): 199; Cooter, *The Cultural Meaning of Popular Science*, 24–28. On the various controversies surrounding the introduction to phrenology, see G. N. Cantor, "A Critique of Shapin's Social Interpretation of the Edinburgh Phrenology Debate," *Annals of Science* 32, no. 3 (1975): 245–256; Cantor, "The Edinburgh Phrenology Debate"; Steven Shapin, "Phrenological Knowledge and the Social Structure of Early Nineteenth-Century Edinburgh," *Annals of Science* 32, no. 3 (1975): 219–243; Steven Shapin, "The Politics of Observation: Cerebral Anatomy and Social Interests

in the Edinburgh Phrenology Disputes," special issue, *Sociological Review* 27 (May 1979): 139–178.

47. On George Combe, see Cooter, *The Cultural Meaning of Popular Science*, 101–133.
48. While the society was preeminent among phrenological societies, it was nevertheless an "outsider' group" relative to other Edinburgh cultural institutions. Shapin, "Phrenological Knowledge and the Social Structure of Early Nineteenth-Century Edinburgh," 228.
49. Cooter, *The Cultural Meaning of Popular Science*, 88–89.
50. Poskett notes that *The Constitution of Man* outsold Charles Darwin's *Origin of Species* by 1900. James Poskett, *Materials of the Mind: Phrenology, Race, and the Global History of Science, 1815–1920* (Chicago: University of Chicago Press, 2019), 2; David Stack, *Queen Victoria's Skull: George Combe and the Mid-Victorian Mind* (London: Hambledon Continuum, 2008), 80. On the development of *The Constitution of Man*, its contents, and its reception, see van Wyhe, *Phrenology and the Origins of Victorian Scientific Naturalism*, 96–164.
51. Stack, *Queen Victoria's Skull*, 80–81.
52. Stack, *Queen Victoria's Skull*, 83.
53. Sherrie Lynne Lyons, *Species, Serpents, Spirits, and Skulls: Science at the Margins in the Victorian Age* (Albany: State University of New York Press, 2009), 78–80.
54. George Combe, *The Constitution of Man Considered in Relation to External Objects*, 3rd ed. (Edinburgh: John Anderson Jr., 1835), 260.
55. Combe, *The Constitution of Man*, 3rd ed., 261; emphasis in the original.
56. Combe, *The Constitution of Man*, 3rd ed., 262.
57. Combe, *The Constitution of Man*, 3rd ed., 262.
58. Combe, *The Constitution of Man*, 3rd ed., 268.
59. George Combe, *Remarks on the Principles of Criminal Legislation and the Practice of Prison Discipline* (London: Simpkin, Marshall & Co., 1854). This pamphlet was an expansion of an earlier article published in the *Westminster Review* the previous year: [George Combe,] "Art. IV—Criminal Legislation and Prison Discipline," *Westminster Review* 5 (April 1854): 409–445. This essay was reprinted in the *American Phrenological Journal* in ten installments through 1855, beginning with: George Combe, "Criminal Legislation and Prison Discipline. Chapter 1," *American Phrenological Journal* 21, no. 2 (February 1855): 31–32. See also George Combe, "Criminal Legislation and Prison Discipline," *The Prisoner's Friend, A Monthly Magazine* 8, no. 8 (April 1856): 211–212.
60. These excerpts were drawn from Combe's *Lectures on Moral Philosophy*. "Art. V—Of the Causes of Pauperism and Criminal Legislation," *American Jurist* 24, no. 47 (October 1840): 79–115; "Art. IV—Of the Duty of Society in Regard to Criminal Legislation and Prison Discipline," *American Jurist* 24, no. 48 (January 1841): 306–328.
61. George Combe, "Criminal Legislation and Prison Discipline," *American Phrenological Journal* 21, no. 3 (March 1855): 58.
62. Reform within phrenological discourse, and the debate on same within the historiography, will be further discussed in chapter 5. See Poskett, *Materials of the Mind*, 116–117; James Poskett, "Phrenology, Correspondence, and the Global Politics of Reform, 1815–1848," *The Historical Journal* 60, no. 2 (2017): 413–414; van Wyhe, "Was Phrenology a Reform Science?"

63. Andrew Combe, *Observations on Mental Derangement* (Edinburgh: John Anderson Jr., 1831).
64. Cooter, *The Cultural Meaning of Popular Science*, 109.
65. Robert Buchanan, "Report on the Development of James Gordon, executed at Dumfries, 6th June 1821, for the murder of John Elliot, a Pedlar Boy," *Transactions of the Phrenological Society* (Edinburgh: John Anderson Jr., 1824): 327–339; G. Combe, "Observations on the Cerebral Development, and Dispositions and Talents, of Mary Macinnes," *Transactions of the Phrenological Society* (Edinburgh: John Anderson Jr., 1824): 362–379; George Combe, "Observations on Evidence in favour of Phrenology, afforded by Reports on the Cerebral Development of Executed Criminals, as indicated by their Skulls," *Transactions of the Phrenological Society* (Edinburgh: John Anderson Jr., 1824): 319–326; Sir George Stewart Mackenzie, "Remarks on the Case of John Bellingham, the Assassin of Mr Perceval," *Transactions of the Phrenological Society* (Edinburgh: John Anderson Jr., 1824): 339–362.
66. For example: "Article XI: Result of an Examination, by Mr James de Ville, of the Heads of 148 Convicts on Board the Convict Ship England, when about to sail for New South Wales in the Spring of 1826," *The Phrenological Journal and Miscellany* 4, no. 15 (1827): 467–471; "Article I. Practical Application of the Phrenological Principles of Criminal Legislation to the Penitentiary System," *The Phrenological Journal and Miscellany* 8, no. 39 (1834): 481–507.
67. Combe's *Essays on Phrenology*, published in 1819, identified the same thirty-three organs as Spurzheim, but in later works, such as *A System of Phrenology*, he expanded this number to thirty-five. See Karl August Blöde, *Dr. F. J. Galls Lehre über die Verrichtungen des Gehirns, nach dessen zu Dresden gehaltenen Vorlesungen in einer fasslichen Ordnung mit gewissenhafter Treue dargestellt* (Dresden: Arnoldischen Buchhandlung, 1805), 101; George Combe, *Essays on Phrenology* (Edinburgh: Bell & Bradfute, 1819), vi; George Combe, *A System of Phrenology*, 3rd ed. (Edinburgh: John Anderson Jr., 1825), xiii; Spurzheim, *The Physiognomical System of Drs. Gall and Spurzheim*, xvi; van Wyhe, *Phrenology and the Origins of Victorian Scientific Naturalism*, 213–215.
68. Nicole Rafter, *The Criminal Brain: Understanding Biological Theories of Crime* (New York: New York University Press, 2008), 49–50.
69. Blöde, *Dr. F. J. Galls Lehre über die Verrichtungen des Gehirns*, 80–81; van Wyhe, *Phrenology and the Origins of Victorian Scientific Naturalism*, 213.
70. H. G. C. von Selpert, *D. Gall's Vorlesungen über die Verrichtungen des Gehirns und die Möglichkeit die Anlagen mehrerer Geistes und Gemüthseigenschaften aus dem Baue des Schädels der Menchen und Thiere zu erkennen* (Berlin: Johann Friedrich Unger, 1805), 92–96; van Wyhe, *Phrenology and the Origins of Victorian Scientific Naturalism*, 213.
71. F. J. Gall, *Vollständige Geisteskunde, oder, Auf Erfahrung gestüzte Darstellung der geistigen und moralischen Fähigkeiten und ihrer Körperlichen Bedingungen* (Nuremberg: Leuchs, 1829), 225–226. Young notes that Gall's exploration of this organ is particularly robust in his writings. Young, *Mind, Brain, and Adaptation in the Nineteenth Century*, 39.
72. Gall, *Vollständige Geisteskunde*, 226–227; C. W. Hufeland, *Some Account of Dr. Gall's New Theory of Physiognomy, Founded upon the Anatomy and Physiology of the Brain, and the Form of the Skull* (London: Longman, Hurst, Rees, and Orme, 1807), 79, 94–98. Though discussing a "penchant au meurtre," in his French texts,

Gall indicated a preference for the name of "l'instinct carnassier" or "l'organe carnassier," as the "instinct du meurtre" was too easily confused with homicide; he further asserted that Spurzheim's "destructivité" was too broad and general. Other French works distinguished between Gall and Spurzheim's systems, including the distinction between Gall's "Instinct carnassier, penchant au meurtre" and Spurzheim's "Destructivité." F. J. Gall, *Anatomie et physiologie du système nerveux en general et du cerveau en particulier*, vol. 3 (Paris, 1818), 246–249; Alexandre David, *Le petit Docteur Gall ou l'art de connaître les hommes par la phrénologie d'après les systèmes de Gall et de Spurzheim* (Paris: Passard, 1859), 22–23.

73. Blöde, *Dr. F. J. Gall's Lehre über die Verrichtungen des Gehirns*, 83–87; van Wyhe, *Phrenology and the Origins of Victorian Scientific Naturalism*, 213; von Selpert, *D. Gall's Vorlesungen über die Verrichtungen des Gehirns*, 97–102.
74. Gall, *Vollständige Geisteskunde*, 238.
75. William Scott, "II. On the Functions of Combativeness, Destructiveness, and Secretiveness—with Illustrations of the effects of different degrees of their endowment on the Characters of Individuals," *Transactions of the Phrenological Society* (Edinburgh: John Anderson Jr., 1824): 134.
76. George Combe, *Notes on the United States of North America, During a Phrenological Visit in 1838–9–40*, vol. 1 (Philadelphia: Carey & Hart, 1841), 135–136.
77. "Rush's Phrenological Development," *American Phrenological Journal* 11, no. 9 (September 1849): 279.
78. "Johnston the Murderer," *American Phrenological Journal* 12, no. 6 (June 1850): 196; "The Lampley Murderers. Hollohan Phrenologically Considered," *The Sun* (Baltimore, MD), June 9, 1873; "The Phrenological Development of the Murderer Wilson," *Leicester Chronicle* (Leicester, UK), September 29, 1849; "Phrenological Characteristics of Ward the Murderer," *Liverpool Mercury* (Liverpool, UK), September 18, 1862; "Phrenological Characteristics of Kohl the Murderer," *Liverpool Mercury* (Liverpool, UK), February 3, 1865; Jno. F. Graff, "Arthur Spring. A Phrenological Sketch," *American Phrenological Journal* 17, no. 6 (June 1853): 126; "John Reed. The Murderer and Suicide. Phrenological Character," *American Phrenological Journal* 28, no. 1 (July 1858): 3; "The Murderer's Phrenological Developments," *The Cheshire Observer and General Advertiser* (Chester, UK), December 27, 1856.
79. Numbering practices varied in phrenological texts. While phrenologists did sometimes include numbers based on measurements by calipers or tape measures of spans of the skull from organ to organ, the numbers assigned to phrenological organs were based on subjective assessment. "Article II. Phrenological developments and character of Peter Robinson, who was executed April 16th, at New Brunswick, N.J., for the murder of A. Suydam, Esq.," *The American Phrenological Journal and Miscellany* 3, no. 10 (July 1841): 453; "Article II. Phrenological Developments and Character of James Eager, Executed for the Murder of Philip Williams, May 9, 1845," *The American Phrenological Journal and Miscellany* 7, no. 8 (August 1845): 264.
80. Fenneke Sysling, "Science and Self-Assessment: Phrenological Charts 1840–1940," *British Journal for the History of Science* 51, no. 2 (2018): 271.
81. "Illustrious Villains," *American Phrenological Journal* 25, no. 3 (March 1857): 50.
82. Gosse, identified only as "an Englishman," was often treated as an exemplar of a higher type of character and used in comparison with opposite types, including murderers. For comparisons between Gosse and Black Hawk, see "Phrenology—Is it a Science?," *American Phrenological Journal and Life Illustrated* 49, no. 10 (October 1869): 371; "Phrenology and Its Foes," *American Phrenological Journal* 31, no. 4

(April 1860): 55–57, at 56. On Gosse, see also "A Shelf in our Cabinet—No. 4," *American Phrenological Journal and Life Illustrated* 35, no. 5 (May 1862): 100–102; "Article XXXVI. Benevolence: Its Definition, Location, Function, Adaptation, and Cultivation," *American Phrenological Journal* 10, no. 6 (June 1848): 179–184; L. N. Fowler, *Phrenological Almanac. 1840* (New York: W. J. Spence, 1839), 27–30, Box 328, Almanac Collection (QC16541), New York State Library. Black Hawk's image also appears as "large destructiveness" elsewhere. See "The New Self-Instructor," *American Phrenological Journal* 30, no. 1 (July 1859): 1–2.

83. Poskett notes that after "Black Hawk was captured in 1832 following his resistance to the Indian Removal Act, he was subject to one final indignity," the taking of a cast of his head by the Fowlers. The Fowlers' ownership of this cast is likely why they made such prolific use of it. Poskett, *Materials of the Mind*, 55.
84. "Article III. Phrenological Developments and Character of the Celebrated Indian Chief and Warrior, Black Hawk; With Cuts," *The American Phrenological Journal and Miscellany* 1, no. 2 (November 1838): 53.
85. "Article III. Phrenological Developments and Character," 55. Claggett also analyzes a version of this article on Black Hawk: Shalyn Claggett, "Putting Character First: The Narrative Construction of Innate Identity in Phrenological Texts," *VIJ: Victorians Institute Journal* 38 (2010): 107–110. On depictions of Indigenous Americans, including Black Hawk, in phrenology, see Charles Colbert, *A Measure of Perfection: Phrenology and the Fine Arts in America* (Chapel Hill: University of North Carolina Press, 1997), 242–253.
86. Poskett notes that Black Hawk was compared favorably by the Fowlers with white men; he was an exemplar of his racial type. Poskett, *Materials of the Mind*, 55.
87. Indeed, as Poskett notes, the large Destructiveness and Combativeness of an Indigenous skull suggested to Combe why North American Indigenous peoples could not be enslaved, whereas the "negro" was "gentler in nature" and therefore more easily enslaved. "Phrenology, therefore, both explained and reinforced racial divisions." Poskett, *Materials of the Mind*, 13.
88. "George Wilson, the Murderer," *American Phrenological Journal* 24, no. 3 (September 1856): 49.
89. Susan Branson, "Phrenology and the Science of Race in Antebellum America," *Early American Studies* 15, no. 1 (2017): 181–182. On abolitionism and antislavery in phrenology, see also Cynthia S. Hamilton, "'Am I Not a Man and a Brother?' Phrenology and Anti-slavery," *Slavery and Abolition* 29, no. 2 (2008): 173–187; Poskett, *Materials of the Mind*, 124–131; Poskett, "Phrenology, Correspondence, and the Global Politics of Reform." On depictions of African Americans within phrenology, see Colbert, *A Measure of Perfection*, 253–257. See also chapter 5 for further discussion of racial theory in phrenology.
90. "Article XLII. John Haggerty, Murderer of Melchoir Fordney—Executed at Lancaster, PA., July 24, 1847," *American Phrenological Journal* 10, no. 7 (July 1848): 212. Karen Halttunen also discusses this case in *Murder Most Foul: The Killer and the American Gothic Imagination* (Cambridge, MA: Harvard University Press, 1998), 218–224, 235–236.
91. "Article LXXIV. George, a Slave, Murderer of Mrs. Foster, with a View of His Skull," *American Phrenological Journal* 11, no. 11 (November 1849): 340–341.
92. Ellis Grosh Lewis and Emanuel Jacob Schaeffer, *Report of The Trial and Conviction of John Haggerty, for The Murder of Melchoir Fordney, Late of The City of Lancaster, Pennsylvania* (Lancaster, PA, 1847), 19.

93. Matthew Frye Jacobson, *Whiteness of a Different Color: European Immigrants and the Alchemy of Race* (Cambridge, MA: Harvard University Press, 1998), 48–53.
94. During the trial, one witness was asked whether they saw a white man or a black man: Haggerty could only be white in this racial binary. Lewis and Schaeffer, *Report of The Trial and Conviction of John Haggerty*, 11.
95. The article notes that when Lorenzo Fowler examined Eustache's bust it was covered from his gaze, so that he "supposed it, of course, belonged to a *white* person, and never knew, till afterwards, that he had been examining the bust of a *negro*." "Article V. Character of Eustache," *The American Phrenological Journal and Miscellany* 2, no 4 (January 1840): 177, 182; emphasis in the original; Poskett, *Materials of the Mind*, 56. On Eustache, see Branson, "Phrenology and the Science of Race in Antebellum America," 181–183; Poskett, *Materials of the Mind*, 51–77.
96. "Article XIX. Destructiveness—Its Definition, Location, Adaptation," *American Phrenological Journal* 10, no. 3 (March 1848): 85.
97. W. B. Powell, "Article IV. Phrenological Developments of Fieschi; Who Attempted to Murder the King of France," *The American Phrenological Journal and Miscellany* 1, no. 11 (August 1839): 439.
98. Pinel's use of "propensity" and "penchant" were primarily focused around suicidal, not homicidal, acts; though he does refer to an "irresistible propensity to commit acts of barbarity and bloodshed," as well as propensities to steal and to incendiarism. Ph. Pinel, *A Treatise on Insanity*, trans. D. D. Davis (Sheffield, UK: W. Todd, 1806), 20–21, 85, 182–183, 231–234; Nicole Hahn Rafter, "The Murderous Dutch Fiddler: Criminology, History, and the Problem of Phrenology," *Theoretical Criminology* 9, no. 1 (2005): 75–76.
99. Rafter, "The Murderous Dutch Fiddler," 75–76.
100. The animal propensities were also sometimes called the "selfish" propensities.
101. *Supplement to the Fourth, Fifth, and Sixth Editions of the Encyclopædia Britannica: With Preliminary Dissertations on the History of the Sciences*, vol. 3 (Edinburgh: Archibald Constable and Company, 1824), s.v. "cranioscopy," 430.
102. *Supplement to the Fourth, Fifth, and Sixth Editions of the Encyclopædia Britannica*; emphasis in the original. This language was likely borrowed from earlier accounts on phrenology, such as an essay in *The Edinburgh Review*, which stated: "GALL called this faculty *murder;* but SPURZHEIM thinks that it produces the propensity to destroy, in general." The same publisher produced both the *Edinburgh Journal* and the *Supplement*. "The Doctrines of Gall and Spurzheim," *The Edinburgh Review, or Critical Journal*, vol. 25 (Edinburgh: Archibald Constable and Company, 1815): 235.
103. *Encyclopædia Londinensis; or, Universal Dictionary of Arts, Sciences, and Literature*, vol. 20 (London, 1825), s.v. "physiognomy," 326.
104. See, for example, P. M. Roget, *Outlines of Physiology: With an Appendix on Phrenology*, 1st American ed. (Philadelphia: Lea and Blanchard, 1839), 475–476.
105. John Fletcher, *The Mirror of Nature, Part I: Presenting a Practical Illustration of the Science of Phrenology* (Boston: Cassady and March, 1839), 27; emphasis in the original.
106. "Phrenology," *Mechanics' Magazine, and Register of Inventions and Improvements* 3, no. 6 (June 1834): 321.
107. "Phrenology," *Boston Traveler*, July 5, 1833.
108. "Moral Insanity," *Salem Gazette*, November 20, 1838; emphasis in the original.
109. "Art. III. The Physiognomical System of Drs. Gall and Spurzheim . . . ," *The Eclectic Review*, vol. 3 (London: Josiah Condler, 1815), 464.

110. "Propensity for Stealing," *Spirit of the Age and Journal of Humanity* 1, no. 35 (January 1834): 4.
111. B. B. T., "The Stealing Propensity," *The Knickerbocker* 4, no. 3 (September 1834): 186.
112. In particular, Rush commented on a "propensity to pilfer." Prichard explored the "Homicidal Propensity," the "Propensity to Arson," the "Propensity to Suicide," and the "Propensity to Theft"; his attention to propensities will be further discussed in chapter 3. [Review of James Cowles Prichard, *On the Different Forms of Insanity*], *The Medico-Chirurgical Review, and Journal of Practical Medicine* 74 (July–October 1842): 527; "A Human Propensity," *Christian Watchman* 25, no. 51 (December 1844): 202.
113. Noel and Carlson, "Origins of the Word 'Phrenology,'" 695.
114. "Monomania, Inducing to Murder," *The Medico-Chirurgical Review, and Journal of Practical Medicine* 44 (January–April 1835): 521.
115. Webb, *The Phrenologist*, 26.

2. Transatlantic Societies and Skulls

1. Though no state was indicated in the letter, it is likely that Kensington refers to the historical area of Philadelphia that was originally its own township, Kensington. The author is unnamed because she signed her letter simply as "C.K," but it is clear from context that this writer was female. C.K. to Anne Nelson, Kensington [PA?], December 15, 1823, Eliza K. Nelson papers, 1823–1867, David M. Rubenstein Rare Book & Manuscript Library, Duke University, Durham, NC.
2. C.K. to Anne Nelson, Kensington [PA?], December 15, 1823; emphasis in the original.
3. The letter-writer refers to "servants" but describes this individual as "a boy who has been bought up for his service & who came from Charleston," which suggests that he may have been enslaved.
4. "For the Literary Magazine: Dr. Gall's System of Craniology," *The Literary Magazine, and American Register* 3, no. 19 (April 1805): 261.
5. "For the Literary Magazine"; "For the Emerald: Some account of Doctor Gall's system of Craniology, condensed from the Monthly Magazine," *The Emerald, or Miscellany of Literature* 1, no. 8 (June 1806): 89–91.
6. "Craniology," *Hampshire Federalist* (Springfield, MA), March 11, 1806.
7. "For the Emerald."
8. Poskett argues that the circulation of material objects, including skulls, plaster casts, letters, texts, periodicals, and photographs, directed the uses of phrenology, framing phrenology itself as a global science of mind. An account of the global nature of phrenological criminal science is beyond the scope of this book. James Poskett, *Materials of the Mind: Phrenology, Race, and the Global History of Science, 1815–1920* (Chicago: University of Chicago Press, 2019).
9. On eighteenth-century "transatlantic cultures of medical improvement," see Simon Finger, *The Contagious City: The Politics of Public Health in Early Philadelphia* (Ithaca, NY: Cornell University Press, 2012), 76–85.
10. Poskett, *Materials of the Mind*, 79.
11. John Hruschka, *How Books Came to America: The Rise of the American Book Trade* (University Park: Pennsylvania State University Press, 2012), 51.
12. Hruschka, *How Books Came to America*, 52.
13. Madeleine B. Stern, *Publishers for Mass Entertainment in Nineteenth Century America* (Boston: G. K. Hall, 1980), 76.

14. Stern, *Publishers for Mass Entertainment*, 76–77. Edward Carey, the younger brother of Henry, also went into publishing with Carey & Hart. The Careys were on equal footing with the prolific New York–based Harper brothers—James, John, Wesley, and Fletcher, of J. & J. Harper and later Harper & Bros. By 1834, the two families published 18 percent of new books. James N. Green, "Part 1: The Rise of Book Publishing," in *A History of the Book in America*, vol. 2: *An Extensive Republic: Print, Culture, and Society in the New Nation, 1790–1840*, ed. Robert A. Gross and Mary Kelly (Chapel Hill: University of North Carolina Press, 2010), 123–125; Stern, *Publishers for Mass Entertainment*, 79, 151–155.
15. Stern, *Publishers for Mass Entertainment*, 76. On John Neal's literary output, see Edward Watts and David J. Carlson, eds., *John Neal and Nineteenth-Century American Literature and Culture* (Lewisburg, PA: Bucknell University Press, 2012).
16. Carey & Lea followed in the footsteps of Mathew Carey, father of Henry Charles Carey, who in the 1790s focused his print enterprises almost entirely on the British reprint trade. Green, "The Rise of Book Publishing," 82–86; Stern, *Publishers for Mass Entertainment*, 74–75.
17. Medicine was a focal point for the press, due to local demand from Philadelphia's medical community. Carey & Lea published 142 titles on medicine between 1822 and 1838, as well as a medical periodical, *The Philadelphia Journal of the Medical and Physical Sciences*. The modern-day successors to the firm, Lea & Febinger, remained a leading medical publisher through the 1950s. David Kaser, *Messrs. Carey & Lea of Philadelphia: A Study in the History of the Booktrade* (Philadelphia: University of Pennsylvania Press, 1957), 119–121.
18. George Combe, *Essays on Phrenology* (Philadelphia: H. C. Carey and I. Lea, 1822); "The History and Progress of Phrenology [Review]," *The Eclectic Journal of Medicine* 4, no. 8 (June 1840): 309. *The Cost Book of Carey & Lea*, edited by David Kaser, begins in 1825, so there is no data on the number of copies produced of Combe's *Essays*. In 1835, they produced 1,500 copies each of Gall's *Manual of Phrenology* and the anonymously authored *Catechism of Phrenology*. David Kaser, ed., *The Cost Book of Carey & Lea, 1825–1838* (Philadelphia: University of Pennsylvania Press, 1963), 167, 177.
19. These works include *A Catechism of Phrenology: Illustrative of the Principles of that Science* (Philadelphia: Carey, Lea, & Blanchard, 1835); Combe, *Essays on Phrenology*; George Combe, *Notes on the United States of North America, During a Phrenological Visit in 1838–9–40*, vols. 1 and 2 (Philadelphia: Carey & Hart, 1841); *Manual of Phrenology: Being an Analytical Summary of the System of Doctor Gall* (Philadelphia: Carey, Lea, & Blanchard, 1835); L. Miles, *Phrenology and the Moral Influence of Phrenology* (Philadelphia: Carey, Lea & Blanchard, 1835).
20. "American Phrenological Journal," *The Boston Medical and Surgical Journal* 19, no. 6 (September 1838): 96. This journal would later move to New York with its new editors, the Fowler brothers.
21. Finger, *The Contagious City*, 79.
22. The Carey & Lea edition of Combe's *Essays* included an inscription by John Bell dedicating the edition to Physick. Physick was also a mentor to Dr. Samuel George Morton. Combe, *Essays on Phrenology*, front matter; Adrian Desmond and James Moore, *Darwin's Sacred Cause: How a Hatred of Slavery Shaped Darwin's Views on Human Evolution* (Boston: Houghton Mifflin Harcourt, 2009), 47.
23. "The History and Progress of Phrenology [Review]," 309; John D. Davies, *Phrenology: Fad and Science; A 19th-Century American Crusade* (Hamden, CT: Archon Books, 1971 [1955]), 13.

24. The oldest American hospital and medical school were in Philadelphia, as well as Benjamin Rush, as signs of its medical preeminence. Walsh identified three key moments for Philadelphia's priority as the site for the beginning of American phrenology: Rush's original use of the term "phrenology"; Nicholas Biddle's phrenological tour in Europe and subsequent return, bearing a human skull marked by Spurzheim; and the 1822 founding of the first American phrenological society. Anthony A. Walsh, "Phrenology and the Boston Medical Community in the 1830s," *Bulletin of the History of Medicine* 50, no. 2 (1976): 261–263. See also W. F. Bynum, *Science and the Practice of Medicine in the Nineteenth Century* (New York: Cambridge University Press, 1994), 51; Kaser, *Messrs. Carey & Lea*, 119; James C. Mohr, *Doctors and the Law: Medical Jurisprudence in Nineteenth-Century America* (Baltimore: Johns Hopkins University Press, 1996 [1993]), 6.
25. Davies, *Phrenology*, 13.
26. George Combe, *Lectures on Phrenology* (New York: Samuel Colman, 1839), 80.
27. Davies, *Phrenology*, 14.
28. Charles Caldwell, *Elements of Phrenology* (Lexington, KY: Thomas T. Skillman, 1824), iii.
29. Charles Caldwell, *Phrenology Vindicated and Antiphrenology Unmasked* (New York: Samuel Colman, 1838); Combe, *Lectures on Phrenology*, 80.
30. Charles Caldwell, *Introductory Address on Independence of Intellect* (Lexington KY, 1825), 36; Combe, *Lectures on Phrenology*, 81.
31. Combe, *Lectures on Phrenology*, 79.
32. George Combe, *The Constitution of Man Considered in Relation to External Objects*, 3rd ed. (Edinburgh: John Anderson Jr., 1835), 270.
33. The preeminence of the Boston Phrenological Society prompted the dismay of the founders of the Central Phrenological Society in Philadelphia, which was often erased in the origins of American phrenology, as was the phrenological society of Washington, DC, founded in 1826. Additional societies likely were founded before Boston, due to Caldwell's purported influence in inciting the formation of societies in the cities in which he lectured. "The History and Progress of Phrenology [Review]," 309; George Combe, *The Constitution of Man Considered in Relation to External Objects*, 8th American ed. (Boston: Marsh, Capen, & Lyon, 1837), 402.
34. On Burke and Hare, see Caroline McCracken-Flesher, *The Doctor Dissected: A Cultural Autopsy of the Burke and Hare Murders* (Oxford: Oxford University Press, 2012); Ruth Richardson, *Death, Dissection and the Destitute*, 2nd ed. (Chicago: University of Chicago Press, 2000 [1987]), 131–158; R. Michael Gordon, *The Infamous Burke and Hare: Serial Killers and Resurrectionists of Nineteenth Century Edinburgh* (Jefferson, NC: McFarland & Company, 2009); Lisa Rosner, *The Anatomy Murders: Being the True and Spectacular History of Edinburgh's Notorious Burke and Hare, and of the Man of Science Who Abetted Them in the Commission of Their Most Heinous Crimes* (Philadelphia: University of Pennsylvania Press, 2019).
35. McCracken-Flesher, *The Doctor Dissected*, 7–8; Richardson, *Death, Dissection and the Destitute*, 132–135; Rosner, *The Anatomy Murders*.
36. Rosner also discusses the phrenological debate between Combe and Stone inspired by the Burke and Hare case. Rosner, *The Anatomy Murders*, 172–186.
37. "Article IV. Phrenological Observations on the Cerebral Development of William Burk [*sic*], Executed for Murder at Edinburgh, on 28th January, 1829, and on the Development of William Hare, His Accomplice," *The Phrenological Journal and Miscellany* 5, no. 20 (May 1828–April 1829): 549–572.

38. "Article IV. Phrenological Observations," 569.
39. G. N. Cantor, "The Edinburgh Phrenology Debate: 1803–1828," *Annals of Science* 32, no. 3 (1975): 202.
40. Steven Shapin, "Phrenological Knowledge and the Social Structure of Early Nineteenth-Century Edinburgh," *Annals of Science* 32, no. 3 (1975): 233.
41. Cantor, Cooter, and Shapin wrote extensively about the meaning and shape of the Edinburgh phrenology debates of the 1810s and 1820s, but only mention the Stone/Combe debate over Burke and Hare in passing. Cantor, "The Edinburgh Phrenology Debate," 202–203; Roger Cooter, *The Cultural Meaning of Popular Science: Phrenology and the Organization of Consent in Nineteenth-Century Britain* (Cambridge: Cambridge University Press, 1984), 24–28, 310n46; Shapin, "Phrenological Knowledge," 224n17.
42. Thomas Stone, *Observations on the Phrenological Development of Burke, Hare, and Other Atrocious Murderers; Measurements of the Heads of the Most Notorious Thieves Confined in the Edinburgh Jail and Bridewell, and of Various Individuals, English, Scotch, and Irish, Presenting an Extensive Series of Facts Subversive of Phrenology* (Edinburgh: Robert Buchanan; William Hunter; and John Stevenson; London: T. and G. Underwood; Glasgow: Robertson and Atkinson; Aberdeen: Alex. Brown & Co.; Dublin: J. Cuming, 1829), 2.
43. Stone, *Observations on the Phrenological Development*, 4.
44. Stone, *Observations on the Phrenological Development*, 5.
45. Stone, *Observations on the Phrenological Development*, 62–73.
46. Stone, *Observations on the Phrenological Development*, 51.
47. Stone, *Observations on the Phrenological Development*, 52.
48. George Combe, *Letter on the Prejudices of the Great in Science and Philosophy against Phrenology; Addressed to the Editor of the Edinburgh Weekly Journal* (Edinburgh: John Anderson Jr.; London: Simpkin & Marshall, 1829), 4.
49. Combe, *Letter on the Prejudices of the Great*, 4–5.
50. George Combe, *Answer to "Observations on the Phrenological Development of Burke, Hare, and Other Atrocious Murderers, &c.—by Thomas Stone, Esq.," &c.* (Edinburgh: John Anderson Jr.; London: Simpkin & Marshall, 1829), 11–12.
51. Thomas Stone, *A Rejoinder to the Answer of George Combe, Esq., to "Observations on the Phrenological Development of Burke, Hare, and Other Atrocious Murderers"* (Edinburgh: Robert Buchanan; William Hunter; and John Stevenson; London: T. and G. Underwood; Glasgow: Robertson and Atkinson; Aberdeen: Alex. Brown & Co., 1829), 4.
52. *A Brief Sketch of the Occurrences on Board the Brig Crawford, on Her Voyage from Matanzas to New-York; Together with an Account of the Trial of the Three Spaniards, Jose Hilario Casares, Felix Barbeito, and Jose Morando . . .* (Richmond: Samuel Shepherd & Co., 1827); *The Life of the Celebrated Mail Robber and Daring Highwayman, Joseph Thompson Hare . . . Also, of the Cruel and Ferocious Pirate, Alexander Tardy* (Philadelphia: J. B. Perry, 1844).
53. J. A. Brereton, *A Report Submitted to the Phrenological Society of the City of Washington, on the 14th of March 1828, and Printed by Order* (Washington, DC: E. De Kraft, Printer, 1828), 2.
54. Brereton, *A Report Submitted to the Phrenological Society*, 3.
55. Brereton, *A Report Submitted to the Phrenological Society*, 7.
56. *A Brief Sketch of the Occurrences on Board the Brig Crawford*, 6.
57. *The Life of the Celebrated Mail Robber*, 72; emphasis and quotation marks in the original.

58. "Article III. Report on the Case of Four Spanish Pirates, by the Phrenological Society of Washington, United States," *The Phrenological Journal and Miscellany* 5, no. 19 (May 1828–April 1829): 364–405.
59. Stone, *Observations on the Phrenological Development*, 42.
60. Stone, *Observations on the Phrenological Development*, 43. Hamilton delivered a series of antiphrenological lectures to the Royal Society of Edinburgh between 1825 and 1829. Cantor, "The Edinburgh Phrenology Debate," 198, 201, 202; Cooter, *The Cultural Meaning of Popular Science*, 28, 285, 310n45; Shapin, "Phrenological Knowledge," 230–231; John van Wyhe, *Phrenology and the Origins of Victorian Scientific Naturalism* (Aldershot, UK: Ashgate, 2004), 85–92.
61. Stone, *Observations on the Phrenological Development*, 43.
62. Combe, *Answer to "Observations,"* 10.
63. Stone, *A Rejoinder to the Answer of George Combe, Esq.*, 12; emphasis in the original.
64. Stone, *A Rejoinder to the Answer of George Combe, Esq.*, 12; emphasis in the original.
65. Stone, *A Rejoinder to the Answer of George Combe, Esq.*, 13; emphasis in the original.
66. Stone, *A Rejoinder to the Answer of George Combe, Esq.*, 14; emphasis in the original.
67. See Walsh, "Phrenology and the Boston Medical Community," 268; Anthony A. Walsh, "The American Tour of Dr. Spurzheim," *Journal of the History of Medicine and Allied Sciences* 27, no. 2 (1972): 187–205.
68. Thomas H. O'Connor, *The Athens of America: Boston, 1825–1845* (Amherst: University of Massachusetts Press, 2006), 23. See also Davies, *Phrenology*, 17; Walsh, "The American Tour of Dr. Spurzheim," 190.
69. O'Connor, *The Athens of America*, 41–65.
70. O'Connor, *The Athens of America*, 101–112.
71. E. Digby Baltzell, *Puritan Boston and Quaker Philadelphia* (New Brunswick, NJ: Transaction Publishers, 1996 [1979]), 282.
72. O'Connor, *The Athens of America*, 111.
73. O'Connor, *The Athens of America*, 111–114.
74. O'Connor, *The Athens of America*, 114–115.
75. O'Connor, *The Athens of America*, 115–120.
76. Angela G. Ray, *The Lyceum and Public Culture in the Nineteenth-Century United States* (East Lansing: Michigan State University Press, 2005), 13–30.
77. Nahum Capen, *Reminiscences of Dr. Spurzheim and George Combe* (New York: Fowler & Wells, 1881), 8–9; Walsh, "The American Tour of Dr. Spurzheim," 189.
78. Capen, *Reminiscences of Dr. Spurzheim and George Combe*, 9; Walsh, "The American Tour of Dr. Spurzheim," 189–90.
79. Capen, *Reminiscences of Dr. Spurzheim and George Combe*, 10; Walsh, "The American Tour of Dr. Spurzheim," 190–193.
80. Quincy was formerly the mayor of Boston; it was under his leadership in the 1820s that Boston's elite came to focus on reform and social improvement. O'Connor, *The Athens of America*, 38–41; Walsh, "The American Tour of Dr. Spurzheim," 190–191.
81. Davies, *Phrenology*, 17; Walsh, "The American Tour of Dr. Spurzheim," 193–195.
82. Capen, *Reminiscences of Dr. Spurzheim and George Combe*, 35–36; Walsh, "The American Tour of Dr. Spurzheim," 195–196.

83. Capen, *Reminiscences of Dr. Spurzheim and George Combe*, 38.
84. Warren audited Spurzheim's lectures in Paris in 1821 and lectured on the subject to his medical students at Harvard. Walsh has argued that Warren was key to the adoption of phrenology by the Boston medical community as one of the earliest American adherents to the science. Capen, *Reminiscences of Dr. Spurzheim and George Combe*, 36; Davies, *Phrenology*, 13, 17; Nathaniel B. Shurtleff, "Article II. Anatomical Report on the Skull of Spurzheim, read before the Boston Phrenological Society," *Annals of Phrenology* 2, no. 1 (May 1835): 73; Stephen Tomlinson, *Head Masters: Phrenology, Secular Education, and Nineteenth-Century Social Thought* (Tuscaloosa: University of Alabama Press, 2005), 222; Walsh, "The American Tour of Dr. Spurzheim," 198n50, 198–201; Walsh, "Phrenology and the Boston Medical Community," 263–265.
85. Capen, *Reminiscences of Dr. Spurzheim and George Combe*, 36, 39–40; Davies, *Phrenology*, 17–18; Charles Follen, *Professor Follen's Funeral Oration Delivered at the Burial of Dr. G. Spurzheim* (Boston: Marsh, Capen & Lyon, 1832); Walsh, "The American Tour of Dr. Spurzheim," 196.
86. Davies, *Phrenology*, 18.
87. Walsh, "The American Tour of Dr. Spurzheim," 196.
88. Capen, *Reminiscences of Dr. Spurzheim and George Combe*, 40. Also quoted in Walsh, "The American Tour of Dr. Spurzheim," 196.
89. Walsh, "Phrenology and the Boston Medical Community," 267.
90. Jonathan Barber, *An Address Delivered Before the Boston Phrenological Society* (Boston: Marsh, Capen & Lyon, 1833), 4.
91. Combe, *Lectures on Phrenology*, 79; "Notices. Boston Phrenological Society," *Annals of Phrenology* 2, no. 4 (February 1836): 510–511.
92. Combe, *Lectures on Phrenology*, 79. The first volume of the *Annals*, for example, contained thirty-one articles; of these, sixteen were republished from the Edinburgh *Phrenological Journal and Miscellany* and three from *The Lancet*. *Annals of Phrenology*, vol. 1 (Boston: Marsh, Capen & Lyon, 1834); Walsh, "Phrenology and the Boston Medical Community," 270.
93. Walsh, "Phrenology and the Boston Medical Community," 268, 272.
94. Marsh, Capen & Lyon also published a series of fifty volumes for use in Boston public schools on behalf of the Massachusetts Board of Education: like Carey & Lea, this firm was not exclusively focused on phrenology. Scott E. Casper, "Part 2. Case Study: Harper & Brothers," in *A History of the Book in America*, vol. 2: *An Extensive Republic: Print, Culture, and Society in the New Nation, 1790–1840*, ed. Robert A. Gross and Mary Kelly (Chapel Hill: University of North Carolina Press, 2010), 132; Massachusetts Board of Education, *First Annual Report of the Board of Education* (Boston: Dutton and Wentworth, 1838), 24–32.
95. G. Spurzheim, *Outlines of Phrenology* (Boston: Marsh, Capen and Lyon, 1832); G. Spurzheim, *Philosophical Catechism of the Natural Laws of Man*, 2nd ed. (Boston: Marsh, Capen and Lyon, 1832); G. Spurzheim, *Phrenology, or the Doctrine of the Mental Phenomena*, 2 vols. (Boston: Marsh, Capen & Lyon, 1832); G. Spurzheim, *A View of the Elementary Principles of Education, Founded on the Study of the Nature of Man* (Boston: Marsh Capen and Lyon, 1832).
96. These works include Andrew Combe, *Observations on Mental Derangement: Being an Application of the Principles of Phrenology to the Elucidation of the Causes, Symptoms, Nature, and Treatment of Insanity* (Boston: Marsh, Capen & Lyon, 1834); George Combe, *Elements of Phrenology*, 4th American ed. (Boston, Marsh, Capen &

Lyon, 1835); George Combe, *A System of Phrenology*, 3rd American ed. (Boston: Marsh, Capen, and Lyon, 1835); François Joseph Gall, *On the Functions of the Brain and of Each of its Parts*, 6 vols. (Boston: Marsh, Capen & Lyon, 1835); Samuel Gridley Howe, *A Discourse on the Social Relations of Man; Delivered Before the Boston Phrenological Society, at the Close of their Course of Lectures* (Boston: Marsh, Capen & Lyon, 1837); Robert Macnish, *An Introduction to Phrenology, in the Form of Question and Answer, with an Appendix, and Copious Illustrative Notes* (Boston: Marsh, Capen & Lyon, 1836); Nathaniel Shurtleff, *An Epitome of Phrenology: Being an Outline of the Science as Taught by Gall Spurzheim and Combe . . .* (Boston: Marsh, Capen & Lyon, 1835); J. G. Spurzheim, *Phrenology, in Connexion with the Study of Physiognomy* (Boston: Marsh, Capen & Lyon, 1833); and others. See also *Annals of Phrenology*, vol. 1 (Boston: Marsh, Capen & Lyon, 1834), n.p. [end pages].

97. Davies, *Phrenology*, 19.
98. Combe, *The Constitution of Man*, 8th American ed., 402.
99. These societies were geographically focused in New England: Hingham, Nantucket, Reading, Leicester, and Worcester, in Massachusetts; Brunswick, Maine; Andover, Amherst, and Hanover, in New Hampshire; Providence, Rhode Island; Hartford, Connecticut; and Oneida, New York. Combe, *The Constitution of Man*, 8th American ed., 402; Walsh, "Phrenology and the Boston Medical Community," 271.
100. Boston physician John McCall was president of the Oneida Phrenological Society in New York; Boston physician Jonathan Barber, a member of the Boston Phrenological Society, was the president of the New York Phrenological Society, in New York City. "Notices. Oneida Phrenological Society," *Annals of Phrenology* 2, no. 4 (February 1836): 511; "Notices. New York," *Annals of Phrenology* 2, no. 2 (August 1835): 260.
101. Poskett, *Materials of the Mind*, 3–8.
102. J. Randolf, *A Memoir on the Life and Character of Philip Syng Physick, M.D.* (Philadelphia: T. K. & P. G. Collins, 1839), 95.
103. Poskett, *Materials of the Mind*, 118.
104. The Nahum Capen papers include over seventy letters to Capen, Samuel Gridley Howe, the Boston Phrenological Society, and Marsh, Capen & Lyon, all predominantly relating to phrenology. Nahum Capen papers, 1783–1885 (inclusive), 1826–1885 (bulk), B MS c23, Boston Medical Library in the Francis A. Countway Library of Medicine, Boston, MA (hereafter cited as Capen Letters).
105. The Boston Phrenological Society in particular was dominated by medical men. Walsh, "Phrenology and the Boston Medical Community," 268.
106. Barber, *An Address Delivered Before the Boston Phrenological Society*, 41. On Samuel Gridley Howe's phrenological leanings, see Harold Schwartz, "Samuel Gridley Howe as Phrenologist," *American Historical Review* 57, no. 3 (1952): 644–651; Tomlinson, *Head Masters*, 224–227.
107. "Notices. Oneida Phrenological Society," 511.
108. Randolf, *A Memoir on the Life and Character of Philip Syng Physick*, 95.
109. *Transactions of the College of Physicians of Philadelphia*, 3rd series, vol. 9 (Philadelphia, 1887), clxii, clxvii, clxviii, clxxv, ccxxii, ccxxviii, ccxxx, ccxxxiii.
110. I owe the identification of this first case to Susan Branson and her paper given at the Newberry Seminar on November 7, 2014 in Chicago, Illinois [Commencement; University of Maryland], *Baltimore Patriot & Mercantile Advertiser*, April 9, 1830. Also cited in Susan Branson, "Phrenology and the Science of Race in Antebellum America," *Early American Studies* 15, no. 1 (2017): 171, 171n11.

111. [Commencement; Transylvania University], *Charleston Courier*, March 31, 1831.
112. Some of these theses may have been critical of phrenology; however, their presence suggests that phrenology was part of the broader content of medical education in this period. "Commencement of the Medical College," *City Gazette & Commercial Daily Advertiser* (Charleston, SC), March 17, 1832; "University of Pennsylvania. Medical Department," *National Gazette and Literary Register* (Philadelphia, PA), April 2, 1835; [Degrees, College of Physicians and Surgeons of the Western District], *Albany Argus*, February 3, 1837; "Jefferson Medical College," *National Gazette & Literary Register* (Philadelphia, PA), March 10, 1838; "Pennsylvania College. Medical Department," *National Gazette and Literary Register* (Philadelphia, PA), March 11, 1841; "Medical College," *New-York Spectator*, February 2, 1842; "Medical College of the State of S. Carolina," *Charleston Courier*, March 18, 1843.
113. "Ohio Reformed Medical College, Worthington," *Ohio Monitor* (Columbus, OH), October 27, 1830.
114. Several examples of this incorporation of phrenological theory and figures appeared in the medical theses of Albany Medical College, which had been founded in 1838 by Amos Dean, a phrenological enthusiast discussed in the next chapter. See, for example, Samuel S. Guy, "Dissertation on the Nature and Some of the Disposing Causes of Insanity" (Medical Theses, Albany Medical College Archives, Albany, NY, 1846); Granville S. Thomas, "The Brain and its Occupant the Mind" (Medical Theses, Albany Medical College Archives, Albany, NY, 1858).
115. The *Boston Medical and Surgical Journal*, for example, published a number of favorable articles on phrenology through the 1830s and early 1840s. Medical texts also sometimes referred to phrenology in passing. Elliotson, for example, incorporated phrenology into his discussion of insanity, including a citation of the phrenological concept of "a propensity to murder." John Elliotson, *Lectures on the Theory and Practice of Medicine* (London: J. F. Moore, 1839), 432.
116. "Article VII. Examination of Heads," *Annals of Phrenology* 2, no. 1 (May 1835): 130.
117. "Article VII. Examination of Heads," 130; emphasis in the original.
118. "Article VII. Examination of Heads," 131; emphasis in the original.
119. "Article VII. Examination of Heads," 132.
120. Combe, *Notes on the United States of North America*, 1:81–82.
121. Combe, *Notes on the United States of North America*, 1:84, 148.
122. Combe, *Notes on the United States of North America*, 1:84.
123. Combe, *Notes on the United States of North America*, 1:100–101.
124. On Combe's American tour, see David Stack, *Queen Victoria's Skull: George Combe and the Mid-Victorian Mind* (London: Hambledon Continuum, 2008), 125–141.
125. Combe, *Notes on the United States of North America*, 1:iii–iv.
126. Despite the support of American medical men, Combe received little support from established physicians in Edinburgh. Cantor, "The Edinburgh Phrenology Debate," 201.
127. Massachusetts Medical Society to George Combe, June 2, 1836, Box 1, Folder 68, Capen Letters.
128. George Henry Calvert to [George Combe?], June 3, 1836, Box 1, Folder 54, Capen Letters.
129. William Mosely Holland to Nahum Capen, June 1, 1836, Box 1, Folder 29, Capen Letters.
130. Some of these American testimonials appeared in a published collection supporting Combe's candidacy. *Testimonials on Behalf of George Combe as a Candidate for the*

Chair of Logic in the University of Edinburgh (Edinburgh: Anderson Jr.; London: Simpkin & Marshall, 1836).

131. Amariah Brigham to Nahum Capen, May 17, 1833, Box 1, Folder 10, Capen Letters; emphasis in the original.
132. Amariah Brigham to Nahum Capen, May 17, 1833.
133. Capen, *Reminiscences of Dr. Spurzheim and George Combe*, 9–10.
134. Nathaniel Shurtleff to Nahum Capen, September 4, 1833, Box 1, Folder 40, Capen Letters.
135. Boston Phrenological Society, *A Catalogue of Phrenological Specimens, Belonging to the Boston Phrenological Society* (Boston: John Ford, 1835), 32–33. Annotated by J. B. S. Jackson, first curator of the Warren Anatomical Museum. Box 10, Folder 1, Warren Anatomical Museum Records, 1835–2010 (inclusive), 1971–1991 (bulk), Harvard Medical Library in the Francis A. Countway Library of Medicine, Boston, MA. See also Silas Jones, *Practical Phrenology* (Boston: Russell, Shattuck, & Williams, 1836), 42.
136. Boston Phrenological Society, *A Catalogue of Phrenological Specimens*, 33.
137. Some racial theorists of the nineteenth century argued that the "subordinate nature" of people of African descent made them "less likely to commit great crimes than the superior white man." J. H. Van Evrie, *Negroes and Negro "Slavery": The First an Inferior Race; The Latter its Normal Condition* (New York: Van Evrie, Horton & Co., 1861), 313. For further discussion, see chapter 5.
138. *Mayors of Boston: An Illustrated Epitome of Who the Mayors Have Been and What They Have Done* (Boston: State Street Trust Company, 1914), 29.
139. "Harvard University. Medical Graduates for the Year 1834," *Medical Magazine* 3, no. 3 (September 1834): 100.
140. Nathaniel Shurtleff to Nahum Capen, September 4, 1833; "Notices. Officers of the Boston Phrenological Society for 1835," *Annals of Phrenology* 1, no. 3 (November 1834): 399.
141. "Pathological Fact," *The American Phrenological Journal and Miscellany* 2, no. 4 (January 1840): 190.
142. Some specimens were listed but not numbered, so the number of specimens was higher than the 416 numbered specimens. On page 21 of the *Catalogue*, for example, sixteen specimens were numbered, but another nine were listed but unnumbered. Boston Phrenological Society, *A Catalogue of Phrenological Specimens*, 21.
143. Boston Phrenological Society, *A Catalogue of Phrenological Specimens*, 18.
144. Boston Phrenological Society, *A Catalogue of Phrenological Specimens*, 5–7. Some "Tattooed" specimens were also included, though what national type they might represent was unclear.
145. On Morton, see Ann Fabian, *The Skull Collectors: Race, Science, and America's Unburied Dead* (Chicago: University of Chicago Press, 2010).
146. "Art. XX.—*Crania Americana* [Review]," *American Journal of Science, &c.* 38, no. 2 (January–March 1840): 341; later reprinted in parts in the *American Phrenological Journal and Miscellany*, beginning with: "Article I: Review of Morton's Crania Americana," *The American Phrenological Journal and Miscellany* 2, no. 9 (June 1840): 385–396; Fabian, *The Skull Collectors*, 95–96.
147. On Combe's relationship with Morton and contributions to *Crania Americana*, see Paul A. Erickson, "Phrenology and Physical Anthropology: The George Combe Connection," *Current Anthropology* 18, no. 1 (1977): 93; Fabian, *The Skull Collectors*, 92–103; Lucile E. Hoyme, "Physical Anthropology and Its Instruments: An Historical Study," *Southwestern Journal of Anthropology* 9, no. 4 (1953): 415.

148. Fabian, *The Skull Collectors*, 92; Hoyme, "Physical Anthropology and Its Instruments," 415.
149. Fabian, *The Skull Collectors*, 93–95; Hoyme, "Physical Anthropology and Its Instruments," 415–416.
150. George Combe to Samuel George Morton, February 7, 1840; Benjamin Silliman to Samuel George Morton, February 19, 1840, with enclosed letter from George Combe to Dr. Morton, February 19, 1840; George Combe to Samuel [George] Morton, February 28, 1840; George Combe to Samuel [George] Morton, March 6, 1840, Series I: Correspondence, April 1838–September 1840, Box 4, Samuel George Morton Papers, Mss.B.M843, American Philosophical Society, Philadelphia, PA (hereafter cited as Morton Papers); Combe, *Notes on the United States of North America*, 1:307–308; Fabian, *The Skull Collectors*, 95–96.
151. "Art. XX.—*Crania Americana*," 352; Erickson, "Phrenology and Physical Anthropology," 92–93; Fabian, *The Skull Collectors*, 97; Hoyme, "Physical Anthropology and Its Instruments," 415; William Stanton, *The Leopard's Spots: Scientific Attitudes toward Race in America 1815–59* (Chicago: University of Chicago Press, 1960), 29, 37–39.
152. See letters from George Combe to Samuel George Morton in Morton Papers. See also Fabian, *The Skull Collectors*, 92–103.
153. "Dr. Morton's Collection of Skulls," *The American Phrenological Journal and Miscellany* 3, no. 4 (January 1841): 191.
154. Boston Phrenological Society, *A Catalogue of Phrenological Specimens*, 7, 8.
155. My estimates of the total number of specimens and the percentage of these specimens relating to criminal types are approximate, due to the inclusion of duplicate specimens.
156. *Transactions of the Phrenological Society* (Edinburgh: John Anderson Jr.; London: Simpkin & Marshall, 1824), xv–xvi.
157. The exact numbers of specimens in this catalogue are hard to determine with certainty, as some are not numbered or are numbered inconsistently. However, I estimate that this collection included at least 350 specimens, of which roughly 12 percent were murderers or other criminals, including those listed as "robber," "pirate," or with other related terms. Catalogue 1, Edinburgh Phrenological Society, Coll-227 (Gen.608/4), Centre for Research Collections, Main Library, University of Edinburgh, Edinburgh, UK.
158. A. A. Royer, "Article III. Catalogue, Numerical and Descriptive, of Heads of Men and Animals, Which Composed the Collection Made by the Late Dr Gall," *The Phrenological Journal and Miscellany* 6, no. 25 (1830): 480–499; A. A. Royer, "Article IV. Catalogue, Numerical and Descriptive, of Heads of Men and Animals, Which Composed the Collection Made by the Late Dr Gall," *The Phrenological Journal and Miscellany* 6, no. 26 (1830): 583–602; A. A. Royer, "Article III. Catalogue, Numerical and Descriptive, of Heads of Men and Animals, Which Composed the Collection Made by the Late Dr Gall," *The Phrenological Journal and Miscellany* 7, no. 27 (1831): 27–36; A. A. Royer, "Article III. Catalogue, Numerical and Descriptive, of Heads of Men and Animals, Which Composed the Collection Made by the Late Dr Gall," *The Phrenological Journal and Miscellany* 7, no. 28 (1831): 181–185; A. A. Royer, "Article III. Catalogue, Numerical and Descriptive, of Heads of Men and Animals, Which Composed the Collection Made by the Late Dr Gall," *The Phrenological Journal and Miscellany* 7, no. 29 (1831): 250–253. Finger and Eling note that at least sixty-nine criminal skulls were included in Ackerknecht's and Vallois's original

count of Gall's cabinet, but many other specimens were of "mixed" types that fit into multiple categories. Stanley Finger and Paul Eling, *Franz Joseph Gall: Naturalist of the Mind, Visionary of the Brain* (New York: New York University Press, 2019), 189–191. See also Erwin H. Ackerknecht and Henri V. Vallois, *François Joseph Gall et sa collection* (Paris: Editions du Muséum, 1955).

159. Samuel Gridley Howe to John Collins Warren, Sr., June 25, 1849; Samuel Gridley Howe to John Collins Warren, Sr., June 27, 1849; Samuel Gridley Howe to John Collins Warren, Sr., September 3, 1849; John Collins Warren, Sr. to Samuel Gridley Howe [probably draft], February 4, 1850, John Collins Warren, Jr., "The Collection of the Boston Phrenological Society—A Retrospect. Original draft of . . . Received by the Museum June 9, 1924," Rare Books 1.Mw.1921.W, Harvard Medical Library in the Francis A. Countway Library of Medicine, Boston, MA.
160. The current curator of the Warren Anatomical Museum, Dominic Hall, believes these annotations and notes were made by J. B. S. Jackson, the first curator of the Warren Museum, and produced when the collection was acquired. The extant collection today amounts to less than half of the original cabinet. Dominic Hall, conversation at the Warren Anatomical Museum, November 1, 2013; email correspondence, November 20, 2019.
161. "Pathological Fact," *The American Phrenological Journal and Miscellany* 2, no. 4 (January 1840): 190.
162. *Catalogue of Busts, Casts, and Skulls in the Phrenological Cabinet, Clinton Hall* (New York: Fowlers and Wells, 1850), 3.
163. *Catalogue of Busts, Casts, and Skulls*, 17.
164. *Catalogue of Busts, Casts, and Skulls*, 35.
165. On scientific collecting practices among amateurs in nineteenth-century America, see Sally Gregory Kohlstedt, "Curiosities and Cabinets: Natural History Museums and Education on the Antebellum Campus," *Isis* 79, no. 3 (1988): 405–426; Sally Gregory Kohlstedt, "Parlors, Primers, and Public Schooling: Education for Science in Nineteenth-Century America," *Isis* 81, no. 3 (1990): 424–445.

3. Phrenology on Trial

1. On the Mitchell case, see Kenneth J. Weiss, "Isaac Ray's Affair with Phrenology," *Journal of Psychiatry & Law* 34, no. 4 (2006): 474; Kenneth J. Weiss, "Isaac Ray at 200: Phrenology and Expert Testimony," *Journal of the American Academy of Psychiatry and Law* 35, no. 3 (2007): 339–345; Christopher J. Beshara, "Moral Hospitals, Addled Brains and Cranial Conundrums: Rationalizations of the Criminal Mind in Antebellum America," *Australasian Journal of American Studies* 29, no. 1 (2010): 45–51.
2. John Neal, "'Signs of Character': Phrenology and Physiognomy," *American Phrenological Journal and Life Illustrated* 44, no. 4 (October 1866): 106.
3. Neal, "'Signs of Character,'" 106.
4. Research suggests that phrenology had not been applied in courts of law in other countries either by this date, making the Mitchell case the first example of phrenological testimony. The last verifiable case of a phrenologist appearing on the witness stand in the United States occurred in 1872, when Dr. Samuel Wells testified for the defense in the case of Lawrence Sullivan, on trial in New York for the murder of John O'Brien. "Maiming," *The Boston Medical and Surgical Journal* 11, no. 25 (January 1835): 404–407; "The Case of Lawrence Sullivan: A Victory for Phrenology," *The Phrenological Journal and Life Illustrated* 54, no. 3 (March 1872): 193–195; "The Murderer Sullivan," *New York Herald*, January 19, 1872.

5. James F. Otis, *Report of the Trial of Major Mitchell, for Felonious Assault and Maiming, on the Person of David H. Crawford: Before the Supreme Judicial Court of the State of Maine, at the Term for the County of Cumberland, Held at Portland, on the First Tuesday of November, 1834; with the Arguments of Counsel* (Portland, ME: Colman & Chisholm, 1834), 13.
6. Otis, *Report of the Trial of Major Mitchell*, 16. About Mighels, Barrett, and Bartlett, little is known. Neal refers to them in a later essay as "three of our leading physicians, and all three believers." Neal, "Signs of Character," 106.
7. "Article IV. The Case of Major Mitchell," *Annals of Phrenology* 2, no. 3 (November 1835): 309; emphasis in the original. This essay excerpts and comments on one published by John Neal in the *New England Galaxy*.
8. On medical jurisprudence in the nineteenth century, see Robert Baker, Dorothy Porter, and Roy Porter, eds., *The Codification of Medical Morality: Historical and Philosophical Studies of the Formalization of Western Medical Morality in the Eighteenth and Nineteenth Centuries* (Dordrecht: Kluwer Academic Publishers, 1993); Susanna L. Blumenthal, *Law and the Modern Mind: Consciousness and Responsibility in American Legal Culture* (Cambridge, MA: Harvard University Press, 2016); Michael Clark and Catherine Crawford, eds., *Legal Medicine in History* (Cambridge: Cambridge University Press, 1994); James C. Mohr, *Doctors and the Law: Medical Jurisprudence in Nineteenth-Century America* (Baltimore: Johns Hopkins University Press, 1996 [1993]).
9. John Harley Warner, *The Therapeutic Perspective: Medical Practice, Knowledge, and Identity in America, 1820–1885* (Princeton, NJ: Princeton University Press, 1997 [1986]), 38.
10. Pierre Schlag, "Law and Phrenology," *Harvard Law Review* 110, no. 4 (1997): 896–897. On the legal profession in the nineteenth century, see Paul D. Carrington, *Stewards of Democracy: Law as a Public Profession* (Boulder, CO: Westview Press, 1999); Morton J. Horwitz, *The Transformation of American Law, 1780–1860* (Cambridge, MA: Harvard University Press, 1977); William P. LaPiana, *Logic and Experience: The Origin of Modern American Legal Education* (Oxford: Oxford University Press, 1994).
11. Schlag, "Law and Phrenology," 896–897.
12. Schlag, "Law and Phrenology," 912.
13. See, for example, favorable commentary appended to the following article by the editors: G. T. C., "Art. VII.—Criminal Law of Insanity," *American Jurist* 15, no. 29 (April 1836): 92–93.
14. Warner, *The Therapeutic Perspective*, 38; William G. Rothstein, *American Physicians in the Nineteenth Century: From Sects to Science* (Baltimore: Johns Hopkins University Press, 1992 [1972]), 125–143, 152–165. On orthodoxy, alternative medicine, and the medical profession in the nineteenth-century United States, see William F. Bynum, *Science and the Practice of Medicine in the Nineteenth Century* (Cambridge: Cambridge University Press, 1994); John S. Haller Jr., *The History of American Homeopathy: From Rational Medicine to Holistic Health Care* (New Brunswick, NJ: Rutgers University Press, 2009); John S. Haller Jr., *The People's Doctor: Samuel Thomson and the American Botanical Movement* (Carbondale: Southern Illinois University Press, 2000); John Harley Warner, *Against the Spirit of System: The French Impulse in Nineteenth-Century American Medicine* (Baltimore: Johns Hopkins University Press, 2003 [1998]); James C. Whorton, *Nature Cures: The History of Alternative Medicine in America* (Oxford: Oxford University Press, 2002).

15. Warner, *The Therapeutic Perspective*, 38.
16. Warner, *The Therapeutic Perspective*, 38; Bruce A. Kimball, *The "True Professional Ideal" in America: A History* (Lanham, MD: Rowman & Littlefield, 1995), 186.
17. Kenneth Allen De Ville, *Medical Malpractice in Nineteenth-Century America: Origins and Legacy* (New York: New York University Press, 1990), 23–24.
18. Theodric Romeyn Beck, *Elements of Medical Jurisprudence*, vol. 1 (Albany, NY: Websters and Skinners, 1823), v.
19. Beck, *Elements of Medical Jurisprudence*, xxiii, xxxiii.
20. Mohr, *Doctors and the Law*, 20.
21. Mohr, *Doctors and the Law*, 42.
22. Mohr, *Doctors and the Law*, 237.
23. Beck, *Elements of Medical Jurisprudence*, vii.
24. "Art. II.—Medical Jurisprudence," *The Law Magazine; or, Quarterly Review of Jurisprudence*, vol. 1, 2nd ed. (London: Saunders and Benning, 1830), 507.
25. [John Hooker] Ashmun, "Art. VI.—Medical Jurisprudence. No. 1," *The American Jurist and Law Magazine* 13, no. 26 (April 1835): 333. Ashmun's work on medical jurisprudence was primarily published postmortem. Joseph Story, "Art. II.—Mr. Justice Story's Funeral Discourse on Professor Ashmun," *The American Jurist and Law Magazine* 10, no. 19 (July 1833): 40–52.
26. Ashmun, "Art. VI.—Medical Jurisprudence," 333.
27. Ashmun, "Art. VI.—Medical Jurisprudence," 335.
28. I. R., "Article III.—Medical Evidence," *The American Jurist and Law Magazine* 24, no. 48 (January 1841): 294.
29. On medical expert witnessing in the nineteenth century, see Joel Peter Eigen, "The Witness Takes the Stand," in *Mad-Doctors in the Dock: Defending the Diagnosis, 1760–1913* (Baltimore: Johns Hopkins University Press, 2016), 89–109; Joel Peter Eigen, "Medical Testimony in Insanity Trials, I: How the Prisoner Met the Doctor," and "Medical Testimony in Insanity Trials, II: What the Mad-Doctor Said in Court," in *Witnessing Insanity: Madness and Mad-Doctors in the English Court* (New Haven, CT: Yale University Press, 1995), 108–132 and 133–160; Mohr, *Doctors and the Law*, 94–108. See also Tal Golan, *Laws of Men and Laws of Nature: The History of Scientific Expert Testimony in England and America* (Cambridge, MA: Harvard University Press, 2004).
30. At Albany Medical College, for example, Chitty's text was taught alongside the works of Beck, Michael Ryan, and Isaac Ray on medical jurisprudence. *Circular of the Trustees and Faculty of Medicine of the Albany Medical College* (Albany, NY: Alfred Southwick, 1838), 19, in *A Collection of Pamphlets and Magazines, from the Press of J. Munsell, Albany, New York*, vol. 4 (Albany, NY: Joel Munsell, 1848), New York State Library, Manuscripts and Archives, Albany, NY.
31. Joseph Chitty, *A Practical Treatise on Medical Jurisprudence: With So Much of Anatomy, Physiology, Pathology, and the Practice of Medicine and Surgery, as Are Essential to Be Known by Members of Parliament, Lawyers, Coroners, Magistrates, Officers in the Army and Navy, and Private Gentlemen; and all the Laws Relating to Medical Practitioners*, Part I (London: Butterworth; Longman, Rees, Orme, Brown, and Green; S. Highley; J. Taylor; Burgess and Hill; Churchill; and H. Renshaw, 1834), 248; emphasis in the original.
32. Chitty, *A Practical Treatise on Medical Jurisprudence*, 253.
33. Chitty, *A Practical Treatise on Medical Jurisprudence*, 255; emphasis in the original.

34. Chitty, *A Practical Treatise on Medical Jurisprudence*, 255.
35. Isaac Ray and his work have been well explored by John Starrett Hughes and Kenneth J. Weiss, including the extent of Ray's attachment to phrenology. John Starrett Hughes, *In the Law's Darkness: Isaac Ray and the Medical Jurisprudence of Insanity in Nineteenth-Century America* (New York: Oceana Publications, 1986); Kenneth J. Weiss, "Epilepsy and Homicide: Issac Ray [*sic*] on Mitigation," *Journal of Psychiatry & Law* 36, no. 2 (2008): 171–209; Weiss, "Isaac Ray's Affair with Phrenology"; Weiss, "Isaac Ray at 200"; Kenneth J. Weiss, "Isaac Ray, Malpractice Defendant," *Journal of the American Academy of Psychiatry and Law* 41, no. 3 (2003): 382–390; Kenneth J. Weiss, "Psychiatry for the General Practitioner: Isaac Ray's Jefferson Lectures, 1871 to 1873," *Journal of Nervous and Mental Disease* 200, no. 12 (2012): 1047–1053.
36. Isaac Ray to John Neal, July 12, 1869, Series 1, Box 3, Folder 3, Isaac Ray letters, Coll. 2125, Maine Historical Society, Portland, ME.
37. Isaac Ray to John Neal, July 12, 1869.
38. This essay was commonly attributed to Ray, although the original journal article does not name Ray as its writer. Hughes, *In the Law's Darkness*, 26, 28.
39. "Article IV. The Case of Major Mitchell," 303.
40. "Article IV. The Case of Major Mitchell," 307.
41. "Article IV. The Case of Major Mitchell," 308.
42. "Article IV. The Case of Major Mitchell," 309.
43. "Medical Institute of Philadelphia," *Philadelphia Journal of the Medical and Physical Sciences* 2, no. 4 (October 1825): 418.
44. Caldwell was one of the earliest American lecturers on medical jurisprudence, beginning in Philadelphia in 1810. Beck, *Elements of Medical Jurisprudence*, xxxii; William Shainline Middleton, "Charles Caldwell, A Biographic Sketch," in *Annals of Medical History*, vol. 3, ed. Francis R. Packard (New York: Paul B. Hoeber, 1921), 171; Mohr, *Doctors and the Law*, 8–9, 29.
45. Charles Caldwell, "Art. I—Phrenology Vindicated, in Remarks on Article III. of the July Number, 1833, of the North American Review, headed 'Phrenology,'" *Annals of Phrenology* 1, no. 1 (October 1833): 88, 89.
46. George Combe, *Notes on the United States of North America, during a Phrenological Visit in 1838–9–10*, vol. 1 (Philadelphia: Carey & Hart, 1841), 71–73.
47. On Dean, see Mohr, *Doctors and the Law*, 35–36.
48. This was an organization that Dean helped to found in 1833 and for which he served as president for the first two years of its existence. Amos Dean, *Lectures on Phrenology* (Albany, NY: Oliver Steele, 1834), vi; New England Historic Genealogical Society, *Memorial Biographies of the New England Historic Genealogical Society*, vol. 6 (Boston: Stanhope Press, 1905), 266; "Article VI. [Review of *The Philosophy of Human Life*]," *The American Phrenological Journal and Miscellany* 2, no. 9 (June 1840): 420.
49. Amos Dean, *The Philosophy of Human Life: Being an Investigation of the Great Elements of Life . . .* (Boston: Marsh, Capen, Lyon and Webb: 1839); "Article VI. [Review of *The Philosophy of Human Life*]."
50. "The Albany Law School," *American Phrenological Journal and Life Illustrated* 44, no. 1 (July 1866): 22.
51. A. Dean, "Article V. Medical Jurisprudence of Insanity," *The American Phrenological Journal and Miscellany* 2, no. 1 (October 1839): 33–41; A. Dean, "Article III. Medical Jurisprudence of Insanity.—No. 2," *The American Phrenological Journal and Miscellany* 2, no. 2 (November 1839): 67–75; Amos Dean, "Article II. Medical

Jurisprudence of Insanity—No. 3," *The American Phrenological Journal and Miscellany* 2, no. 3 (December 1839): 111–116.

52. Dean also corresponded with Nahum Capen. Capen Letters. Amos Dean to Nahum Capen, September 29, 1838, Box 1, Folder 20, Nahum Capen papers, 1783–1885 (inclusive), 1826–1885 (bulk), B MS c23, Boston Medical Library, Francis A. Countway Library of Medicine, Boston, MA (hereafter cited as Capen Letters).
53. In 1851, Dean founded Albany Law School, and he later became the first president of the University of Iowa. Beck was not a member of the faculty or staff in the original 1838 circular of the college. In the 1840 circular, he was listed as a curator, and in 1843 he was both the college librarian and Professor of Materia Medica. While his book was assigned in the medical jurisprudence course, it was Amos Dean who taught this course. *Circular of the Trustees and Faculty of Medicine of the Albany Medical College* (1838), 10, 19; *Catalogue and Circular of the Albany Medical College* (Albany, NY: Joel Munsell, 1840): n.p. [front matter]; *Catalogue and Circular of the Albany Medical College* (Albany, NY: J. Munsell, 1843), n.p. [front matter], 12, in *A Collection of Pamphlets and Magazines, from the Press of J. Munsell, Albany, New York*, vol. 4 (Albany, NY: Joel Munsell, 1848), New York State Library, Manuscripts and Archives, Albany, NY. See also John C. Gerber, *A Pictorial History of the University of Iowa* (Iowa City: University of Iowa Press, 2005), 10; Mohr, *Doctors and the Law*, 36.
54. Dean to Capen, September 29, 1838, Capen Letters.
55. Amos Dean, *Principles of Medical Jurisprudence: Designed for the Professions of Law and Medicine* (Albany, NY: Banks & Brothers, 1850); Mohr, *Doctors and the Law*, 37. John S. Haller Jr. has noted that at the Worcester Medical Institution in 1851–1852, the two authors taught on medical jurisprudence were T. R. Beck and Amos Dean; the author suggests this curriculum "did not deviate to any great degree from other colleges—both regular and sectarian." John S. Haller Jr., *Kindly Medicine: Physio-Medicalism in America, 1836–1911* (Kent, OH: Kent State University Press, 1997), 56–57.
56. For an overview of the development of the medical jurisprudence of insanity, see Blumenthal, *Law and the Modern Mind*, 59–86. See also Joel Peter Eigen, *Unconscious Crime: Mental Absence and Criminal Responsibility in Victorian London* (Baltimore: Johns Hopkins University Press, 2003); Eigen, *Witnessing Insanity*; Roger Smith, *Trial by Medicine: Insanity and Responsibility in Victorian Trials* (Edinburgh: Edinburgh University Press, 1981); Charles E. Rosenberg, *The Trial of the Assassin Guiteau: Psychiatry and the Law in the Gilded Age* (Chicago: University of Chicago Press, 1976 [1968]).
57. Eric T. Carlson and Norman Dain, "The Meaning of Moral Insanity," *Bulletin of the History of Medicine* 36, no. 2 (1962): 132; Hughes, *In the Law's Darkness*, 43. On moral insanity, see also Lawrence B. Goodheart, "Murder and Madness: The Ambiguity of Moral Insanity in Nineteenth-Century Connecticut," in *Murder on Trial, 1620–2002*, ed. Robert Asher, Lawrence B. Goodheart, and Alan Rogers (Albany, NY: State University of New York Press, 2005), 135–154.
58. Carlson and Dain, "The Meaning of Moral Insanity," 132–133.
59. Hughes, *In the Law's Darkness*, 43; J. G. Spurzheim, *Observations on the Deranged Manifestations of the Mind, or Insanity* (London: Baldwin, Cradock, and Joy, 1817); [Johann] G. Spurzheim, *Observations sur la folie* (Paris: Treuttel et Würtz, 1818).
60. Carlson and Dain, "The Meaning of Moral Insanity," 134.

61. James Cowles Prichard, *Treatise on Insanity and Other Disorders Affecting the Mind* (London: Sherwood, Gilbert, and Piper, 1835).
62. Hughes, *In the Law's Darkness*, 42–43.
63. After his death, Prichard was remembered far more fondly, if somewhat disingenuously, by the *American Phrenological Journal*. "Phrenology: Dr. Prichard and Phrenology," *American Phrenological Journal* 19, no. 3 (March 1854): 49–51.
64. Andrew Combe, "I. Remarks on Dr. Prichard's Third Attack on Phrenology, in his 'Treatise on Insanity,'" *The Phrenological Journal and Magazine of Moral Science* 9, no. 57 (London: Simpkin, Marshall, and Co., 1838): 345.
65. Combe, "I. Remarks on Dr. Prichard's Third Attack," 345.
66. David Hoffman, *A Course of Legal Study, Addressed to Students and the Professional Generally*, vol. 2, 2nd ed. (Baltimore: Joseph Neal, 1836), 702; emphasis in the original.
67. "Moral Insanity," *Salem Gazette*, November 11, 1838.
68. G. P., "Insanity," *The Boston Medical and Surgical Journal* 14, no. 16 (May 1836): 1–8.
69. Hughes, *In the Law's Darkness*, 42.
70. Hughes, *In the Law's Darkness*, 42–44.
71. Hughes, *In the Law's Darkness*, 20–26.
72. Hughes, *In the Law's Darkness*, 21–23.
73. Hughes, *In the Law's Darkness*, 19.
74. Weiss, "Isaac Ray's Affair with Phrenology"; Weiss, "Isaac Ray at 200," 344.
75. Hughes, *In the Law's Darkness*, 31–32.
76. Others have framed Ray's theories as influenced by phrenology. See, for example, Andrew W. Arpey, *The William Freeman Murder Trial: Insanity, Politics, and Race* (Syracuse, NY: Syracuse University Press, 2003), 46; Nicole Rafter, *The Criminal Brain: Understanding Biological Theories of Crime* (New York: New York University Press, 2008), 55.
77. Hughes, *In the Law's Darkness*, 44.
78. I. Ray, *A Treatise on the Medical Jurisprudence of Insanity* (Boston: Charles C. Little and James Brown, 1838), 68.
79. Ray, *A Treatise on the Medical Jurisprudence of Insanity*, 74–75.
80. Ray, *A Treatise on the Medical Jurisprudence of Insanity*, 75.
81. Ray, *A Treatise on the Medical Jurisprudence of Insanity*, 77, 104.
82. Ray, *A Treatise on the Medical Jurisprudence of Insanity*, 187–190.
83. Ray, *A Treatise on the Medical Jurisprudence of Insanity*, 197; emphasis in the original.
84. Ray, *A Treatise on the Medical Jurisprudence of Insanity*, 199.
85. Ray, *A Treatise on the Medical Jurisprudence of Insanity*, 201–204, 212–213, 216–217.
86. Ray, *A Treatise on the Medical Jurisprudence of Insanity*, 207, 218.
87. Ray, *A Treatise on the Medical Jurisprudence of Insanity*, 229, 230.
88. Ray, *A Treatise on the Medical Jurisprudence of Insanity*, 231, 232.
89. Ray, *A Treatise on the Medical Jurisprudence of Insanity*, 229; emphasis in the original.
90. Ray, *A Treatise on the Medical Jurisprudence of Insanity*, 207.
91. Dr. J. [*sic*] Ray, "Art. I—Criminal Law of Insanity," *The American Jurist and Law Magazine* 14, no. 28 (October 1835): 253–274.
92. G. T. C., "Art. VII.—Criminal Law of Insanity," 92.

93. G. T. C., "Art. VII.—Criminal Law of Insanity," 93.
94. G. T. C., "Art. VII.—Criminal Law of Insanity," 94.
95. J. R., "Art. II—Criminal Law of Insanity. Reply to the remarks of G.T.C. in the Jurist No. XXIX. on a 'Lecture on the Criminal Law of Insanity,' by Dr. J. Ray, in No. XXVIII," *The American Jurist and Law Magazine* 16, no. 31 (October 1836): 58.
96. The expert witnesses who used phrenology as a component of their testimony were typically physicians, though some practical phrenologists also served as expert witnesses, as will be addressed in the next chapter.
97. Haggerty also murdered Fordney's wife and injured one of their four children during his attack, while the oldest son ran for help, but he was only tried for the murder of Melchoir Fordney. Ellis Grosh Lewis and Emanuel Jacob Schaeffer, *Report of The Trial and Conviction of John Haggerty, for The Murder of Melchoir Fordney, Late of The City of Lancaster, Pennsylvania* (Lancaster, PA, 1847), 7.
98. On the insanity defense, see Andrea L. Alden, *Disorder in the Court: Morality, Myth, and the Insanity Defense* (Tuscaloosa: University of Alabama Press, 2018); Richard Moran, "The Modern Foundation for the Insanity Defense: The Cases of James Hadfield (1800) and Daniel McNaughtan (1843)," *Annals of the American Academy of Political and Social Science* 477, no. 1 (1985): 31–42; Daniel N. Robinson, *Wild Beasts & Idle Humours: The Insanity Defense from Antiquity to the Present* (Cambridge, MA: Harvard University Press, 1996); Alan Rogers, "Mad Men and Wronged Women: Murder and the Insanity Defense in Massachusetts, 1844–2000," in *Murder on Trial, 1620–2002*, ed. Robert Asher, Lawrence B. Goodheart, and Alan Rogers (Albany: State University of New York Press, 2005), 155–182; Smith, *Trial by Medicine.*
99. Lewis and Schaeffer, *Report of The Trial and Conviction of John Haggerty*, 18; emphasis in the original.
100. Lewis and Schaeffer, *Report of The Trial and Conviction of John Haggerty*, 19.
101. Lewis and Schaeffer, *Report of The Trial and Conviction of John Haggerty*, 19.
102. Lewis and Schaeffer, *Report of The Trial and Conviction of John Haggerty*, 19.
103. Lewis and Schaeffer, *Report of The Trial and Conviction of John Haggerty*, 19; emphasis in the original.
104. The closest analogy to this case for this time period would be that of Phineas Gage, the railway worker who, after an iron rod entered through his skull and brain, experienced a massive change of personality, veering towards aggression. However, Gage's accident (and his subsequent fame in both popular culture and scientific theory) occurred in September 1848, a year and a half *after* Haggerty's trial: the defense attorney did not have the benefit of a famous case to support his claims. To my knowledge, the Haggerty case was not cited in accounts of Phineas Gage or similar brain injuries. Malcolm Macmillan, *An Odd Kind of Fame: Stories of Phineas Gage* (Cambridge, MA: MIT Press, 2000), 11–13.
105. Lewis and Schaeffer, *Report of The Trial and Conviction of John Haggerty*, 41.
106. Lewis and Schaeffer, *Report of The Trial and Conviction of John Haggerty*, 42.
107. In 1848, the *American Phrenological Journal* published an account by an unknown author of the phrenological developments of John Haggerty. However, this short profile made no mention of the injury to the skull or of the use of phrenology in the trial. "Article XLII. John Haggerty, Murderer of Melchoir Fordney—Executed at Lancaster, PA., July 24, 1847," *American Phrenological Journal* 10, no. 7 (July 1848): 212.
108. *Nancy Farrer v. The State of Ohio*, 2 Ohio St. 54 (1853).
109. *Nancy Farrer v. The State of Ohio.*
110. *Nancy Farrer v. The State of Ohio.*

111. *Nancy Farrer v. The State of Ohio.*
112. Parker's use of phrenological language seems to tie him politically to American phrenologists, who were commonly associated with reformist causes. However, other newspaper articles described Parker as "the great apologist for slavery" and a prominent pro-slavery advocate. See H. W. Davison, "Ecclesiastical Juggling," *The Liberator* (Boston, MA), October 5, 1838.
113. The context of these charges to the jury was never made clear in these articles, nor were the details of the trial at hand addressed in this long discourse.
114. "Court of Common Pleas. Charge," *New Hampshire Patriot and State Gazette* (Concord, NH), October 15, 1838.
115. "Court of Common Pleas. Charge."
116. "Court of Common Pleas. Charge."
117. "Charge to the Grand Jury," *New Hampshire Patriot and State Gazette* (Concord, NH), October 22, 1838.
118. While Prichard did, at times, make use of the language of propensity in his text, it was primarily as a citation of other authors. Moreover, Spurzheim's use of the language of propensity predates the publication of Prichard's work. This was part of the reason why phrenological critics of Prichard assessed him as a phrenologist, even though he was openly hostile to phrenology. "Charge to the Grand Jury," *New Hampshire Patriot and State Gazette* (Concord, NH), October 29, 1838.
119. Combe, *Notes on the United States of North America*, 1:125. Correspondence suggests that Woodward also published on the subject of insanity with Marsh, Capen & Lyon in the 1830s, although it is possible that the project never came to fruition, given the difficulty of finding a copy of one of his works with this imprint. Samuel Bayard Woodward to Marsh, Capen & Lyon, April 6, 1835, Capen Letters.
120. "Charge to the Grand Jury," October 29, 1838.
121. "Charge to the Grand Jury," October 29, 1838.
122. "Criminal Jurisprudence," *The American Phrenological Journal and Miscellany* 3, no. 6 (March 1841): 288.
123. "Criminal Jurisprudence."
124. Combe, *Notes on the United States of North America*, 1:124–125; Charles Gibbon, *The Life of George Combe, author of the "Constitution of Man," in two volumes*, vol. 2 (London: Macmillan and Co., 1878), 101, 113.
125. Combe, *Notes on the United States of North America*, 1:124.
126. Combe, *Notes on the United States of North America*, 1:125.
127. *Brock, Appellant, v. Luckett's Executors*, 5 Miss. 459 (1840).
128. *Brock, Appellant, v. Luckett's Executors.*
129. *Brock, Appellant, v. Luckett's Executors.*
130. *Brock, Appellant, v. Luckett's Executors.*
131. While I have identified a number of cases that cite Ray or use the language of propensity, court cases were not regularly transcribed in the nineteenth century. The records that exist were often published at the behest of counsel or were based on newspaper accounts; personal interest, profit, and sensationalism all informed these records. It is possible that many more cases made use of Ray or phrenological theories than those discussed here.
132. On the M'Naghten trial and Rules, see Alden, *Disorder in the Court*, 32–47; Moran, "The Modern Foundation for the Insanity Defense," 37–41; Richard Moran, *Knowing Right from Wrong: The Insanity Defense of Daniel McNaughtan* (New York: Free Press, 1981); Rogers, "Mad Men and Wronged Women," 156–157; Rosenberg, *The*

Trial of the Assassin Guiteau, 54–56; Smith, *Trial by Medicine*, 14–18; Donald J. West and Alexander Walk, eds., *Daniel McNaughton: His Trial and the Aftermath* (Ashford, UK: Headley for the "British Journal of Psychiatry," 1977). I have chosen to spell the name "M'Naghten," following Rosenberg. Rosenberg, *Trial of the Assassin Guiteau*, 54.

133. Bernard L. Diamond, "Isaac Ray and the Trial of Daniel M'Naghten," *American Journal of Psychiatry* 112, no. 8 (1956): 652–654.
134. Benjamin F. Hall, *The Trial of William Freeman for the Murder of John G. Van Nest, Including the Evidence and the Arguments of Counsel . . .* (Auburn, NY: Derby, Miller & Co. Publishers, 1848), 219–222.
135. Hall, *The Trial of William Freeman*, 497–500, 502–506. On the Freeman trial, see Arpey, *The William Freeman Murder Trial.*
136. C. W. Crozier and A. R. M'Kee, *Life and Trial of Dr. Abner Baker, Jr., (A Monomaniac,) Who Was Executed October 3, 1845 . . .* (Louisville, KY: Prentice and Weissinger, 1846), vi.
137. Crozier and M'Kee, *Life and Trial of Dr. Abner Baker, Jr.*, 56.
138. Crozier and M'Kee, *Life and Trial of Dr. Abner Baker, Jr.*, 57–60.
139. This discussion also included some references to Lexington (i.e., "Lexington Doctors"), the site of Transylvania University, Charles Caldwell's institution, as the cause for accusations of phrenological sympathy. Crozier and M'Kee, *Life and Trial of Dr. Abner Baker, Jr.*, 50–51.
140. Crozier and M'Kee, *Life and Trial of Dr. Abner Baker, Jr.*, 56.
141. T. C. Leland, *Trial of John Metcalf Thurston, Convicted of the Murder of Anson Garrison . . .* (Owego, NY: Hiram A. Beebe, 1851), 13–14.
142. Defendant's Counsel, *Trial of Charles B. Huntington for Forgery: Principle Defence: Insanity* (New York: John S. Voorhies, 1857), 244.
143. Defendant's Counsel, *Trial of Charles B. Huntington for Forgery*, ix, 324, 338–341, 420, 424.
144. M. Gonzalez Echeverria, *The Trial of "John Reynolds," Medico-legally Considered* (New York: Baker & Godwin, Printers, 1870), 10.
145. John Delafield, *The Law of Circumstantial Evidence and of Insanity: A Report in Full of the Trial of Edward D. Worrell, Indicted for the Murder of Basil H. Gordon . . .* (St. Louis: M. Niedner, 1857), 65.
146. Delafield, *The Law of Circumstantial Evidence and of Insanity*, 65.
147. I. Ray, "Hints to the Medical Witness in Questions of Insanity," *American Journal of Psychiatry* 8, no. 1 (April 1851): 53–67.
148. H. H. McFarland, *Report of the Trial of Willard Clark, Indicted for the Murder of Richard W. Wight . . .* (New Haven, CT: Thomas H. Pease, 1855), 76.
149. McFarland, *Report of the Trial of Willard Clark*, 214; emphasis in the original.
150. Coventry also testified in the Freeman murder trial, alongside other medical witnesses, including John McCall and Amariah Brigham, who also used phrenology in their testimony. Arpey, *The William Freeman Murder Trial*, 75–76.
151. Bowen Whiting, *Report of the Trial of Henry Wyatt, a Convict in the State Prison at Auburn, Indicted for the Murder of James Gordon, Another Convict within the Prison* (New York: J. C. Derby & Co., 1846), 27.
152. Benn Pitman, *The Assassination of President Lincoln and the Trial of the Conspirators* (New York: Moore, Wilstach & Baldwin, 1865), 162.
153. J. H. Balfour Browne, *The Medical Jurisprudence of Insanity*, 2nd ed. (Philadelphia: Lindsay & Blakiston, 1876), 347.

154. Recent examples of phrases like "propensity to commit a crime," "propensity to steal," and "propensity for violence," appear in newspapers from the *New York Times* to my local newspaper. There are also many examples in popular media, particularly crime dramas and true crime novels. For example, see Dan Bilefsky and Ian Austen, "Toronto Van Attack Suspect Expressed Anger at Women," *New York Times*, April 24, 2018.

4. The Prison as Laboratory

1. "Article V. Phrenological Developments and Character of William Miller, Who Was Executed at Williamsport, PA., July 27th, 1838 for the Murder of Solomon Hoffman," *The American Phrenological Journal and Miscellany* 1, no. 8 (1839): 272–286.
2. "Article V. Phrenological Developments and Character of William Miller," 278.
3. "Article V. Phrenological Developments and Character of William Miller," 273.
4. "Article V. Phrenological Developments and Character of William Miller," 274; emphasis in the original.
5. "Article V. Phrenological Developments and Character of William Miller," 274.
6. "Article V. Phrenological Developments and Character of William Miller," 277; emphasis in the original.
7. "Article V. Phrenological Developments and Character of William Miller," 278; emphasis in the original.
8. *The American Law Register* addressed this case two decades later, for example, as part of a discussion of the insanity plea and the difficulty of assessing it in court. "The Plea of Insanity," *The American Law Register* 4, no. 12 (October 1856): 709–710.
9. For an overview of the history of this dispute, see Fenneke Sysling, "Science and Self-Assessment: Phrenological Charts 1840–1940," *British Journal for the History of Science* 51, no. 2 (2018): 262–265, 262n4. See also Roger Cooter, *The Cultural Meaning of Popular Science* (Cambridge: Cambridge University Press, 1984); Cynthia Eagle Russett, *Sexual Science: The Victorian Construction of Womanhood* (Cambridge, MA: Harvard University Press, 1989), 19–22; Steven Shapin, "Phrenological Knowledge and the Social Structure of Early Nineteenth-Century Edinburgh," *Annals of Science* 32, no. 3 (1975): 219–243.
10. John van Wyhe, "Was Phrenology a Reform Science? Towards a New Generalization for Phrenology," *History of Science* 42, no. 3 (2004): 316, 318.
11. James Poskett, *Materials of the Mind: Phrenology, Race, and the Global History of Science, 1815–1920* (Chicago: University of Chicago Press, 2019), 116–117.
12. "Article VII: The Phrenological Character of John C. Colt.—Capital Punishment," *The American Phrenological Journal and Miscellany* 4, no. 10 (October 1842): 314.
13. Frank Morn, *Forgotten Reformer: Robert McClaughry and Criminal Justice Reform in Nineteenth-Century America* (Lanham, MD: University Press of America, 2011), xi–xiv; David J. Rothman, *The Discovery of the Asylum: Social Order and Disorder in the New Republic* (New York: Aldine de Gruyter, 2002 [1971]), 48–56.
14. Morn, *Forgotten Reformer*, xiv; Steven Mintz, *Moralists and Modernizers: America's Pre–Civil War Reformers* (Baltimore: Johns Hopkins University Press, 1995), 86–87.
15. On the emergence of the penitentiary and debates about the Auburn versus Pennsylvania system in this period, see Thomas G. Blomberg and Karol Lucken, "Age of the Penitentiary in Nineteenth-Century America (1830–1870s)," in *American Penology: A History of Control*, 2nd ed. (New Brunswick, NJ: Transaction Publishers, 2017 [2010]), 48–57; Scott Christianson, *With Liberty for Some: 500 Years of Imprisonment in*

America (Boston: Northeastern University Press, 1998), 110–120, 132–138, 141–149; Mark Colvin, *Penitentiaries, Reformatories, and Chain Gangs: Social Theory and the History of Punishment in Nineteenth-Century America* (New York: St. Martin's Press, 1997), 82–99; Jennifer Lawrence Janofsky, "'Hopelessly Hardened': The Complexities of Penitentiary Discipline at Philadelphia's Eastern State Penitentiary," in *Buried Lives: Incarcerated in Early America*, ed. Michele Lise Tarter and Richard Bell (Athens: University of Georgia Press, 2012), 106–123; Norman Johnston, "Great Expectations: Prison Reform in North America until the Mid-Nineteenth Century," in *Forms of Constraint: A History of Prison Architecture* (Urbana: University of Illinois Press, 2000), 67–87; Paul Kahan, "The Pennsylvania System, 1829–1866," in *Seminary of Virtue: The Ideology and Practice of Inmate Reform at Eastern State Penitentiary, 1829–1971* (New York: Peter Lang, 2012), 21–52; Mark E. Kann, "Penitentiary Punishment," in *Punishment, Prisons, and Patriarchy: Liberty and Power in the Early American Republic* (New York: New York University Press, 2005), 130–150; W. David Lewis, "The Auburn System and Its Champions," in *From Newgate to Dannemora: The Rise of the Penitentiary in New York, 1796–1848* (Ithaca, NY: Cornell University Press, 2009 [1965]), 81–110; Michael Meranze, *Laboratories of Virtue: Punishment, Revolution, and Authority in Philadelphia, 1760–1835* (Williamsburg, VA: The Institute of Early American History and Culture, 1996), 254–265; Martin B. Miller, "Sinking Gradually into the Proletariat: The Emergence of the Penitentiary in the United States," *Crime and Social Justice* 14 (1980): 37–43; Mintz, *Moralists and Modernizers*, 86–88; Janet Miron, *Prisons, Asylums, and the Public: Institutional Visiting in the Nineteenth Century* (Toronto: University of Toronto Press, 2011), 45–47; Rothman, *The Discovery of the Asylum*, 79–108; David J. Rothman, "Perfecting the Prison: United States, 1789–1865," in *The Oxford History of the Prison: The Practice of Punishment in Western Society*, ed. Norval Morris and David J. Rothman (New York: Oxford University Press, 1998): 100–116; Negley K. Teeters and John D. Shearer, *The Prison at Philadelphia, Cherry Hill: The Separate System of Penal Discipline, 1829–1913* (New York: Columbia University Press, 1957), 3–32, 201–212.

16. Mintz, *Moralists and Modernizers*, 86–87; Morn, *Forgotten Reformer*, xiv–xv.
17. Mintz, *Moralists and Modernizers*, 80.
18. Meranze, *Laboratories of Virtue*, 254–255. Rothman notes that the most famous European reports on these systems were Gustave de Beaumont and Alexis de Tocqueville's *Du système pénitentiaire aux États-Unis et de son application en France* [On the penitentiary system in the United States and its application in France] (1833) and Charles Dickens's *American Notes* (1850): Rothman, "Perfecting the Prison," 116. Poskett addresses the global nature of this debate: Poskett, *Materials of the Mind*, 131–136; James Poskett, "Phrenology, Correspondence, and the Global Politics of Reform, 1815–1848," *The Historical Journal* 60, no. 2 (2017): 409–442.
19. Meranze, *Laboratories of Virtue*, 255–265.
20. Blomberg and Lucken, *American Penology*, 44.
21. On phrenology and prison reform, see also Nicole Rafter, *The Criminal Brain: Understanding Biological Theories of Crime* (New York: New York University Press, 2008), 53–55.
22. Samuel Gridley Howe, a phrenological enthusiast, for example, wrote on the distinctions between the two systems, advocating in particular for the Pennsylvania system. Samuel Gridley Howe, *An Essay on Separate and Congregate Systems of Prison Discipline* (Boston: William D. Ticknor and Co., 1846), xi.

23. "What is the Use of It?," *American Phrenological Journal and Life Illustrated* 47, no. 2 (February 1868): 69.
24. "Are Murderers All Bad?," *American Phrenological Journal and Life Illustrated* 37, no. 3 (March 1863): 65.
25. "Responsibility. Cranial Defects in Criminal Classes," *American Phrenological Journal and Life Illustrated* 49, no. 11 (November 1869): 426–427.
26. "Morbid Activity of Destructiveness," *The American Phrenological Journal and Miscellany* 2, no. 8 (May 1840): 378.
27. "Palmer's Phrenological Developments. Examination by Mr. Bridges," *Liverpool Mercury* (Liverpool, UK), June 16, 1856.
28. Cooter, *The Cultural Meaning of Popular Science*, 124–125; Ronald G. Walters, *American Reformers 1815–1860* (New York: Hill and Wang, 1978), 196–200.
29. James Haughton, "Statistics of Crime," *The Prisoner's Friend, A Monthly Magazine* 4, no. 1 (September 1851): 16.
30. "Treatment of the Criminal," *The Hangman* 1, no. 33 (November 1845): 129.
31. L. Maria Child, *Letters from New-York* (New York: Charles S. Francis and Company, 1843), 55. Child herself was phrenologically examined by Lorenzo Fowler. Madeleine B. Stern, *Heads & Headlines: The Phrenological Fowlers* (Norman: University of Oklahoma Press, 1971), 21.
32. On Farnham, see Anne A. Clothier, "Prisons, Petticoats and Phrenology: Eliza Farnham and Reform at Sing Sing Prison, 1844–1848" (MA thesis, State University of New York College at Oneonta, 2007); Janet Floyd, "Dislocations of the Self: Eliza Farnham at Sing Sing Prison," *Journal of American Studies* 40, no. 2 (2006): 311–325.
33. Floyd, "Dislocations of the Self," 313–314.
34. Floyd, "Dislocations of the Self," 313–314.
35. Floyd, "Dislocations of the Self," 314.
36. "Phrenology in the United States Prisons," *The Phrenological Journal and Magazine of Moral Science* 19, no. 87 (Edinburgh, April 1846): 198–199; Stern, *Heads & Headlines*, 40–41.
37. Floyd, "Dislocations of the Self," 323.
38. Spear did not specify which Fowler brother this was. Charles Spear, "Letter from the Senior Editor," *Prisoner's Friend* 1, no. 21 (May 1846): 82.
39. Stanley Finger, *Minds Behind the Brain: A History of the Pioneers and their Discoveries* (Oxford: Oxford University Press, 2000), 132–135; Stanley Finger, *Origins of Neuroscience: A History of Explorations into Brain Function* (New York: Oxford University Press, 1994), 34–36; Stanley Finger and Paul Eling, *Franz Joseph Gall: Naturalist of the Mind, Visionary of the Brain* (New York: New York University Press, 2019), 454–462.
40. Finger, *Minds Behind the Brain*, 132–135; Finger, *Origins of Neuroscience*, 34–36.
41. Finger, *Origins of Neuroscience*, 34–36, 52.
42. See W. F. Bynum, *Science and the Practice of Medicine in the Nineteenth Century* (Cambridge: Cambridge University Press, 1994), 46–54; John Harley Warner, *Against the Spirit of System: The French Impulse in Nineteenth-Century American Medicine* (Baltimore: Johns Hopkins University Press, 2003 [1998]), 3–5; James C. Mohr, *Doctors and the Law: Medical Jurisprudence in Nineteenth-Century America* (Baltimore: Johns Hopkins University Press, 1996 [1993]), 49. On the Paris clinic, see also Erwin H. Ackerknecht, *Medicine at the Paris Hospital, 1794–1848* (Baltimore: Johns Hopkins University Press, 1967); Michel Foucault, *The Birth of the Clinic: An*

Archeology of Medical Perception, trans. A. M. Sheridan Smith (New York: Vintage Books, 1994 [1973]).

43. The Society faded from view around 1840. The sale of the cabinet and its subsequent donation to Harvard in the late 1840s signaled its definitive end. Stephen Tomlinson, *Head Masters: Phrenology, Secular Education, and Nineteenth-Century Social Thought* (Tuscaloosa: University of Alabama Press, 2005), 226.
44. Stern, *Heads & Headlines*, 29–30.
45. Stern, *Heads & Headlines*, 29–30.
46. Stern, *Heads & Headlines*, 29–32.
47. Andrew W. Arpey, *The William Freeman Murder Trial: Insanity, Politics, and Race* (Syracuse, NY: Syracuse University Press, 2003), 47; John D. Davies, *Phrenology, Fad and Science: A 19th-Century American Crusade* (Hamden, CT: Archon Books, 1971 [1955]), 60.
48. "Article I. The American Phrenological Journal for 1849," *The American Phrenological Journal and Miscellany* 11, no. 1 (January 1849): 10. Also cited in Stern, *Heads & Headlines*, 35.
49. "Article IV. Existing Evils and Their Remedy,*—No. I," *The American Phrenological Journal and Miscellany* 4, no. 2 (February 1842): 41; emphasis in the original. Also cited in Daniel Patrick Thurs, *Science Talk: Changing Notions of Science in American Popular Culture* (New Brunswick, NJ: Rutgers University Press, 2007), 29.
50. "Article IV. Existing Evils and Their Remedy," 43; emphasis in the original.
51. The antebellum United States witnessed a broad-based culture of reform on matters as varied as poverty, crime, illiteracy, sex work, and care of the Deaf and blind. For an overview of antebellum reform efforts, see Mintz, *Moralists and Modernizers*.
52. Stern, *Heads & Headlines*, 34–52, 174–176, 228–230; Thurs, *Science Talk*, 29.
53. *Transactions of the Edinburgh Phrenological Society*, vol. 1 (Edinburgh: John Anderson Jr., 1824).
54. "Signs of Civilization," *American Phrenological Journal* 11, no. 11 (November 1849): 355.
55. "Execution in New-York," *American Phrenological Journal* 14, no. 3 (September 1851): 68.
56. The author also highlighted the relationship between John C. Colt and his brother, Samuel Colt, the gun manufacturer, whose "inventions are all destructive—*death-dealing* weapons." "The Phrenological Character of John C. Colt," 313, 314.
57. J. Kenny, "Article V. The Law of Love a Far More Effectual Preventive of Crime Than Punitive Measures, Capital Punishment Included. No. 1," *The American Phrenological Journal and Miscellany* 7, no. 2 (February 1845): 56.
58. Kenny, "Article V. The Law of Love," 57.
59. Other articles in the *American Phrenological Journal* used Christian doctrine to argue against the practice of hanging. This Christian "law of love" itself was also described elsewhere as "founded in *a law of mind*," connecting Christian theology to phrenology. "'Hang Him,'" *American Phrenological Journal* 10, no. 7 (July 1848): 225; "The Law of Kindness," *The American Phrenological Journal and Miscellany* 6, no. 12 (December 1845): 413–414. Thurs notes that American phrenologists often used religious language to talk about science, including phrenology. Thurs, *Science Talk*, 43–46.
60. "Article IV. The Law of Love a Far More Effectual Preventive of Crime Than Punitive Measures, Capital Punishment Included. No. 2," *The American Phrenological*

Journal and Miscellany 7, no. 3 (March 1845): 81–86; B. J. G., "Article IV. The Law of Love a Far More Effectual Preventive of Crime Than Punitive Measures, Capital Punishment Included. No. 3," *The American Phrenological Journal and Miscellany* 7, no. 6 (June 1845): 174–177; The Friend of Virtue, "Article III. The Law of Love a Far More Effectual Preventive of Crime Than Punitive Measures, Capital Punishment Included. No. 4," *The American Phrenological Journal and Miscellany* 7, no. 8 (August 1845): 269–273; Lydia M. Child, "Article III. The Law of Love a Far More Effectual Preventive of Crime Than Punitive Measures, Capital Punishment Included. No. V," *The American Phrenological Journal and Miscellany* 6 [*sic*], no. 12 (December 1845): 400–403.

61. L. N. F. [Lorenzo Fowler], [No Title—Reformation of Criminals], *American Phrenological Journal and Life Illustrated* 12, no. 8 (August 1850): 262.
62. "Lecture XIV. Duty of Society in Regard to the Treatment of Criminals," *American Phrenological Journal and Life Illustrated* 34, no. 1 (July 1861): 9–11, 18–19. See also George Combe, *The Constitution of Man Considered in Relation to External Objects*, 3rd ed. (Edinburgh: John Anderson Jr., 1835), 262–263.
63. Combe, *The Constitution of Man*, 3rd ed., 262–263; "Practical Essays. Phrenology, as Applied to the Professions," *American Phrenological Journal* 19, no. 3 (March 1854): 58–59.
64. "Practical Essays," 59.
65. "Moral Responsibility. The Idiotic, Insane, and Violent," *American Phrenological Journal and Life Illustrated* 44, no. 2 (August 1866): 35.
66. "Miscellany. Capital Punishment. Is it so?," *American Phrenological Journal* 12, no. 8 (August 1850): 258.
67. "Practical Essays," 59.
68. "Practical Essays," 59.
69. L. N. F., [No Title—Reformation of Criminals], 262.
70. "Article XXIII. A New, but Effectual Preventive of Crime," *American Phrenological Journal* 12, no. 4 (April 1850): 111.
71. On the influence of phrenology on American religious experimentation during the early to mid-nineteenth century, see Christopher G. White, "Minds Intensely Unsettled: Phrenology, Experience, and the American Pursuit of Spiritual Assurance, 1830–1880," *Religion and American Culture* 16, no. 2 (2006): 227–261.
72. Nahum Capen, *Reminiscences of Dr. Spurzheim and George Combe* (New York: Fowler and Wells, 1881), 23–24.
73. [George Combe], "Article VII. Report of Mr. Combe's Visit to Dublin," in *Illustrations of Phrenology; Being a Selection of Articles from the Edinburg Phrenological Journal, and the Transactions of the Edinburg Phrenological Society*, ed. George H. Calvert (Baltimore: William and Joseph Neal, 1832), 150–176. Among the nine essays reprinted in this collection from the *Transactions* or the Edinburgh *Phrenological Journal*, six were on the subject of murderers, criminals, or prison visits, including accounts of Burke and Hare and the visits of both Combe and Gall to different prisons.
74. George Combe, *Notes on the United States of North America, during a Phrenological Visit in 1838–9–10*, vol. 1 (Philadelphia: Carey & Hart, 1841), 116–117.
75. Combe, *Notes on the United States of North America*, 1:140, 217–227; Poskett, *Materials of the Mind*, 135.
76. Poskett, *Materials of the Mind*, 131–136.

77. "Article IX. Result of an Examination, by Mr. James De Ville, on the Heads of 148 Convicts on Board the Convict Ship England, When About to Sail for New South Wales in the Spring of 1826," in *Illustrations of Phrenology; Being a Selection of Articles from the Edinburg Phrenological Journal, and the Transactions of the Edinburg Phrenological Society*, ed. George H. Calvert (Baltimore: William and Joseph Neal, 1832), 188–189.
78. "Article IX. Result of an Examination," 192.
79. Hubert Lauvergne, *Les forçats considérés sous le rapport physiologique, moral et intellectuel, observés au bagne de Toulon* (Paris: J.-B. Baillière, 1841).
80. L. N. Fowler, Collection of Phrenological Cards, 1834–1835 (B MS b215.1), Boston Medical Library in the Francis A. Countway Library of Medicine, Boston, MA (hereafter cited as Fowler Phrenological Cards).
81. L. N. Fowler, Phrenological Reading of W. V. Leggette, Penn. Penitentiary, Philadelphia, PA, c. April 1835, Fowler Phrenological Cards.
82. L. N. Fowler, Phrenological Reading of Margaret Montgomery, Penn. Penitentiary, Philadelphia, PA, c. April 1835, Fowler Phrenological Cards; L. N. Fowler, Phrenological Reading of Henry Fitz, Indiana Penitentiary, Jeffersonville, IN, July 20, 1835, Fowler Phrenological Cards.
83. Fowler, Phrenological Reading of W. V. Leggette, Fowler Phrenological Cards; L. N. Fowler, Phrenological Reading of Haggerty, Louisville Jail, Louisville, KY, June 8, 1835, Fowler Phrenological Cards. This is not likely the same Haggerty as discussed in chapters 1 and 3.
84. "Article IV. Phrenological Examination of Prisoners," *The American Phrenological Journal and Miscellany* 3, no. 2 (November 1840): 83.
85. N. Sizer, "Article LXVII. L.N. Fowler's Visit to the Tombs," *American Phrenological Journal* 11, no. 9 (October 1849): 317.
86. Sizer, "Article LXVII. L.N. Fowler's Visit to the Tombs," 317
87. "Article IV. Phrenological Examination of Prisoners," 84.
88. F. Coombs, Lecture Broadside (1841), Louise M. Darling Biomedical Library, University of California, Los Angeles, CA.
89. F. Coombs, *Coombs's Popular Phrenology* (Boston, 1841), 114; F. Coombs, Lecture Broadside (1841).
90. Alternately spelled Moselman or Moselmann.
91. "Art. I. Report of a Series of Experiments made by the Medical Faculty of Lancaster, upon the body of Henry Cobler Moselmann, executed in the Jail Yard of Lancaster County, Pa., on the 20th of December, 1839," *The American Journal of the Medical Sciences* 26, no. 51 (May 1840): 27.
92. "Art. I. Report of a Series of Experiments," 29.
93. William B. Fahnestock, "Article V. Phrenological Developments of Henry Cobler Moselman," *The American Phrenological Journal and Miscellany* 2, no. 11 (August 1840): 516–527.
94. Arpey discusses the William Freeman case in great detail, but includes little analysis of the postmortem examination and nothing on Fosgate's findings. Arpey, *The William Freeman Murder Trial*, 139–140.
95. Brigham had been a member of the Boston Phrenological Society and founded the Hartford Phrenological Society in Connecticut. McCall was the president of the Oneida Phrenological Society as well as the president of the Medical Society of the State of New York. Benjamin F. Hall, *The Trial of William Freeman for the Murder of*

John G. Van Nest, including the evidence and the arguments of counsel . . . (Auburn, NY: Derby, Miller & Co. Publishers, 1848), 417, 450, 497; Amariah Brigham to Nahum Capen, May 17, 1833; Amariah Brigham to Nahum Capen, July 11, 1833; Box 1, Folder 10, Nahum Capen papers, 1783–1885 (inclusive), 1826–1885 (bulk), B MS c23, Boston Medical Library, Francis A. Countway Library of Medicine, Boston, MA.

96. Hall, *The Trial of William Freeman*, 504.
97. Hall, *The Trial of William Freeman*, 504; L. N. Fowler, *Phrenological and Physiological Almanac for 1848* (New York: Fowlers and Wells, 1847), 47.
98. Blanchard Fosgate, "Art. XI.—Case of William Freeman, the Murderer of the Van Nest Family," *The American Journal of the Medical Sciences* 28 (October 1847): 409–414; Hall, *The Trial of William Freeman*, 506.
99. "James Stephens. Phrenological Character and Biography," *American Phrenological Journal* 31, no. 3 (March 1860): 33.
100. "Article II. Phrenological Developments and Character of Peter Robinson, Who Was Executed April 16th, at New Brunswick, N.J., for the Murder of A. Suydam, Esq.," *The American Phrenological Journal and Miscellany* 3, no. 10 (July 1841): 452.
101. "George Wilson, the Murderer," *American Phrenological Journal* 24, no. 3 (September 1856): 49.
102. M. C. Tracy, "Article X: Facts Relative to Harris Bell, Executed at Honesdale, Pennsylvania, in 1848," *American Phrenological Journal* 12, no. 2 (February 1850): 56–59.
103. "Character of Arthur Spring," *American Phrenological Journal* 24, no. 6 (December 1856): 132.
104. W. Byrd Powell, "A Phrenological Exposition of John A. Murel," *Alabama Intelligencer and States Rights Expositor* (Tuscaloosa, AL), October 17, 1835.
105. Fowler's reading of Murrell was reprinted in a number of different publications, alternately attributed to Orson and Lorenzo. See *The Life and Adventures of John A. Murrell, the Great Western Land Pirate* (New York: H. Long & Brother, [1848]), iv; L. N. Fowler, *The Phrenological and Physiological Almanac for 1849* (New York: Fowlers and Wells, 1849), 37, Box 328, Almanac Collection (QC16541), New York State Library, Albany, NY; "Likeness of Murrell. Sketch of the Phrenological Developments of John A. Murrell, as given by L. N. Fowler, in the State Prison at Nashville, Dec. 1835," *National Police Gazette* 2, no. 13 (December 1846): 100; P. P., "Uses and Abuses of Lynch Law, no. 111," *The American Whig Review* 7, no. 3 (March 1851): 217.
106. James Lal Penick Jr., *The Great Western Land Pirate: John A. Murrell in Legend and History* (Columbia: University of Missouri Press, 1981), 31; Bertram Wyatt-Brown, *Southern Honor: Ethics & Behavior in the Old South* (Oxford: Oxford University Press, 1982), 49.
107. "Executions," *The Sun* (Baltimore, MD), February 19, 1844.
108. "Organ of Destructiveness," *Charleston Courier*, May 17, 1831.
109. [Chastine Cox; Prof. Fowler], *The Daily Picayune* (New Orleans, LA), July 16, 1879. On Chastine Cox, see Courtney E. Thompson, "The Curious Case of Chastine Cox: Murder, Race, Medicine and the Media in the Gilded Age," *Social History of Medicine* 32, no. 3 (August 2019): 481–501.
110. "The Gallows. Triple Execution at Cincinnati," *New York Herald*, May 1, 1867.
111. "Additions to Our Cabinet," *The American Phrenological Journal and Life Illustrated* 44, no. 4 (October 1866): 117.
112. "Article II. Phrenological Developments and Character of James Eager, Executed for the Murder of Philip Williams, May 9, 1845," *The American Phrenological Journal and Miscellany* 7, no. 8 (August 1845): 263–268.

113. "Article II. Phrenological Developments and Character of James Eager," 265; emphasis in the original.
114. "Article II. Phrenological Developments and Character of James Eager," 265.
115. "Article II. Phrenological Developments and Character of James Eager," 268; emphasis in the original.
116. This essay focused on the possibility of the innocence of the prisoner and the factor of intoxication in inciting criminal acts. "The Law of Love . . . No. 4," 269.
117. This was most frequently the case with accounts of foreign criminals. For example, see W. B. Powell, "Article IV. Phrenological Developments of Fieschi; Who Attempted to Murder the King of France," *The American Phrenological Journal and Miscellany* 1, no. 11 (August 1839): 438–440.
118. "Selected Summary," *American Traveller* (Boston, MA), May 22, 1835.
119. "Selected Summary."
120. "Phrenology," *The Sun* (Baltimore, MD), January 11, 1849.
121. Le Blanc's first name was sometimes given as Antonio. A cast of his head was collected by the Boston Phrenological Society.
122. "Article VI. Character of Le Blanc, the Murderer of Judge Sayre and Family, of Morristown, N.J.; with Cuts," *The American Phrenological Journal and Miscellany* 1, no. 3 (December 1838): 92; emphasis in the original.
123. "Article II. Case in Which Character Was Inferred from Cerebral Development," *The American Phrenological Journal and Miscellany* 1, no. 12 (September 1839): 456.
124. "Article II. Case in Which Character Was Inferred from Cerebral Development," 456.
125. The author did not specify whether this was Orson or Lorenzo.
126. "Phrenology. Hugh Carrigan the Murderer. Examination of his Skull," *American Phrenological Journal* 25, no. 3 (March 1857): 50.
127. "Phrenology. Hugh Carrigan the Murderer."
128. D. P. Butler, "A Skull. A Test Examination," *American Phrenological Journal* 19, no. 2 (February 1854): 42–43.
129. Butler, "A Skull," 42.
130. L. N. Fowler, "Article V. Examination, by the Editor, of Casts of Skulls, Numbered 1 and 2, Illustrated with Engravings, and of A. and B.," *The American Phrenological Journal and Miscellany* 8, no. 7 (July 1846): 224.
131. Fowler, "Article V. Examination, by the Editor," 224.
132. Bittel notes that practical phrenologists framed encounters with their science, including lectures, debates, and private readings, as investigative and experimental. Carla Bittel, "Testing the Truth of Phrenology: Knowledge Experiments in Antebellum American Cultures of Science and Health," *Medical History* 63, no. 3 (2019): 366–367.
133. [Miscellaneous], *New York Tribune*, September 10, 1870.
134. The corpses dissected in early modern public anatomies were typically those of executed criminals. For discussion of the origins of this relationship between the criminal and the atomized cadaver, see Andrea Carlino, *Books of the Body: Anatomic Ritual and Renaissance Learning* (Chicago: University of Chicago Press, 1999), 92–108; Katharine Park, "The Criminal and the Saintly Body: Autopsy and Dissection in Renaissance Italy," *Renaissance Quarterly* 47, no. 1 (1994): 1–33; Katharine Park, *Secrets of Women: Gender, Generation, and the Origins of Human Dissection* (New York: Zone Books, 2006), 211–214; Jonathan Sawday, *The Body Emblazoned: Dissection and the Human Body in Renaissance Culture* (London: Routledge, 1995), 54–84.
135. As Richardson discusses in *Death, Dissection and the Destitute*, the increased need for cadavers for medical education was met in part by the Anatomy Act of 1832 in

Britain, which provided the unclaimed pauper dead from workhouses for medical uses. This aspect of the New Poor Law was controversial, leading to sometimes bloody protests. This also resulted in decreased need for the corpses of executed criminals, a sign of changing attitudes about such usage in the nineteenth century. Ruth Richardson, *Death, Dissection and the Destitute*, 2nd ed. (Chicago: University of Chicago Press, 2000 [1987]). See also Michael Sappol, *A Traffic of Dead Bodies: Anatomy and Embodied Social Identity in Nineteenth-Century America* (Princeton, NJ: Princeton University Press, 2002).

136. "Horrible Fate of a Ghoul," *Macon Weekly Telegraph*, April 16, 1880. Noted as reprinted from the *Hagerstown Globe* (Hagerstown, MD).
137. "Horror of Horrors. The Most Terrible Tale Ever Told," *Wheeling Register* (Wheeling, WV), March 29, 1880. Noted as reprinted from the *Cincinnati Enquirer*; also reprinted as: "A Sickening Horror," *The Standard* (Clarksdale, TX), April 16, 1880.
138. "Horror of Horrors."
139. "Horror of Horrors."
140. "Horror of Horrors."
141. Michel Foucault, *Discipline and Punish: The Birth of the Prison*, trans. Alan Sheridan (New York: Vintage Books, 1995 [1977]), 195–228.
142. Foucault, *Discipline and Punish*, 203.
143. Foucault, *Discipline and Punish*, 204.
144. Tom McGlamery, *Protest and the Body in Melville, Dos Passos, and Hurston* (New York: Routledge, 2004), 30–32.
145. McGlamery, *Protest and the Body*, 31.
146. McGlamery, *Protest and the Body*, 32.
147. Foucault, *Discipline and Punish*, 202.
148. Foucault, *Discipline and Punish*, 207.
149. Foucault, *Discipline and Punish*, 195.

5. Policing the Self and the Stranger

1. Martha L. P. to Miss Abby F. Newall, June 8, 1839, Ms. Coll. No. 504.048, Louise M. Darling Biomedical Library, University of California, Los Angeles, CA; emphasis in the original.
2. Miller and Melvin suggest that by 1860, New York held 1 million people, compared to Boyer's estimate of 800,000. Paul Boyer, *Urban Masses and Moral Order in America, 1820–1920* (Cambridge, MA: Harvard University Press, 1992 [1978]), 67; Zane L. Miller and Patricia Mooney Melvin, *The Urbanization of Modern America: A Brief History*, 2nd ed. (New York: Harcourt Brace Jovanovich, 1987 [1973]), 32.
3. Miller and Melvin, *The Urbanization of Modern America*, 31–32.
4. Boyer, *Urban Masses and Moral Order in America*, 67; Miller and Melvin, *The Urbanization of Modern America*, 40–41.
5. Karen Halttunen, *Confidence Men and Painted Women: A Study of Middle-Class Culture in America, 1830–1870* (New Haven, CT: Yale University Press, 1982), 35, citing Lyn H. Lofland, *A World of Strangers: Order and Action in Urban Public Space* (New York: Basic Books, 1973), 8–12. See also Alan I Marcus, *Plague of Strangers: Social Groups and the Origins of City Services in Cincinnati, 1819–1870* (Columbus: Ohio State University Press, 1991), 9–12.
6. Boyer, *Urban Masses and Moral Order in America*, 68.
7. Boyer, *Urban Masses and Moral Order in America*, 67–70.
8. Marcus, *Plague of Strangers*, 12–14.

9. Robert C. Wadman and William Thomas Allison, *To Protect and Serve: A History of Police in America* (Upper Saddle River, NJ: Pearson Prentice Hall, 2004), 1–2, 8–12; Elizabeth Hinton and DeAnza Cook, "The Mass Criminalization of Black Americans: A Historical Overview," *Annual Review of Criminology* 4, no. 1 (January 2021; preprint June 22, 2020): 1–26, at 6.
10. David R. Johnson, *Policing the Urban Underworld: The Impact of Crime on the Development of the American Police, 1800–1887* (Philadelphia: Temple University Press, 1979), 8–15; Wadman and Allison, *To Protect and Serve*, 8, 14–15.
11. Hereward Senior, *Constabulary: The Rise of Police Institutions in Britain, the Commonwealth and the United States* (Toronto: Dundurn Press, 1997), 50–52; Wadman and Allison, *To Protect and Serve*, 20–22.
12. Marcus, *Plague of Strangers*, 14.
13. Frank Morn, *"The Eye that Never Sleeps": A History of the Pinkerton National Detective Agency* (Bloomington: Indiana University Press, 1982), 11–14.
14. Wadman and Allison, *To Protect and Serve*, 22–26; Sidney L. Harring, *Policing a Class Society: The Experience of American Cities, 1865–1915* (New Brunswick, NJ: Rutgers University Press, 1983), 13–18.
15. Halttunen, *Confidence Men and Painted Women*, xv.
16. Sharrona Pearl, *About Faces: Physiognomy in Nineteenth-Century Britain* (Cambridge, MA: Harvard University Press, 2010), 28.
17. Pearl, *About Faces*, 5, 191.
18. Great men were also occasionally considered in the aggregate. For example, "The Phrenological Developments of the Busts of Distinguished Men," *The American Phrenological Journal and Miscellany* 8, no. 4 (April 1846): 123–124; S. G. H. [Samuel Gridley Howe], "Article VI. The Heads of Our Great Men," *The American Phrenological Journal and Miscellany* 1, no. 8 (May 1839): 286–294.
19. On phrenological explorations of great men and men of genius in the nineteenth century, see Charles Colbert, *A Measure of Perfection: Phrenology and the Fine Arts in America* (Chapel Hill: University of North Carolina Press, 1997), 218–242.
20. Historical conceptions of "idiocy" can be broadly defined by two features: "firstly, the lack of, or failure to develop, intellectual functions to a normal degree. Secondly, that this situation is apparent early in life." These assumptions were often linked to "physical manifestations or deformities," particularly of the head, in the nineteenth century. I use the term "idiot" in this book as an actors' category. Edgar Miller, "Idiocy in the Nineteenth Century," *History of Psychiatry* 7, no. 27 (1996): 361–363.
21. L. N. Fowler, *The Phrenological Almanac for 1842* (New York: Vincent L. Dill, 1841): 39, Box 328, Almanac Collection, QC16541, New York State Library, Albany, New York (hereafter cited as Almanac Collection).
22. The facial angle, though often lumped in with racialized studies of intelligence, was originally intended by Camper to only have bearing on issues of aesthetics and racial difference. The facial angle was adopted by Lavater in his physiognomy, which might have influenced its use by phrenologists. Contemporaries of the Fowlers considered Camper's facial angle to be primarily concerned with intelligence. Miriam Claude Meijer, *Race and Aesthetics in the Anthropology of Petrus Camper (1722–1789)* (Amsterdam: Editions Rodopi bv, 1999), 120–121, 170–176; Daniel Noble, *The Brain and its Physiology* (London: John Churchill, 1846), 53; Melissa Percival, *The Appearance of Character: Physiognomy and Facial Expression in Eighteenth-Century France* (London: W. S. Maney & Son, 1999), 20.

23. O. S. Fowler, *Fowler's Practical Phrenology* (Philadelphia, 1840), 33.
24. L. N. Fowler, *Phrenological Almanac for 1841* (New York: W. J. Spence, 1840), Almanac Collection.
25. This name has been anglicized from "Pierre Jeannin." "The Good Man and the Murderer. A Contrast," *American Phrenological Journal* 17, no. 1 (January 1853): 4.
26. The catalogue of the Boston Phrenological Society also includes a description of a murderer named Martin, who may be the same person. Boston Phrenological Society, *A Catalogue of Phrenological Specimens, Belonging to the Boston Phrenological Society* (Boston: John Ford, 1835), 31.
27. "The Good Man and the Murderer," 4; emphasis in the original.
28. Despite this, many women were phrenologists or participated in phrenology; the Fowler-Wells firm itself was a "mixed gender professional setting." Carla Bittel, "Woman, Know Thyself: Producing and Using Phrenological Knowledge in Nineteenth-Century America," *Centaurus* 55, no. 2 (2013): 112.
29. William H. A. F. Strathern, Commonplace Book, 480. James Marshall and Marie-Louise Osborn Collection, Beinecke Rare Book and Manuscript Library, Yale University, New Haven, CT; emphasis in the original.
30. Strathern, Commonplace Book, 481; emphasis in the original.
31. Strathern, Commonplace Book, 487; emphasis in the original.
32. J. St. John, "Lecture on Phrenology: Or, How to 'Raise the Wind,'" *The Mystic Pioneer* (Mystic, CT), May 14, 1859.
33. "A List of Specimens Designed for Phrenological Societies," *American Phrenological Journal* 10, no. 4 (April 1848): 129–130.
34. This collection also includes figure 2, which depicts small and large Destructiveness.
35. L. N. Fowler, *The Phrenological Almanac for 1843* (New York: O. S. & L. N. Fowler, 1842), 19. Almanac Collection; emphasis in the original.
36. James Poskett, *Materials of the Mind: Phrenology, Race, and the Global History of Science, 1815–1920* (Chicago: University of Chicago Press, 2019), 193.
37. O. S. and L. N. Fowler, *Phrenology Proved, Illustrated, and Applied*, 2nd ed. (New York, 1837), 372.
38. Bittel, "Woman, Know Thyself," 117; Carla Bittel, "Testing the Truth of Phrenology: Knowledge Experiments in Antebellum American Cultures of Science and Health," *Medical History* 63, no. 3 (2019): 353.
39. On phrenology as psychological counseling, see Michael M. Sokal, "Practical Phrenology as Psychological Counseling in the 19th-Century United States," in *The Transformation of Psychology: Influences of 19th-Century Philosophy, Technology, and Natural Science*, ed. Christopher D. Green, Marlene Shore, and Thomas Teo (Washington, DC: American Psychological Association, 2001), 21–44. On phrenology as self-improvement, see Bittel, "Woman, Know Thyself"; Fenneke Sysling, "Science and Self-Assessment: Phrenological Charts 1840–1940," *British Journal for the History of Science* 51, no. 2 (2018): 261–280.
40. Spurzheim noted that the inscription over the door on the temple of Delphi was γνῶθι σεαυτόν, translated to "know thyself." J. Spurzheim, *Phrenology, or, the Doctrine of the Mind; and of the Relations between its Manifestations and the Body*, 3rd ed. (London: Charles Knight, 1835), 2. See also Bittel, "Woman, Know Thyself," 105–106.
41. O. S. and L. N. Fowler, *The Illustrated Self-Instructor in Phrenology and Physiology* (New York: Fowlers and Wells, 1855), 9; emphasis in the original.
42. O. S. Fowler, *The Practical Phrenologist; and Recorder and Delineator of the Character and Talents . . .* (Boston: O. S. Fowler, 1869), n.p. [back matter].

43. Bittel, "Woman, Know Thyself," 105.
44. Sysling, "Science and Self-Assessment," 278.
45. O. S. and L. N. Fowler, *The Illustrated Self-Instructor*, 127–134.
46. For example, see C. Donovan, *A Handbook of Phrenology* (London: Longmans, Green, Reader, and Dyer, 1870), n.p. [plate 1, and two unlabeled plates], 130–137; R. B. D. Wells, *A New Illustrated Hand-Book of Phrenology, Physiology, and Physiognomy* (London: H. Vickers, [1878?]), 63–66.
47. Donovan, *A Handbook of Phrenology*, 130.
48. Nelson Sizer, *Forty Years in Phrenology; Embracing Recollections of History, Anecdote, and Experience* (New York: Fowler & Wells Co., 1888), 58.
49. "Article VI. Practical Phrenology—No. 2," *The American Phrenological Journal and Miscellany* 4, no. 2 (February 1842): 54.
50. "Article IV. Signs of Character as Indicated by Phrenology, Physiology, Physiognomy, Natural Language, Manners, Conversation, &c. Illustrated by a Likeness of Harrahwaukay, the New-Zealand Chief, No. 2," *The American Phrenological Journal and Miscellany* 8, no. 2 (February 1846): 55.
51. "Article IV. Signs of Character," 55.
52. Poskett notes that the Fowlers' phrenological enterprise, including publications, was a business, and the *APJ* reached 30,000 subscribers by midcentury. Poskett, *Materials of the Mind*, 154–155.
53. These calculations make use of John McCusker's Composite Consumer Price Index, which I used to convert the prices to 1990 currency, and then used the inflation calculator to convert the January 1990 figures to the January 2020 equivalent. Interestingly, though Ferguson paid more in 1865 for the second reading, six dollars reflects a decline in cost, due to deflation; the second reading cost $96.87 in 2020 currency. Diary, Book 1, entry dated November 2, 1858, Mary Ferguson Diaries, #6405, Division of Rare and Manuscript Collections, Cornell University Library, Ithaca, NY (hereafter cited as Ferguson Diaries); Diary, Book 1, entry dated February 8, 1865, Ferguson Diaries, 1855–1881; L. N. Fowler, Collection of Phrenological Cards, 1834–1835, B MS b215.1, Boston Medical Library in the Francis A. Countway Library of Medicine, Boston, MA (hereafter cited as Fowler Phrenological Cards); John J. McCusker, "How Much Is That in Real Money? A Historical Price Index for Use as a Deflator of Money Values in the Economy of the United States," *Proceedings of the American Antiquarian Society* 106, no. 2 (1997): 327–334; "CPI Inflation Calculator," U.S. Bureau of Labor Statistics, accessed June 17, 2020, http://www.bls.gov/data/inflation_calculator.htm.
54. Some charts are extant for notable individuals. Both Mark Twain and Walt Whitman had readings done by the Fowler brothers (Twain on more than one occasion), and both incorporated or mentioned phrenology in their writings; Twain in his autobiography and *Huckleberry Finn*, and Whitman in *Leaves of Grass*. Edward Hungerford, "Walt Whitman and His Chart of Bumps," *American Literature* 2, no. 4 (1931): 350–384; Madeleine B. Stern, "Mark Twain Had His Head Examined," *American Literature* 41, no. 2 (1969): 207–218; Arthur Wrobel, "Whitman and the Phrenologists: The Divine Body and the Sensuous Soul," *PMLA* 89, no. 1 (1974): 17–23.
55. On phrenological charts, see Sysling, "Science and Self-Assessment."
56. Bittel, "Testing the Truth of Phrenology," 359.
57. This reading was possibly transcribed: while the front page stated that the reading was performed by Fowler, the final page of the document read, "reported by James H. Wilson." L. N. Fowler, "Phrenological Character of Miss Emily Sawyer,"

February 8, 1861, RL.10470, David M. Rubenstein Rare Book & Manuscript Library, Duke University, Durham, NC.

58. Sysling notes that most clients' scores were above average, as phrenological readings in aggregate tended to convey positive messages. Sysling, "Science and Self-Assessment," 273.
59. Nelson Sizer, Phrenological Character of Mr. Samuel P. Leeds, August 19, 1864, Ms. Coll. No. 504.026, Louise M. Darling Biomedical Library, University of California, Los Angeles, CA; emphasis in the original.
60. Nelson Sizer, Phrenological Character of Mrs. Robert A. Phillips, December 30, 1880, Ms. Coll. No. 504.031, Louise M. Darling Biomedical Library, University of California, Los Angeles, CA.
61. Fowler, "Phrenological Character of Miss Emily Sawyer."
62. Sally Gregory Kohlstedt, "Parlors, Primers, and Public Schooling: Education for Science in Nineteenth-Century America," *Isis* 81, no. 3 (1990): 428.
63. Kohlstedt, "Parlors, Primers, and Public Schooling," 428–429, 432.
64. Katherine Pandora, "Popular Science in National and Transnational Perspective: Suggestions from the American Context," *Isis* 100, no. 2 (2009): 351, 353. On popular science in nineteenth-century Britain, see Bernard Lightman, *Victorian Popularizers of Science: Designing Nature for New Audiences* (Chicago: University of Chicago Press, 2007).
65. "Educational Department. Ignorance and Crime," *American Phrenological Journal* 14, no. 6 (December 1851): 129.
66. Bittel, "Woman, Know Thyself," 110, 115, 117–118; Cynthia Eagle Russett, *Sexual Science: The Victorian Construction of Womanhood* (Cambridge, MA: Harvard University Press, 1989), 20–22. On the cult of true womanhood, see Barbara Welter, "The Cult of True Womanhood: 1820–1860," *American Quarterly* 18, no. 2 (1966): 151–174.
67. Mrs. J. H. Hanaford, "The Mother and the Lecturer," *American Phrenological Journal* 14, no. 6 (December 1851): 129.
68. Hanaford, "The Mother and the Lecturer," 130.
69. Lydia Folger Fowler, *Familiar Lessons on Physiology, Designed for the Use of Children and Youth in Schools and Families*, vol. 1 (New York: Fowlers and Wells, 1847); Lydia Folger Fowler, *Familiar Lessons on Phrenology, Designed for the Use of Children and Youth in Schools and Families*, vol. 2 (New York: Fowlers and Wells, 1847); Bittel, "Woman, Know Thyself," 112–113; John Harley Warner, *Against the Spirit of System: The French Impulse in Nineteenth-Century American Medicine* (Baltimore: Johns Hopkins University Press, 2003 [1998]), 51. Bittel notes that phrenological advice directed toward parents about childrearing, particularly Lydia Fowler's works, could be viewed as representative of the development of scientific motherhood in the mid-nineteenth century. On scientific motherhood, see Rima D. Apple, "Constructing Mothers: Scientific Motherhood in the Nineteenth and Twentieth Centuries," *Social History of Medicine* 8, no. 2 (1995): 161–178; Rima D. Apple, *Perfect Motherhood: Science and Childrearing in America* (New Brunswick, NJ: Rutgers University Press, 2006), 11–33.
70. The first excerpt published in the *APJ* from Lydia Fowler's work was specifically focused on Destructiveness, suggesting its relevance to the instruction of children. Mrs. L. N. Fowler, "Article XXIX. 'Phrenology for the Use of Children in Schools and Families,'" *The American Phrenological Journal and Miscellany* 9, no. 5 (May 1847): 163–165.

71. On the influence of phrenology on American education, see Stephen Tomlinson, *Head Masters: Phrenology, Secular Education, and Nineteenth-Century Social Thought* (Tuscaloosa: University of Alabama Press, 2005).
72. L. N. Fowler, Phrenological Reading of Lucy Cutter, Miss Bliss Infant School, Louisville, KY, June 26, 1835, L. N. Fowler, Collection of Phrenological Cards, 1834–1835 (B MS b215.1), Boston Medical Library in the Francis A. Countway Library of Medicine, Boston, MA (hereafter cited as Fowler Phrenological Cards); L. N. Fowler, Phrenological Reading of Mariah Pettet, Miss Bliss Infant School, Louisville, KY, c. June 1835, Fowler Phrenological Cards; L. N. Fowler, Phrenological Reading of George Eldridge, Louisville, KY, June 26, 1835, Fowler Phrenological Cards; L. N. Fowler, Phrenological Reading of Miss H. M. Burke, Pittsburgh, PA, April 22, 1835, Fowler Phrenological Cards.
73. Sokal, "Practical Phrenology as Psychological Counseling," 35–37.
74. L. N. Fowler, Phrenological Reading of Mrs. De Hart, Louisville, KY, July 3, 1835, Fowler Phrenological Cards.
75. L. N. Fowler, Phrenological Reading of Mr. Wilson, Louisville, KY, August 15, 1835, Fowler Phrenological Cards; L. N. Fowler, Phrenological Reading of Mrs. Wilson, Louisville, KY, August 15, 1835, Fowler Phrenological Cards; L. N. Fowler, Phrenological Reading of Miss Wilson, Louisville, KY, August 15, 1835, Fowler Phrenological Cards.
76. Ferguson does not specify whether this was Orson or Lorenzo.
77. Bittel also discusses the Mary Ferguson diaries and this phrenological encounter. Bittel, "Woman, Know Thyself," 117–118.
78. Diary, Book 1, entry dated November 2, 1858, Ferguson Diaries.
79. Diary, Book 1, entry dated November 4, 1858, Ferguson Diaries. Bittel has argued that phrenological clients did not always accept their readings at face value, but instead "assessed them and determined their utility and validity," as Ferguson does here. Bittel, "Testing the Truth of Phrenology," 358.
80. Diary, Book 1, entry dated February 8, 1865, Ferguson Diaries.
81. Diary, Book 1, entry dated February 8, 1865, Ferguson Diaries.
82. Diary, Book 1, entry dated October 29, 1858, Ferguson Diaries.
83. O. S. Fowler, Phrenological Character of M. Wm. H. Davis, Cincinnati, February 15, 1851, Ms. Coll. No. 504.046, Louise M. Darling Biomedical Library, University of California, Los Angeles, CA.
84. O. S. Fowler, Phrenological Character of M. Wm. H. Davis.
85. Ed., "Article III. On the Training of the Infant Mind. An Appeal to Woman," *The American Phrenological Journal and Miscellany* 4, no. 5 (May 1842): 136; emphasis in the original; Bittel, "Woman, Know Thyself," 115.
86. A Father, "Article III. Woman—Her Character, Influence, Sphere, and Consequent Duties and Rducation. No. II," *The American Phrenological Journal and Miscellany* 6, no. 11 (November 1845): 373, 370.
87. A Father, "Article III. Woman—Her Character," 373.
88. "Two Paths of Life," *The American Phrenological Journal* 21, no. 1 (January 1855): 12.
89. "Good and Bad Heads," *American Phrenological Journal* 15, no. 3 (March 1852): 61.
90. Ira Wilcox, "A Fact for Phrenology," *The American Phrenological Journal and Miscellany* 12, no. 3 (March 1850): 99.
91. Wilcox, "A Fact for Phrenology," 99.
92. L. N. Fowler, Phrenological Reading of Master Adam Tailor, Jeffersonville, IN, July 23, 1835, Fowler Phrenological Cards.

93. L. N. Fowler, Phrenological Reading of Wm. Buchanan, Jeffersonville, IN, July 23, 1835, Fowler Phrenological Cards.
94. L. N. Fowler, Phrenological Reading of Miss M. E. Walker, Cincinnati, OH, May 13, 1835, Fowler Phrenological Cards.
95. L. N. Fowler, Phrenological Reading of Miss M. E. Walker.
96. Jane Roberts, Diary, vol. 1, entry dated [January] 6, 1837, Jane Roberts, diary and notebook, 1833–1839 and 1851, David M. Rubenstein Rare Book & Manuscript Library, Duke University, Durham, NC.
97. Roberts, Diary, vol. 1, entry dated [January] 6, 1837.
98. "A 'Corned' Phrenologist," *Wabash Courier* (Terre-Haute, IN), July 24, 1841.
99. "An Enthusiastic Phrenologist," *The People's Advocate* (Alexandria, VA), November 25, 1840.
100. [Phrenologist; combativeness], *Idaho Tri-Weekly Statesman* (Boise, ID), June 21, 1873.
101. Poe was also interested in phrenology and took on the subject satirically in some of his stories, including "The Imp of the Perverse" (1845), "The System of Dr. Tarr and Prof. Fether" (1856), and "The Business Man" (1850), among other writings. See Edward Hungerford, "Poe and Phrenology," *American Literature* 2, no. 3 (1930): 209–231; Madeleine B. Stern, *Heads & Headlines: The Phrenological Fowlers* (Norman: University of Oklahoma Press, 1971), 73–77; Madeleine B. Stern, "Poe: 'The Mental Temperament' for Phrenologists," *American Literature* 40, no. 2 (1968): 155–163.
102. LeRoy Lad Panek, *Before Sherlock Holmes: How Magazines and Newspapers Invented the Detective Story* (Jefferson, NC: McFarland & Company, 2011), 1–7; Heather Worthington, *The Rise of the Detective in Early Nineteenth-Century Popular Fiction* (New York: Palgrave Macmillan, 2005), 3–4.
103. Hungerford, "Poe and Phrenology," 223–224; Edgar Allan Poe, "The Murders in the Rue Morgue," in Edgar Allan Poe, *The Pit and the Pendulum and Other Tales*, ed. David Van Leer (Oxford: Oxford University Press, 1998; 2018), 94.
104. Sokal compares phrenological methodology with Sherlock Holmes's method of observation. Sokal, "Practical Phrenology as Psychological Counseling," 37–39.
105. "An Incident in the Travels of a Phrenologist," *Daily Evening Traveller* (Boston, MA), May 4, 1857; "An Incident in the Travels of a Phrenologist," *American Traveller* (Boston, MA), May 8, 1857; "An Incident in the Travels of a Phrenologist. From the *Boston Traveller*," *Alexandria Gazette*, May 9, 1857; "An Incident in the Travels of a Phrenologist," *True Flag* (Boston, MA), May 23, 1857; "Incident in the Travels of a Phrenologist," *The Humboldt Times* (Arcata, CA), October 24, 185; "Incident in the Travels of a Phrenologist," *American Phrenological Journal* 26, no. 5 (November 1857): 109; "Incident in the Travels of a Phrenologist," *Lowell Daily Citizen & News* (Lowell, MA), December 31, 1857.
106. "An Incident in the Travels of a Phrenologist," *Daily Evening Traveller*.
107. "An Incident in the Travels of a Phrenologist," *Daily Evening Traveller*.
108. "An Incident in the Travels of a Phrenologist," *Daily Evening Traveller*.
109. "An Incident in the Travels of a Phrenologist," *Daily Evening Traveller*.
110. "A Thief Discovered," *American Phrenological Journal* 27, no. 2 (August 1857): 44. Noted as having been translated and reprinted from *Le Journal de Maine et Loire*, France.
111. "A Thief Discovered," 44.
112. "A Thief Discovered," 44.
113. Identified as "James H—" and therefore most likely James Harper, mayor in 1844–1845, and the only James H. to be mayor of New York in the nineteenth century. The

article implied that the mayor practiced as a phrenologist. The city's first municipal police force was established during Harper's short term as mayor. "Detecting a Thief. A Phrenological Fact," *American Phrenological Journal and Life Illustrated* (*APJ*) 37, no. 2 (February 1863): 40–41; "Detecting a Thief. A Phrenological Fact," *California Farmer and Journal of Useful Sciences* (Sacramento, CA), June 26, 1963; Moses King, *King's Handbook of New York City: An Outline, History, and Description of the American Metropolis* (Boston: Moses King, 1892), 232–234, 484.

114. "Detecting a Thief," *APJ*, 41.
115. H. R. Addison, "The Phrenologist," *The Albion* 7, no. 42 (October 1848): 496; H. R. Addison, "The Phrenologist," *Home Journal* 44, no. 142 (October 1848): 1; H. R. Addison, "The Phrenologist," *Coldwater Sentinel* (Coldwater, MI), November 10, 1848; H. R. Addison, "The Phrenologist," *The Bee* (Boston, MA), November 14, 1848; H. R. Addison, "The Phrenologist," *The Concordia Intelligencer* (Vidalia, LA), November 18, 1848; H. R. Addison, "The Phrenologist," *Supplement to the Courant* [*Connecticut Courant*] (Hartford, CT), November 24, 1848; H. R. Addison, "Miscellaneous: The Phrenologist," *Vermont Watchman & State Journal* (Montpelier, VT), November 30, 1848; H. R. Addison, "The Phrenologist," *The Spirit of the Times* 18, no. 39 (November 1848): 460; H. R. Addison, "The Phrenologist," *The Hudson River Chronicle* (Ossining, NY), December 5, 1848; "Miscellaneous Selections. The Phrenologist," *Connecticut Courant* (Hartford, CT), December 16, 1848; H. R. Addison, "Miscellany. The Phrenologist," *The Semi-Weekly Eagle* (Brattleboro, VT), December 21, 1848; H. R. Addison, "Miscellany. The Phrenologist," *St. Albans Messenger* (St. Albans, VT), December 28, 1848; H. R. Addison, "Miscellany. The Phrenologist," *The New Hampshire Gazette* (Portsmouth, NH), May 29, 1849; H. R. Addison, "The Phrenologist," *American Phrenological Journal* 24, no. 5 (November 1856): 104–105.
116. Addison, "The Phrenologist," *The Albion*, 496; emphasis in the original.
117. Addison, "The Phrenologist," *The Albion*, 496; emphasis in the original.
118. "The Phrenologist's Prophecy," *American Phrenological Journal* 49, no. 10 (October 1869): 375. It does not appear that Gall met Klemens von Metternich, the Prince of Metternich-Winneberg zu Beilstein, so this story is likely entirely fictional. Stanley Finger and Paul Eling, *Franz Joseph Gall: Naturalist of the Mind, Visionary of the Brain* (New York: New York University Press, 2019), 271n70.
119. "The Phrenologist's Prophecy," 375.
120. "The Phrenologist's Prophecy," 375.
121. "The King and the Phrenologist," *Wheeling Register* (Wheeling, WV), October 24, 1879; "King Frederick and the Phrenologist," *Daily Bulletin Supplement* (San Francisco, CA), November 1, 1879; "How a King Tested Phrenology," *Springfield Republican* (Springfield, MA), November 2, 1879; "King Frederick and the Phrenologist," *The Indianapolis Daily Sentinel*, November 6, 1879; "King Frederick and the Phrenologist," *Daily Territorial Enterprise* (Virginia City, NV), November 13, 1879; "The Two Notables. How a King Tested the Science of a Phrenologist," *Times-Picayune* (New Orleans, LA), November 30, 1879.
122. Unlike the tale of Gall meeting Metternich, this account seems to have been based on actual events, as Gall was invited to the court of Friedrich Wilhelm III to present his theories to Queen Louise. Finger and Eling indicate that the king did, in fact, test Gall as the story suggests. However, in the original story, Gall won, not the skeptical king. This shift in the story likely reflects changing attitudes towards phrenology. Finger and Eling, *Franz Joseph Gall*, 235–236.

123. The effects of the Civil War and Reconstruction on medicine and science in the United States have been well explored by historians. See for example: Andrew McIlwaine Bell, *Mosquito Soldiers: Malaria, Yellow Fever, and the Course of the American Civil War* (Baton Rouge: Louisiana State University Press, 2010); Jim Downs, *Sick from Freedom: African-American Illness and Suffering During the Civil War and Reconstruction* (Oxford: Oxford University Press, 2012); Margaret Humphreys, *Intensely Human: The Health of the Black Soldier in the American Civil War* (Baltimore: Johns Hopkins University Press, 2008); Margaret Humphreys, *Marrow of Tragedy: The Health Crisis of the American Civil War* (Baltimore: Johns Hopkins University Press, 2013); Lisa A. Long, *Rehabilitating Bodies: Health, History, and the American Civil War* (Philadelphia: University of Pennsylvania Press, 2004).
124. On racial science, see Michael Banton, *Racial Theories*, 2nd ed. (Cambridge: Cambridge University Press, 1998 [1987]); David Bindman, *Ape to Apollo: Aesthetics and the Idea of Race in the 18th Century* (Ithaca, NY: Cornell University Press, 2002); Joyce E. Chaplin, *Subject Matter: Technology, the Body, and Science on the Anglo-American Frontier, 1500–1676* (Cambridge, MA: Harvard University Press, 2001); Alice L. Conklin, *In the Museum of Man: Race, Anthropology, and Empire in France, 1850–1950* (Ithaca, NY: Cornell University Press, 2013); Andrew S. Curran, *The Anatomy of Blackness: Science & Slavery in an Age of Enlightenment* (Baltimore: Johns Hopkins University Press, 2011); Bruce Dain, *A Hideous Monster of the Mind: American Race Theory in the Early Republic* (Cambridge, MA: Harvard University Press, 2002); Ann Fabian, *The Skull Collectors: Race, Science, and America's Unburied Dead* (Chicago: University of Chicago Press, 2010); Rana A. Hogarth, *Medicalizing Blackness: Making Racial Difference in the Atlantic World, 1780–1840* (Chapel Hill: University of North Carolina Press, 2017); Samuel J. Redman, *Bone Rooms: From Scientific Racism to Human Prehistory in Museums* (Cambridge, MA: Harvard University Press, 2016); Londa Schiebinger, *Nature's Body: Gender in the Making of Modern Science* (Boston: Beacon Press, 1993); Suman Seth, *Difference and Disease: Medicine, Race, and the Eighteenth-Century British Empire* (Cambridge: Cambridge University Press, 2018); William Stanton, *The Leopard's Spots: Scientific Attitudes Toward Race in America 1815–59* (Chicago: University of Chicago Press, 1960); Melissa N. Stein, *Measuring Manhood: Race and the Science of Masculinity, 1830–1934* (Minneapolis: University of Minnesota Press, 2015); Nancy Stepan, *The Idea of Race in Science: Great Britain 1800–1960* (Hamden, CT: Archon Books, 1982); Tracy Teslow, *Constructing Race: The Science of Bodies and Cultures in American Anthropology* (Cambridge: Cambridge University Press, 2014); Christopher D. Willoughby, "'His Native, Hot Country': Racial Science and Environment in Antebellum American Medical Thought," *Journal of the History of Medicine and Allied Sciences* 72, no. 3 (2017): 328–351.
125. Samuel A. Cartwright, "I.—Report on the Diseases and Physical Peculiarities of the Negro Race," *The New Orleans Medical and Surgical Journal* 7, no. 6 (May 1851): 696. On Cartwright, see Christopher D. E. Willoughby, "Running Away from Drapetomania: Samuel A. Cartwright, Medicine, and Race in the Antebellum South," *Journal of Southern History* 84, no. 3 (2018): 579–614.
126. Cynthia S. Hamilton, "'Am I Not a Man and a Brother?' Phrenology and Antislavery," *Slavery and Abolition* 29, no. 2 (2008): 181–182. Susan Branson similarly notes that both pro- and antislavery advocates made use of phrenology in the service of their causes. Susan Branson, "Phrenology and the Science of Race in Antebellum America," *Early American Studies* 15, no. 1 (2017): 165.

127. Hamilton, "'Am I Not a Man and a Brother?,'" 176; Poskett, *Materials of the Mind*, 124–131.
128. Branson, "Phrenology and the Science of Race in Antebellum America," 168; Fabian, *The Skull Collectors*, 93.
129. Fabian, *The Skull Collectors*, 97–102; Poskett, *Materials of the Mind*, 118–124. On Combe's complex approach to race, see David Stack, *Queen Victoria's Skull: George Combe and the Mid-Victorian Mind* (London: Hambledon Continuum, 2008), 217–230.
130. Hamilton, "'Am I Not a Man and a Brother?,'" 177.
131. Branson, "Phrenology and the Science of Race in Antebellum America," 177.
132. Branson, "Phrenology and the Science of Race in Antebellum America," 181.
133. Branson, "Phrenology and the Science of Race in Antebellum America," 181–182.
134. J. H. Van Evrie, *Negroes and Negro "Slavery": The First an Inferior Race; The Latter Its Normal Condition* (New York: Van Evrie, Horton & Co., 1861), 313.
135. Van Evrie, *Negroes and Negro "Slavery,"* 150.
136. Van Evrie, *Negroes and Negro "Slavery,"* 167.
137. Van Evrie's assertion that "hybrids" were more dangerous than the "pure-blooded negro" counters the assumptions of other racial theorists, like Josiah Nott, who framed mixed-race individuals as "weak, sexually compromised hybrids." Stein, *Measuring Manhood*, 56.
138. For an overview of this history, see Hinton and Cook, "The Mass Criminalization of Black Americans."
139. Hinton and Cook, "The Mass Criminalization of Black Americans," 7–8; Khalil Gibran Muhammad, *The Condemnation of Blackness: Race, Crime, and the Making of Modern Urban America* (Cambridge, MA: Harvard University Press, 2010), 1, 282n4.
140. Estelle B. Freedman, *Redefining Rape: Sexual Violence in the Era of Suffrage and Segregation* (Cambridge, MA: Harvard University Press, 2013), 89–103.
141. Muhammad, *The Condemnation of Blackness*, 4.
142. R. W. Shufeldt, *America's Greatest Problem: The Negro* (Philadelphia: F. A. Davis Company, 1915), 148–149.
143. Britt Rusert, "The Science of Freedom: Counterarchives of Racial Science on the Antebellum Stage," *African American Review* 45, no. 3 (2012): 302. See also Britt Rusert, *Fugitive Science: Empiricism and Freedom in Early African American Culture* (New York: New York University Press, 2017), 121–126.
144. Buchanan's theories, though originating in phrenology, were more broad-based, so this interpretation of phrenology was not fully representative of contemporaneous practical phrenology. Edward Bliss Foote, *Sammy Tubbs, the Boy Doctor, and "Sponsie," The Troublesome Monkey*, vol. 4 (New York: Murray Hill Publishing, 1874), 103–108, 113–135, 163. On Sammy Tubbs, see Michael Sappol, *A Traffic of Dead Bodies: Anatomy and Embodied Social Identity in Nineteenth-Century America* (Princeton, NJ: Princeton University Press, 2002), 245–271.
145. Sappol, *A Traffic of Dead Bodies*, 253, 254–255.
146. Rusert, "The Science of Freedom," 302–303.
147. *White's New Illustrated Melodeon Song Book* (New York: H. Long & Brother, 1848), 81–82.
148. *White's New Illustrated Melodeon Song Book*, 81–82.
149. J. Barnes, *The Darkey Phrenologist: A Nigger Absurdity in One Act* (New York: Dick & Fitzgerald, 1899.

150. To be played by a man.
151. Barnes, *The Darkey Phrenologist*, 6–7.
152. Josiah C. Nott and George R. Gliddon, *Indigenous Races of the Earth; or, New Chapters of Ethnological Inquiry* (Philadelphia: J. B. Lippincott & Co., 1857), 212n15.
153. The *APJ*, which promoted an abolitionist stance, published a number of articles during the Civil War on the national crisis, including a series of essays on the phrenological characteristics of U.S. Army officers, including Sherman and McClellan, and the occasional piece on Confederate leaders like Robert E. Lee. Poskett notes that the Civil War forced the Fowlers to be more upfront about their pro-Union and abolitionist leanings, yet they also saw potential for expanding their business empire even with the disruptions of war and continued to pursue topics of perennial interest, including crime. For example, in 1863, at the height of the Civil War, the *APJ* was still asking, "Are Murderers All Bad?" Poskett, *Materials of the Mind*, 163–164; "Are Murderers All Bad?," *American Phrenological Journal and Life Illustrated* 37, no. 3 (March 1863): 64–65.
154. L. A. Vaught, *Vaught's Practical Character Reader* (Chicago: L. A. Vaught, 1902), 39.
155. Vaught, *Vaught's Practical Character Reader*, 11.

6. A Victory for Phrenology?

1. "The Murderer Sullivan," *New York Herald*, January 19, 1872.
2. "The Murderer Sullivan."
3. "The Case of Lawrence Sullivan: A Victory for Phrenology," *The Phrenological Journal and Life Illustrated* 54, no. 3 (March 1872): 195.
4. "The Case of Lawrence Sullivan," 193. This was one of several variations of the name of the *American Phrenological Journal*, which rebranded several times in the last decades of the century, before landing on *The Phrenological Journal and Science of Health*.
5. "The Case of Lawrence Sullivan," 195.
6. "The Murderer Sullivan."
7. "The Murderer Sullivan—A Phrenological Plea," *New-York Tribune*, April 22, 1871.
8. Wells served as a witness for the prosecution in an earlier case, in which his phrenological testimony was permitted in court, though there was little documentation of this trial. "Charles Quinn Sentenced for Life," *San Francisco Bulletin*, August 12, 1870.
9. "The Case of Lawrence Sullivan," 195.
10. In 1890, the *Philadelphia Inquirer* reported that a French murder trial used hypnotism and phrenology unsuccessfully in defense of two murderers, but French sources cannot be found to corroborate this. "Curious Features of a French Criminal Trial," *Philadelphia Inquirer*, December 2, 1890.
11. On the trial, see Charles E. Rosenberg, *The Trial of the Assassin Guiteau: Psychiatry and the Law in the Gilded Age* (Chicago: University of Chicago Press, 1976 [1968]).
12. H. H. Alexander and Edward D. Easton, *Report of the Proceedings in the Case of the United States vs. Charles J. Guiteau . . .*, Part 2 (Washington, DC: Government Printing Office, 1882), 974.
13. Alexander and Easton, *Report of the Proceedings*, 975; Rosenberg, *The Trial of the Assassin Guiteau*, 160.
14. Stanley Finger, *Origins of Neuroscience: A History of Explorations into Brain Function* (New York: Oxford University Press, 1994), 34–36.

15. On neurology and particularly localization in the nineteenth century, see Jason W. Brown and Karen L. Chobar, "Phrenological Studies of Aphasia before Broca: Broca's Aphasia or Gall's Aphasia?," *Brain and Language* 43, no. 3 (1992): 475–486; Stephen T. Casper, *The Neurologists: A History of a Medical Specialty in Modern Britain, c. 1789–2000* (Manchester, UK: Manchester University Press, 2014); Stanley Finger, *Minds Behind the Brain: A History of the Pioneers and Their Discoveries* (Oxford: Oxford University Press, 2000); Finger, *Origins of Neuroscience*, 32–62; Mitchell Glickstein, *Neuroscience: A Historical Introduction* (Cambridge, MA: MIT Press, 2014); Charles G. Gross, *Brain, Vision, Memory: Tales in the History of Neuroscience* (Cambridge, MA: MIT Press, 1998); Katja Guenther, *Localization and Its Discontents: A Genealogy of Psychoanalysis & the Neuro Disciplines* (Chicago: University of Chicago Press, 2015); Anne Harrington, *Medicine, Mind, and the Double Brain: A Study in Nineteenth-Century Social Thought* (Princeton, NJ: Princeton University Press, 1989 [1987]); Leonard L. LaPointe, *Paul Broca and the Origins of Language in the Brain* (San Diego: Plural Publishing, 2013); Robert M. Young, *Mind, Brain, and Adaptation in the Nineteenth Century: Cerebral Localization and Its Biological Context from Gall to Ferrier* (New York: Oxford University Press, 1990 [1970]).
16. The literature on the asylum and psychiatry is too vast to be fully explicated here. On the asylum and psychiatry in nineteenth-century America, see Gerald N. Grob, *The Mad among Us: A History of the Care of America's Mentally Ill* (New York: Free Press, 1994); Lawrence B. Goodheart, "From Cure to Custodianship of the Insane Poor in Nineteenth-Century Connecticut," *Journal of the History of Medicine and Allied Sciences* 65, no. 1 (2010): 106–130; Lawrence B. Goodheart, *Mad Yankees: The Hartford Retreat for the Insane and Nineteenth-Century Psychiatry* (Amherst: University of Massachusetts Press, 2003); Janet Miron, *Prisons, Asylums, and the Public: Institutional Visiting in the Nineteenth Century* (Toronto: University of Toronto Press, 2011); Benjamin Reiss, *Theaters of Madness: Insane Asylums & Nineteenth-Century American Culture* (Chicago: University of Chicago Press, 2008); Edward Shorter, "The Asylum Era," in *A History of Psychiatry: From the Era of the Asylum to the Age of Prozac* (New York: John Wiley & Sons, 1997), 33–68; Nancy Tomes, *A Generous Confidence: Thomas Story Kirkbride and the Art of Asylum-Keeping, 1840–1883* (Cambridge: Cambridge University Press, 1984); Katherine Ziff, *Asylum on the Hill: History of a Healing Landscape* (Athens: Ohio University Press, 2012).
17. On the influence of laboratory science and scientific medicine on American medicine, see Thomas Neville Bonner, "The Spread of Laboratory Teaching, 1850–1870," in *Becoming a Physician: Medical Education in Britain, France, Germany, and the United States, 1750–1945* (New York: Oxford University Press, 1995), 231–250; W. F. Bynum, "Medicine in the Laboratory," in *Science and the Practice of Medicine in the Nineteenth Century* (Cambridge: Cambridge University Press, 1994), 92–117; John Harley Warner, "The Fall and Rise of Professional Mystery: Epistemology, Authority and the Emergence of Laboratory Medicine in Nineteenth-Century America," in *The Laboratory Revolution in Medicine*, ed. Andrew Cunningham and Perry Williams (Cambridge: Cambridge University Press, 1992), 110–141; John S. Haller Jr., *American Medicine in Transition, 1840–1910* (Urbana: University of Illinois Press, 1981), 216–217; William G. Rothstein, "Bacteriology and the Medical Profession," in *American Physicians in the Nineteenth Century: From Sects to Science* (Baltimore: Johns Hopkins University Press, 1992 [1972]), 261–281; John Harley Warner, "Americans and Paris in an Age of German Ascendancy," in *Against the*

Spirit of System: The French Impulse in Nineteenth-Century American Medicine (Baltimore: Johns Hopkins University Press, 2003 [1998]), 291–329; John Harley Warner, "Physiological Therapeutics and the Dissipation of Therapeutic Gloom," in *The Therapeutic Perspective: Medical Practice, Knowledge, and Identity in America, 1820–1885* (Princeton, NJ: Princeton University Press, 1997 [1986]), 235–257.

18. Tabea Cornel, "Something Old, Something New, Something Pseudo, Something True: Pejorative and Deferential References to Phrenology since 1840," *Proceedings of the American Philosophical Society* 161, no. 4 (2017): 301.
19. Including J. G. Spurzheim, who entitled his first English text *The Physiognomical System of Drs. Gall and Spurzheim* (London: Baldwin, Cradock, and Joy, 1815); Sharrona Pearl, *About Faces: Physiognomy in Nineteenth-Century Britain* (Cambridge, MA: Harvard University Press, 2010), 186, 189–191.
20. J. Stanley Grimes, *A New System of Phrenology* (Buffalo, NY: Oliver G. Steele, 1839).
21. "Article I. My Proposed Course," *The American Phrenological Journal and Miscellany* 4, no. 1 (January 1842): 2; emphasis in the original.
22. Cornel, "Something Old, Something New," 305–306.
23. Cornel, "Something Old, Something New," 306.
24. Cornel, "Something Old, Something New," 306.
25. Cornel, "Something Old, Something New," 313–314.
26. Cornel, "Something Old, Something New," 314.
27. "Critic Gossip," *Daily Critic* (Washington, DC), February 14, 1873.
28. Finger, *Origins of Neuroscience*, 34–36; Cornel, "Something Old, Something New," 307.
29. These claims by phrenologists were explored by Jason W. Brown and Karen L. Chobar, who contend that while Gall "provided the first complete descriptions of an expressive aphasia with a proposed brain localization," this was "the correct result of a mixed set of arguments." Further, they suggest that if Gall had stopped after localizing language, his status would likely be more secure in the history of neurology. Brown and Chobar, "Phrenological Studies of Aphasia before Broca," 481–482.
30. "What the Savans are Doing for Phrenology," *The Phrenological Journal and Life Illustrated* 59, no. 6 (December 1874): 13.
31. "The Motor Centre Controversy," *Phrenological Journal and Life Illustrated* 82, no. 6 (June 1886): 349.
32. The *Phrenological Magazine* was a British publication, but its publisher was L. N. Fowler. J. W., "Is Phrenology a Science?," *The Phrenological Magazine* 1 (July 1880): 214.
33. J. W., "Is Phrenology a Science?," 214.
34. J. W., "Is Phrenology a Science?," 214.
35. J. W., "Is Phrenology a Science?," 214.
36. Geelossapuss E. O'Dell, "What Phrenology Is," in *Phrenology: Essays and Studies*, ed. Stackpool E. O'Dell and Geelossapuss E. O'Dell (London: The London Phrenological Institution, 1899), 4.
37. O'Dell, "What Phrenology Is," 4.
38. "The Human Brain. A Scientist Waking Up.," *The Phrenological Journal and Life Illustrated* 58, no. 2 (February 1874): 114–115.
39. "The Human Brain," 115.
40. Similarly, a biographical notice published in the *Phrenological Journal and Life Illustrated* as a memorial after Broca's death did not discuss his dispute with phrenology, even though most other articles addressing Broca in this era made this point central to their discussion of his work. "Paul Broca, the Eminent French Physiologist," *Phrenological Journal and Life Illustrated* 74, no. 2 (February 1882): 75–76.

41. This was not the first article published in the *Popular Science Monthly* with this title. Andrew Wilson, "The Old Phrenology and the New," *The Popular Science Monthly* 14 (February 1879): 475–491.
42. Peter Gay, *Freud: A Life for Our Time* (New York: W. W. Norton, 2006 [1998]), 196; Horace Winchell Magoun, *American Neuroscience in the Twentieth Century: Confluence of the Neural, Behavioral, and Communicative Streams* (Leiden: A. A. Balkema, 2003), 379–380; Jonathan W. Marshall, *Performing Neurology: The Dramaturgy of Dr Jean-Martin Charcot* (New York: Palgrave Macmillan, 2016), 75.
43. M. Allen Starr, "The Old and the New Phrenology," *The Popular Science Monthly* 35, no. 6 (October 1889): 730.
44. Starr, "The Old and the New Phrenology," 730.
45. The phrase "new phrenology," along with the similar phrase "scientific phrenology," was used several times throughout the latter part of the century in the *Popular Science Monthly* in articles that described or explained scientific studies of the motor functions and other localization efforts. See Bernard Hollander, "Centers of Ideation in the Brain," *The Popular Science Monthly* 37 (August 1890): 514; Henry de Varigny, "Cerebral Localization; or, the New Phrenology," *The Popular Science Monthly* 18 (March 1881): 599–531; Wilson, "The Old Phrenology and the New."
46. Starr, "The Old and the New Phrenology," 748. Also quoted in Cornel, "Something Old, Something New," 299.
47. R., "The Old and the New Phrenology," *The Phrenological Journal and Science of Health* 89, no. 5 (November 1889): 204.
48. The article in question was Wilson, "The Old Phrenology and the New."
49. R., "The Old and the New Phrenology," 205.
50. R., "The Old and the New Phrenology," 206.
51. Prof. H. S. Drayton, "Old and New Phrenology," *The Phrenological Journal and Science of Health* 6 (December 1892): 278.
52. Drayton, "Old and New Phrenology," 279.
53. Drayton, "Old and New Phrenology," 279.
54. Drayton, "Old and New Phrenology," 279.
55. Drayton, "Old and New Phrenology," 280.
56. H. S. Drayton, "A Defense of Phrenology," *The Sunday Inter Ocean* (Chicago, IL), February 28, 1892. Drayton was responding to "Bumps and Feelers," *The Daily Inter Ocean* (Chicago, IL), January 18, 1892.
57. Drayton, "A Defense of Phrenology."
58. "Our Subject and its Correlatives," *The Phrenological Journal and Science of Health* 4 (October 1892): 190–191.
59. "Who are Phrenologists?," *The Phrenological Journal and Life Illustrated* 75, no. 4 (October 1882): 220.
60. "Who are Phrenologists?," 221.
61. "Who are Phrenologists?," 221.
62. Mary Gibson, *Born to Crime: Cesare Lombroso and the Origins of Biological Criminology* (Westport, CT: Praeger, 2002), 20.
63. On Lombroso, see Piers Beirne, *Inventing Criminology: Essays on the Rise of* Homo Criminalis (Albany: State University of New York Press, 1993), 147–155; Michael Dow Burkhead, *The Search for the Causes of Crime: A History of Theory in Criminology* (Jefferson, NC: McFarland & Company, 2006), 72–81; Arthur E. Fink, *Causes of Crime: Biological Theories in the United States, 1800–1915* (Philadelphia: University of Pennsylvania Press, 1938), 101–103, 112–113, 118–120; Gibson, *Born to Crime*;

David G. Horn, *The Criminal Body: Lombroso and the Anatomy of Deviance* (New York: Routledge, 2003); David A. Jones, *History of Criminology: A Philosophical Perspective* (Westport, CT: Greenwood Press, 1986), 82–93; Nicole Hahn Rafter, *Creating Born Criminals* (Urbana: University of Illinois Press, 1997), 113–114, 120–126; Ysabel Rennie, *The Search for Criminal Man: A Conceptual History of the Dangerous Offender* (Lexington, MA: Lexington Books, 1978), 67–78.

64. Rennie, *The Search for Criminal Man*, 68.
65. Hilts has argued that phrenology encapsulated and promoted a strongly hereditarian view, pre-Darwin and late-century discourse on degeneration and eugenics. Victor L. Hilts, "Obeying the Laws of Hereditary Descent: Phrenological Views on Inheritance and Eugenics," *Journal of the History of the Behavioral Sciences* 18, no. 1 (1982): 63.
66. *L'uomo delinquente* was first published in 1876 and went through five editions, each expanding on the original work. An abridged edition was published posthumously in 1911 by Lombroso's daughter, Gina Lombroso Ferrero; this was the only edition of the work to be translated into English. As Mary Gibson has observed, many readers in the Anglo-American context would have accessed Lombroso's theories secondhand or through commentaries and critiques. However, the companion work, *La donna delinquente*, published in 1893, was swiftly translated into English in 1895, with both American and British editions. Gibson, *Born to Crime*, 18–30, 212–213, 249; C. Lombroso and E. G. Ferrero, *La donna delinquente, la prostituta e la donna normale* (Turin: Editori L. Roux e C., 1893); Cæsar Lombroso and William Ferrero, *The Female Offender* (New York: D. Appleton and Company, 1895); Cesare Lombroso, *L'uomo delinquente* (Milan: Hoepli, 1876); Cesare Lombroso and Gina Lombroso Ferrero, *Criminal Man* (New York; London: G. P. Putnam's Sons, 1911).
67. This process accelerated after the second International Congress of Criminal Anthropology in 1889. Gibson, *Born to Crime*, 43–45, 249–250.
68. Rafter, *Creating Born Criminals*, 111.
69. Rafter, *Creating Born Criminals*, 111.
70. Daniel Patrick Thurs, *Science Talk: Changing Notions of Science in American Popular Culture* (New Brunswick, NJ: Rutgers University Press, 2007), 24.
71. On specialization in nineteenth-century medicine, see George Weisz, *Divide and Conquer: A Comparative History of Medical Specialization* (Oxford: Oxford University Press, 2006).
72. Burton Peter Thom, "The Science of Crime. Part I," *The Phrenological Journal and Science of Health* 108, no. 10 (October 1899): 314.
73. Thom, "The Science of Crime," 314.
74. Thom, "The Science of Crime," 314.
75. A. Boardman, *A Defence of Phrenology* (New York: Fowler and Wells, 1847), 118–120; Finger, *Minds Behind the Brain*, 127.
76. Gibson, *Born to Crime*, 21.
77. Cesare Lombroso, "Why Criminals of Genius Have No Type," *The International Quarterly* 6, no. 1 (September–December 1903): 229–240.
78. "Criminal Woman [Review]," *The Speaker* (London), October 12, 1895, 398.
79. "Criminal Anthropology," *The Phrenological Journal and Science of Health* 100, no. 4 (October 1895): 195.
80. "Criminal Anthropology," 195.
81. Thomas Wilson, "Criminal Anthropology," in *Annual Report of the Board of Regents of the Smithsonian Institution . . .* (Washington, DC: Government Printing Office, 1891), 619, 622–623.

82. Gibson, *Born to Crime*, 39–40.
83. "Notes in Science and Industry. From the Congress on Criminal Anthropology," *The Phrenological Journal and Science of Health* 89, no. 5 (November 1889): 231–232.
84. "The New Debtor to the Old," *The Phrenological Journal and Science of Health* 89, no. 5 (November 1889): 236.
85. "The New Debtor to the Old," 236.
86. The translation suggested within the article, "let the credit be awarded without envy or prejudice," differs from the traditional translation of the Latin, "Let he who merited the palm bear it." "The New Debtor to the Old," 237. Latin translation is thanks to Scott DiGiulio.
87. "A More Cheerful View," *The Phrenological Journal and Science of Health* 4 (April 1893): 194.
88. "A More Cheerful View," 195.
89. Bernard Hollander, "Centers of Ideation in the Brain," *The Popular Science Monthly* 37, no. 32 (August 1890): 514–528.
90. Hollander, "Centers of Ideation in the Brain," 527.
91. Hollander, "Centers of Ideation in the Brain," 527–528.
92. Gibson, *Born to Crime*, 43.
93. "A Merry Christmas to All Our Friends and a Basketful of Good Cheer. Dr. Lombroso, the Criminologist," *The Phrenological Journal and Science of Health* 122, no. 12 (December 1909): 401.
94. "A Merry Christmas to All Our Friends," 401.
95. George Combe, *Elements of Phrenology* (Edinburgh: John Anderson Jr., 1824), 225–227; Lucile E. Hoyme, "Physical Anthropology and Its Instruments: An Historical Study," *Southwestern Journal of Anthropology* 9, no. 4 (1953): 413–414.
96. George Combe, *Elements of Phrenology*, 5th ed. (Edinburgh: Maclachlan, Stewart, & Co., 1841), 196.
97. Samuel George Morton, *Crania Americana; or, A Comparative View of the Skulls of Various Aboriginal Nations of North and South America* (Philadelphia: J. Dobson; London: Simpkin, Marshall & Co., 1839), 262. See also discussion of Morton and Combe in chapter 2.
98. Alphonse Bertillon, *Identification anthropométrique: Instructions signalétiques* (Melun, France: Typographie-Lithographie Administrative, 1885); Alphonse Bertillon, *Signaletic Instructions, Including the Theory and Practice of Anthropometrical Identification* (Chicago: Werner Company, 1896).
99. Simon A. Cole, *Suspect Identities: A History of Fingerprinting and Criminal Identification* (Cambridge, MA: Harvard University Press, 2001), 33–34. On Bertillon and his system, see also Jonathan Finn, *Capturing the Criminal Image: From Mug Shot to Surveillance Society* (Minneapolis: University of Minnesota Press, 2009), 23–28.
100. "To Identify Criminals. A French Method Better than Photographs," *New York Times*, May 18, 1890.
101. Cole, *Suspect Identities*, 63–69, 74–80.
102. Cole, *Suspect Identities*, 75.
103. "To Identify Criminals"; Cole, *Suspect Identities*, 49.
104. Cole, *Suspect Identities*, 51–58.
105. During the 1920s, American law enforcement agencies phased out anthropometric files in favor of fingerprint-based files, although in some cases Bertillonage cards were still being used into the 1930s, as in the records of prisons and reformatories in

New York State. Cole, *Suspect Identities*, 217; Male inmate identification file (Bertillon ledger), 1921–1936 (B0059), New York State Archives, Albany, NY; Admission registers, 1877–1950, Elmira Reformatory (B0140), New York State Archives, Albany, NY; Female inmate identification file, 1909–1933, (B0054), New York State Archives, Albany, NY.

106. "To Identify Criminals"; "Bertillon System Taught," *New York Times*, July 16, 1896.
107. "The Bertillon Identification Scheme," *Scientific American* 91, no. 25 (1904): 433.
108. "The Bertillon Identification Scheme," 432.
109. "To Identify Criminals"; "The Bertillon Identification Scheme," 433.
110. "The New Debtor to the Old," 236.
111. Henry Clark, "Some Notes on a Rogue's Gallery," *The Phrenological Journal and Life Illustrated* 88, no. 4 (October 1888): 183–185; H. S. Drayton, "Phrenotypes and Side-Views, No. 21: In a Gallery of Rogues," *The Phrenological Journal and Science of Health* 105, no. 3 (March 1898): 73–76.
112. Drayton, "Phrenotypes and Side-Views," 74.
113. Drayton, "Phrenotypes and Side-Views," 73.
114. D., "The Identification of Criminals," *The Phrenological Journal and Science of Health* 103, no. 4 (April 1897): 188.
115. D., "The Identification of Criminals," 188.
116. D., "The Identification of Criminals," 188–189.
117. Cole, *Suspect Identities*, 34.
118. Pasi Falk, *The Consuming Body* (London: Sage Publications, 1997 [1994]), 53.
119. Cole, *Suspect Identities*, 34.
120. Patricia Cline Cohen, *A Calculating People: The Spread of Numeracy in Early America* (Chicago: University of Chicago Press, 1982); Theodore M. Porter, *Trust in Numbers: The Pursuit of Objectivity in Science and Public Life* (Princeton, NJ: Princeton University Press, 1995).
121. "Not Bumps, but Calipers. Miss Fowler Talks about Skulls and Upsets a Popular Notion about Phrenology," *The Sunday News* (Charleston, SC), January 21, 1906.
122. See, for example, Finger, *Minds Behind the Brain*; Finger, *Origins of Neuroscience*; Glickstein, *Neuroscience*; Gross, *Brain, Vision, Memory*; Guenther, *Localization and Its Discontents*; Harrington, *Medicine, Mind, and the Double Brain*; Rafter, *Creating Born Criminals*; Nicole Hahn Rafter, "The Murderous Dutch Fiddler: Criminology, History, and the Problem of Phrenology," *Theoretical Criminology* 9, no. 1 (2005): 65–96; Young, *Mind, Brain, and Adaptation in the Nineteenth Century*. The covers of a number of books in this field also depict the phrenological bust, including Harrington, *Medicine, Mind, and the Double Brain*; LaPoint, *Paul Broca and the Origins of Language in the Brain*; and Rafter, *Creating Born Criminals*.

Epilogue

1. J. D. Gehring, "Utility of Phrenology: A Dream of Fifty Years Forward," *The Phrenological Journal and Science of Health* 5 (May 1892): 215.
2. R. T. Webb, *The Phrenologist; A Farce, in Two Acts: Containing a Popular Summary of That Pseudo, or Real Science* (London: Printed for the author, by C. Slater, 1824), 30.
3. John Collins Warren Jr., "The Collection of the Boston Phrenological Society—A Retrospect," *Annals of Medical History* 3, no. 1 (1921): 1, in John Collins Warren Jr., "The Collection of the Boston Phrenological Society—A Retrospect. Original draft

of . . . Received by the Museum June 9, 1924," Rare Books 1.Mw.1921.W, Harvard Medical Library in the Francis A. Countway Library of Medicine, Boston, MA.

4. Samuel Gridley Howe to John Collins Warren Sr., June 25, 1849; Samuel Gridley Howe to John Collins Warren Sr., June 27, 1849; Samuel Gridley Howe to John Collins Warren Sr., September 3, 1849; and John Collins Warren Sr. to Samuel Gridley Howe [probably draft], February 4, 1850, in Warren, "The Collection of the Boston Phrenological Society."
5. Warren, "The Collection of the Boston Phrenological Society," 1.
6. Warren, "The Collection of the Boston Phrenological Society," 1.
7. Warren, "The Collection of the Boston Phrenological Society," 11.
8. See Robert N. Smith, *An Evil Day in Georgia: The Killing of Coleman Osborn and the Death Penalty in the Progressive-Era South* (Knoxville: University of Tennessee Press, 2015).
9. "Georgia Slayers Executed; Wife's Confession Fails," *Times-Picayune* (New Orleans, LA), August 4, 1928.
10. James F. Cook, *The Governors of Georgia, 1754–2004*, 3rd ed. (Macon, GA: Mercer University Press, 2005), 228–229; Smith, *An Evil Day in Georgia*, 97.
11. Cook, *The Governors of Georgia*, 229; Smith, *An Evil Day in Georgia*, 97.
12. Eula Mae Thompson was the first woman sentenced to the electric chair in Georgia. After the sentence was commuted to life in prison, she served eight years before a later governor, Eugene Talmadge, pardoned her. Harold Martin, "State's First Woman Sentenced to Chair Tells Her Life Story," *Atlanta Constitution*, August 17, 1941.
13. Smith, *An Evil Day in Georgia*, 105, 129–130, 139–140.
14. "Judge Relies on Phrenology," *Daily Herald* (London), August 21, 1928, Marshall Phrenological Collection: News Cuttings, scrapbook, 1929–1939. Box 1, Folder 33, Series IV. Publications about Phrenology, B. News Clippings, News Cuttings, scrapbook, 1929–1939, Marshall Phrenological Collection, 1876–1958, BMS c99, Boston Medical Library in the Francis A. Countway Library of Medicine, Boston, MA.
15. Whitner Cary, "With Plea for Life of Wife, Thompson Goes to His Death," *Atlanta Constitution*, August 4, 1928.
16. Martin, "State's First Woman Sentenced to Chair Tells Her Life Story."
17. "Hardman Asked to Study Photo in Death Penalty," *Atlanta Constitution*, August 17, 1928.
18. "Hardman Asked to Study Photo in Death Penalty."
19. "High Court Upholds 3 Death Sentences," *Atlanta Constitution*, March 15, 1929.
20. Much of the work on criminal and forensic science in the twentieth and twenty-first centuries has been published outside of the academic press, with by far the majority focusing on the "true crime" genre. See for example: Suzanne Bell, *Crime and Circumstance: Investigating the History of Forensic Science* (Westport, CT: Praeger, 2008); Deborah Blum, *The Poisoner's Handbook: Murder and the Birth of Forensic Medicine in Jazz Age New York* (New York: Penguin, 2010); James O'Brien, *The Scientific Sherlock Holmes: Cracking the Case with Science and Forensics* (Oxford: Oxford University Press, 2013); Katherine Ramsland, *Beating the Devil's Game: A History of Forensic Science and Criminal Investigation* (New York: Berkley Books, 2007).
21. J. Tiihonen et al., "Genetic Background of Extreme Violent Behavior," *Molecular Psychiatry* 20, no. 6 (2015): 792.

22. For a small sample of the coverage of this report, see Agata Blaszczak-Boxe, "Two Genes May Contribute to Violent Crime, Study Says," CBS News, October 29, 2014, http://www.cbsnews.com/news/two-genes-may-contribute-to-violent-crime-study-says/; Justin Glawe, "Identifying 'Criminal' Genes Will Never Prevent Violence But Might Help Explain It," *Vice*, November 13, 2014, http://www.vice.com/read/identifying-criminal-genes-will-never-prevent-violence-but-might-help-explain-it-1113; Melissa Healy, "For Some, Violent Criminality May Be Written in Their Genes," *Los Angeles Times*, October 29, 2014, http://www.latimes.com/science/sciencenow/la-sci-violent-criminality-genes-20141028-story.html; Sarah Knapton, "Violence Genes May Be Responsible for One in 10 Serious Crimes," *Telegraph*, October 28, 2014, http://www.telegraph.co.uk/news/science/science-news/11192643/Violence-genes-may-be-responsible-for-one-in-10-serious-crimes.html; Mariette Le Roux, "What Makes a Criminal? Gene Trawl Raises Questions," Business Insider, October 28, 2014, http://www.businessinsider.com/afp-what-makes-a-criminal-gene-trawl-raises-questions-2014-10.
23. Megan Scudellari, "Extreme Violent Crimes Tied to Gene in Study of Criminals," Bloomberg, October 28, 2014, http://www.bloomberg.com/news/2014-10-28/extreme-violent-crimes-tied-to-gene-in-study-of-criminals.html.
24. Sarah Griffiths, "Are Criminals Born with a MURDER GENE? Scientists Identify Cause of Violent Behaviour," *Daily Mail Online*, October 28, 2014, http://www.dailymail.co.uk/sciencetech/article-2810667/Are-thugs-BORN-not-Genes-associated-violent-behaviour-identified.html.
25. Anthony Rivas, "Genes May Predict Violent Criminal Behavior, But This Isn't Minority Report," *Medical Daily*, October 29, 2014, http://www.medicaldaily.com/two-genes-may-predict-violent-criminal-behavior-isnt-minority-report-308434.
26. TNO Staff, "Scientists Find that Nazis were Correct about Heredity and Criminality," *The New Observer*, October 30, 2014, http://newobserveronline.com/scientists-find-that-nazis-were-correct-about-heredity-and-criminality/.
27. Marc Lallanilla, "Genetics May Provide Clues to Newtown Shooting," Live Science, December 28, 2012, http://www.livescience.com/25853-newtown-shooter-dna.html; Julia Llewellyan Smith, "Studying Adam Lanza: Is Evil in Our Genes?," *Telegraph*, April 10, 2013, http://www.telegraph.co.uk/news/science/science-news/9968753/Studying-Adam-Lanza-is-evil-in-our-genes.html.
28. For example: Eyal Aharoni et al., "Neuroprediction of Future Rearrest," *Proceedings of the National Academy of Sciences of the United States of America* 110, no. 15 (2013): 6223–6228; Sarah Gregory et al., "The Antisocial Brain: Psychopathy Matters: A Structural MRI Investigation of Antisocial Male Violent Offenders," *Archives of General Psychiatry* 69, no. 9 (2012): 962–972.
29. Tim Adams, "How to Spot a Murderer's Brain," *Guardian*, May 11, 2013, http://www.theguardian.com/science/2013/may/12/how-to-spot-a-murderers-brain.
30. Michael P. Haselhuhn and Elaine M. Wong, "Bad to the Bone: Facial Structure Predicts Unethical Behavior," *Proceedings of the Royal Society B* 279, no. 1728 (2012): 571–576.
31. Michael P. Haselhuhn, Elaine M. Wong, and Margaret E. Ormiston, "Self-Fulfilling Prophecies as a Link between Men's Facial Width-to-Height Ratio and Behavior," *PLOS One* 8, no. 8 (2013): e72259, https://doi.org/10.1371/journal.pone.0072259.
32. Justin M. Carré, Cheryl M. McCormick, and Catherine J. Mondloch, "Facial Structure Is a Reliable Cue for Aggressive Behavior," *Psychological Science* 20, no. 10 (2009): 1194–1198; Justin M. Carré and Cheryl M. McCormick, "In Your Face: Facial

Metrics Predict Aggressive Behaviour in the Laboratory and in Varsity and Professional Hockey Players," *Proceedings of the Royal Society B: Biological Sciences* 275, no. 1651 (2008): 2651–2656; Michael P. Haselhuhn, Margaret E. Ormiston, and Elaine M. Wong, "Men's Facial Width-to-Height Ratio Predicts Aggression: A Meta-Analysis," *PLOS One* 10, no. 4 (2015): e0122637, https://doi.org/10.1371/journal.pone.0122637; Ian S. Penton-Voak et al., "Personality Judgments from Natural and Composite Facial Images: More Evidence for a 'Kernel of Truth' in Social Perception," *Social Cognition* 24, no. 5 (2006): 607–640.

33. Shawn N. Geniole et al., "Evidence from Meta-Analyses of the Facial Width-to-Height Ratio as an Evolved Cue of Threat," *PLOS One* 10, no. 7 (2015): e0132726, https://doi.org/10.1371/journal.pone.0132726.
34. Jorge Gómez-Valdés et al., "Lack of Support for the Association between Facial Shape and Aggression: A Reappraisal Based on a Worldwide Population Genetics Perspective," *PLOS One* 8, no. 1 (2013): e52317, https://doi.org/10.1371/journal.pone.0052317.
35. University of California–Riverside, "Wide-Faced Men Make Others Act Selfishly," ScienceDaily, September 16, 2013, www.sciencedaily.com/releases/2013/09/130916140451.htm; University of California–Riverside, "Wide-Faced Men Make Others Act Selfishly," Medical Xpress, https://medicalxpress.com/news/2013-09-wide-faced-men-selfishly.html. The image is no longer included in the ScienceDaily version of the press release.
36. The phrase is used throughout this essay. Carré, McCormick, and Mondloch, "Facial Structure Is a Reliable Cue for Aggressive Behavior," 1194, 1196, 1197, 1198.
37. This association is sometimes acknowledged directly, particularly in essays in which these findings are disputed, as in the Gómez-Valdés et al. essay, which begins with Gall, though it incorrectly dates Gall's work. See Gómez-Valdés et al., "Lack of Support for the Association between Facial Shape and Aggression."
38. Tom Whyman, "People Keep Trying to Bring Back Phrenology," *The Outline*, October 15, 2019, https://theoutline.com/post/8104/phrenology-hirevue-quillette?zd=1&zi=fo6j2djm.

Bibliography

Archives

Albany Medical College Archives, Albany, NY
American Philosophical Society, Philadelphia, PA
Beinecke Rare Book and Manuscript Library, Yale University, New Haven, CT
Centre for Research Collections, Main Library, University of Edinburgh, Edinburgh, UK
David M. Rubenstein Rare Book & Manuscript Library, Duke University, Durham, NC
Division of Rare and Manuscript Collections, Cornell University Library, Cornell University, Ithaca, NY
Francis A. Countway Library of Medicine, Harvard University, Boston, MA
Harvey Cushing/John Hay Whitney Medical Library, Yale University, New Haven, CT
Louise M. Darling Biomedical Library, University of California, Los Angeles, CA
Maine Historical Society, Portland, ME
New York Academy of Medicine, New York, NY
New York State Archives, Albany, NY
New York State Library, Albany, NY
Wellcome Collection, London, UK

Periodicals

The Albion
American Journal of Science
The American Journal of the Medical Sciences
The American Jurist and Law Magazine
The American Law Register
American Phrenological Journal (by various titles)
The American Whig Review
Annals of Phrenology
Atkinson's Casket or Gems of Literature, Wit and Sentiment
The Boston Medical and Surgical Journal
Christian Watchman
The Eclectic Journal of Medicine
The Eclectic Review
The Edinburgh Review, or Critical Journal
The Emerald, or Miscellany of Literature
Foreign Quarterly Review
The Hangman
Home Journal
The International Quarterly
The Knickerbocker
The Law Magazine; or, Quarterly Review of Jurisprudence
The Literary Magazine, and American Register
Mechanics' Magazine, and Register of Inventions and Improvements
Medical Magazine

The Medico-Chirurgical Review, and Journal of Practical Medicine
National Police Gazette
The New Orleans Medical and Surgical Journal
Philadelphia Journal of the Medical and Physical Sciences
The Phrenological Journal and Magazine of Moral Science
The Phrenological Journal and Miscellany
The Phrenological Magazine
The Popular Science Monthly
The Prisoner's Friend, A Monthly Magazine
Scientific American
Spirit of the Age and Journal of Humanity
Transactions of the College of Physicians of Philadelphia
Transactions of the Phrenological Society
Westminster Review

Printed Primary Sources

Alexander, H. H., and Edward D. Easton. *Report of the Proceedings in the Case of the United States vs. Charles J. Guiteau . . .* Washington, DC: Government Printing Office, 1882.

Annual Report of the Board of Regents of the Smithsonian Institution . . . Washington, DC: Government Printing Office, 1891.

Barber, Jonathan. *An Address Delivered Before the Boston Phrenological Society.* Boston: Marsh, Capen & Lyon, 1833.

Barnes, J. *The Darkey Phrenologist: A Nigger Absurdity in One Act.* New York: Dick & Fitzgerald, 1899.

Beck, Theodric Romeyn. *Elements of Medical Jurisprudence.* Vol. 1. Albany, NY: Websters and Skinners, 1823.

Bertillon, Alphonse. *Identification anthropométrique: Instructions signalétiques.* Melun, France: Typographie-Lithographie Administrative, 1885.

———. *Signaletic Instructions, Including the Theory and Practice of Anthropometrical Identification.* Chicago: Werner Company, 1896.

Blöde, Karl August. *Dr. F. J. Galls Lehre über die Verrichtungen des Gehirns, nach dessen zu Dresden gehaltenen Vorlesungen in einer fasslichen Ordnung mit gewissenhafter Treue dargestellt.* Dresden: Arnoldischen Buchhandlung, 1805.

Boardman, A. *A Defence of Phrenology.* New York: Fowler and Wells, 1847.

Boston Phrenological Society. *A Catalogue of Phrenological Specimens, Belonging to the Boston Phrenological Society.* Boston: John Ford, 1835.

Brereton, J. A. *A Report Submitted to the Phrenological Society of the City of Washington, on the 14th of March 1828, and Printed by Order.* Washington, DC: E. De Kraft, Printer, 1828.

A Brief Sketch of the Occurrences on Board the Brig Crawford, on Her Voyage from Matanzas to New-York; Together with an Account of the Trial of the Three Spaniards, Jose Hilario Casares, Felix Barbeito, and Jose Morando . . . Richmond, VA: Samuel Shepherd & Co., 1827.

Brock, Appellant, v. Luckett's Executors. 5 Miss. 459. 1840.

Browne, J. H. Balfour. *The Medical Jurisprudence of Insanity.* 2nd ed. Philadelphia: Lindsay & Blakiston, 1876.

Caldwell, Charles. *Elements of Phrenology.* Lexington, KY: Thomas T. Skillman, 1824.

———. *Introductory Address on Independence of Intellect.* Lexington, KY: Printed at the Office of the Kentucky Whig, 1825.

———. *Phrenology Vindicated and Antiphrenology Unmasked.* New York: Samuel Colman, 1838.

Calvert, George H., ed. *Illustrations of Phrenology; Being a Selection of Articles from the Edinburg Phrenological Journal, and the Transactions of the Edinburg Phrenological Society.* Baltimore: William and Joseph Neal, 1832.

Capen, Nahum. *Reminiscences of Dr. Spurzheim and George Combe.* New York: Fowler & Wells, 1881.

Catalogue of Busts, Casts, and Skulls in the Phrenological Cabinet, Clinton Hall. New York: Fowlers and Wells, 1850.

A Catechism of Phrenology: Illustrative of the Principles of that Science. Philadelphia: Carey, Lea, & Blanchard, 1835.

Child, L. Maria. *Letters from New-York.* New York: Charles S. Francis and Company, 1843.

Chitty, Joseph, *A Practical Treatise on Medical Jurisprudence: With So Much of Anatomy, Physiology, Pathology, and the Practice of Medicine and Surgery, as Are Essential to Be Known by Members of Parliament, Lawyers, Coroners, Magistrates, Officers in the Army and Navy, and Private Gentlemen; and all the Laws Relating to Medical Practitioners.* Part I. London: Butterworth; Longman, Rees, Orme, Brown, and Green; S. Highley; J. Taylor; Burgess and Hill; Churchill; and H. Renshaw, 1834.

A Collection of Pamphlets and Magazines, from the Press of J. Munsell, Albany, New York. Vol. 4. Albany, NY: Joel Munsell, 1848.

Combe, Andrew. *Observations on Mental Derangement.* Edinburgh: John Anderson Jr., 1831.

———. *Observations on Mental Derangement: Being an Application of the Principles of Phrenology to the Elucidation of the Causes, Symptoms, Nature, and Treatment of Insanity.* Boston: Marsh, Capen & Lyon, 1834.

Combe, George. *Answer to "Observations on the Phrenological Development of Burke, Hare, and Other Atrocious Murderers, &c.—by Thomas Stone, Esq.," &c.* Edinburgh: John Anderson Jr.; London: Simpkin & Marshall, 1829.

———. *The Constitution of Man Considered in Relation to External Objects.* 3rd ed. Edinburgh: John Anderson Jr., 1835.

———. *The Constitution of Man Considered in Relation to External Objects.* 8th American ed. Boston: Marsh, Capen, & Lyon, 1837.

———. *Elements of Phrenology.* Edinburgh: John Anderson Jr., 1824.

———. *Elements of Phrenology.* 4th American ed. Boston: Marsh, Capen & Lyon, 1835.

———. *Elements of Phrenology.* 5th ed. Edinburgh: Maclachlan, Stewart, & Co., 1841.

———. *Essays on Phrenology.* Edinburgh: Bell & Bradfute, 1819.

———. *Essays on Phrenology.* Philadelphia: H. C. Carey and I. Lea, 1822.

———. *Lectures on Phrenology.* New York: Samuel Colman, 1839.

———. *Letter on the Prejudices of the Great in Science and Philosophy against Phrenology; Addressed to the Editor of the Edinburgh Weekly Journal.* Edinburgh: John Anderson Jr.; London: Simpkin & Marshall, 1829.

———. *Notes on the United States of North America, During a Phrenological Visit in 1838–9–40.* Vols. 1 and 2. Philadelphia: Carey & Hart, 1841.

———. *Remarks on the Principles of Criminal Legislation and the Practice of Prison Discipline.* London: Simpkin, Marshall & Co., 1854.

———. *A System of Phrenology.* 3rd ed. Edinburgh: John Anderson Jr., 1825.

———. *A System of Phrenology.* 3rd American ed. Boston: Marsh, Capen, and Lyon, 1835.

Coombs, F. *Coombs's Popular Phrenology.* Boston, 1841.

Crozier, C. W., and A. R. M'Kee. *Life and Trial of Dr. Abner Baker, Jr., (A Monomaniac,) Who Was Executed October 3, 1845* . . . Louisville, KY: Prentice and Weissinger, 1846.

Cureau de la Chambre, Marin. *L'art de connoistre les hommes*. Paris: Chez Iacques d'Allin, 1667.

David, Alexandre. *Le petit Docteur Gall ou l'art de connaître les hommes par la phrénologie d'après les systèmes de Gall et de Spurzheim*. Paris: Passard, 1859.

Dean, Amos. *Lectures on Phrenology*. Albany, NY: Oliver Steele, 1834.

———. *The Philosophy of Human Life: Being an Investigation of the Great Elements of Life* . . . Boston: Marsh, Capen, Lyon and Webb, 1839.

———. *Principles of Medical Jurisprudence: Designed for the Professions of Law and Medicine*. Albany, NY: Banks & Brothers, 1850.

Defendant's Counsel. *Trial of Charles B. Huntington for Forgery. Principle Defence: Insanity*. New York: John S. Voorhies, 1857.

Delafield, John. *The Law of Circumstantial Evidence and of Insanity: A Report in Full of the Trial of Edward D. Worrell, Indicted for the Murder of Basil H. Gordon* . . . St. Louis: M. Niedner, 1857.

Donovan, C. *A Handbook of Phrenology*. London: Longmans, Green, Reader, and Dyer, 1870.

Echeverria, M. Gonzalez. *The Trial of "John Reynolds," Medico-legally Considered*. New York: Baker & Godwin, Printers, 1870.

Elliotson, John, *Lectures on the Theory and Practice of Medicine*. London: J. F. Moore, 1839.

Encyclopædia Londinensis; or, Universal Dictionary of Arts, Sciences, and Literature. Vol. 20. London, 1825.

Fletcher, John. *The Mirror of Nature, Part I: Presenting a Practical Illustration of the Science of Phrenology*. Boston: Cassady and March, 1839.

Follen, Charles. *Professor Follen's Funeral Oration Delivered at the Burial of Dr. G. Spurzheim*. Boston: Marsh, Capen & Lyon, 1832.

Foote, Edward Bliss. *Sammy Tubbs, the Boy Doctor, and "Sponsie," The Troublesome Monkey*. Vol. 4. New York: Murray Hill Publishing, 1874.

Fowler, Lydia Folger. *Familiar Lessons on Physiology, Designed for the Use of Children and Youth in Schools and Families*. 2 vols. New York: Fowlers and Wells, 1847.

Fowler, L. N. *Phrenological Almanac. 1840*. New York: W. J. Spence, 1839.

———. *Phrenological Almanac for 1841*. New York: W. J. Spence, 1840.

———. *The Phrenological Almanac for 1842*. New York: Vincent L. Dill, 1841.

———. *Phrenological and Physiological Almanac for 1848*. New York: Fowlers and Wells, 1847.

———. *The Phrenological and Physiological Almanac for 1849*. New York: Fowlers and Wells, 1849.

Fowler, O. S. *Fowler's Practical Phrenology*. Philadelphia: O. S. Fowler, 1840.

———. *The Practical Phrenologist; and Recorder and Delineator of the Character and Talents* . . . Boston: O. S. Fowler, 1869.

Fowler, O. S., and L. N. Fowler. *The Illustrated Self-Instructor in Phrenology and Physiology*. New York: Fowlers and Wells, 1855.

———. *Phrenology Proved, Illustrated, and Applied*. 2nd ed. New York, 1837.

Gall, F. J. *Anatomie et physiologie du système nerveux en general et du cerveau en particulier*. Vol. 3. Paris, 1818.

———. *On the Functions of the Brain and of Each of Its Parts*. 6 vols. Translated by Winslow Lewis Jr. Boston: Marsh, Capen & Lyon, 1835.

———. *Sur les fonctions du cerveau et sur celles de chacune de ses parties, avec des observations sur la possibilité de reconnaitre les instincts, les penchans, les talens, ou les dispositions morales et intellectuelles des hommes et des animaux, par la configuration de leur cerveau et de leur tête.* 6 vols. Paris: J.-B. Ballière, 1825.

———. *Vollständige Geisteskunde, oder, Auf Erfahrung gestüzte Darstellung der geistigen und moralischen Fähigkeiten und ihrer Körperlichen Bedingungen.* Nuremberg: Leuchs, 1829.

Gall, F. J., and [Johann] G. Spurzheim. *Anatomie et physiologie du système nerveux en général, et du cerveau en particulier, avec des observations sur la possibilité de reconnoître plusieurs dispositions intellectuelles et morales de l'homme et des animaux, par la configuration de leurs têtes.* Vol. 1. Paris: F. Schoell, 1810.

Gibbon, Charles. *The Life of George Combe, author of the "Constitution of Man," in two volumes.* Vol. 2. London: Macmillan and Co., 1878.

Grimes, J. Stanley. *A New System of Phrenology.* Buffalo, NY: Oliver G. Steele, 1839.

Hall, Benjamin F. *The Trial of William Freeman for the Murder of John G. Van Nest, Including the Evidence and the Arguments of Counsel . . .* Auburn, NY: Derby, Miller & Co. Publishers, 1848.

Hoffman, David. *A Course of Legal Study, Addressed to Students and the Professional Generally.* Vol. 2. 2nd ed. Baltimore: Joseph Neal, 1836.

Howe, Samuel Gridley. *A Discourse on the Social Relations of Man; Delivered Before the Boston Phrenological Society, at the Close of Their Course of Lectures.* Boston: Marsh, Capen & Lyon, 1837.

———. *An Essay on Separate and Congregate Systems of Prison Discipline.* Boston: William D. Ticknor and Co., 1846.

Hufeland, C. W. *Some Account of Dr. Gall's New Theory of Physiognomy, Founded upon the Anatomy and Physiology of the Brain, and the Form of the Skull.* London: Longman, Hurst, Rees, and Orme, 1807.

Jones, Silas. *Practical Phrenology.* Boston: Russell, Shattuck, & Williams, 1836.

King, Moses. *King's Handbook of New York City: An Outline, History, and Description of the American Metropolis.* Boston: Moses King, 1892.

Lauvergne, Hubert. *Les forçats considérés sous le rapport physiologique, moral et intellectuel, observés au bagne de Toulon.* Paris: J.-B. Baillière, 1841.

Leland, T. C. *Trial of John Metcalf Thurston, Convicted of the Murder of Anson Garrison . . .* Owego, NY: Hiram A. Beebe, 1851.

Lewis, Ellis Grosh, and Emanuel Jacob Schaeffer. *Report of The Trial and Conviction of John Haggerty, for The Murder of Melchoir Fordney, Late of The City of Lancaster, Pennsylvania.* Lancaster, PA, 1847.

The Life and Adventures of John A. Murrell, the Great Western Land Pirate. New York: H. Long & Brother, [1848].

The Life of the Celebrated Mail Robber and Daring Highwayman, Joseph Thompson Hare . . . Also, of the Cruel and Ferocious Pirate, Alexander Tardy. Philadelphia: J. B. Perry, 1844.

Lombroso, Cesare. *L'uomo delinquent.* Milan: Hoepli, 1876.

Lombroso, Cesare, and E. G. Ferrero. *La donna delinquente, la prostituta e la donna normale.* Turin: Editori L. Roux e C., 1893.

Lombroso, Cesare, and Gina Lombroso Ferrero. *Criminal Man.* New York: G. P. Putnam's Sons, 1911.

Lombroso, Cesare, and William Ferrero. *The Female Offender.* New York: D. Appleton and Company, 1895.

Macnish, Robert. *An Introduction to Phrenology, in the Form of Question and Answer, with an Appendix, and Copious Illustrative Notes*. Boston: Marsh, Capen & Lyon, 1836.

Manual of Phrenology: Being an Analytical Summary of the System of Doctor Gall. Philadelphia: Carey, Lea, & Blanchard, 1835.

Massachusetts Board of Education. *First Annual Report of the Board of Education*. Boston: Dutton and Wentworth, 1838.

Mayors of Boston: An Illustrated Epitome of Who the Mayors Have Been and What They Have Done. Boston: State Street Trust Company, 1914.

McFarland, H. H. *Report of the Trial of Willard Clark, Indicted for the Murder of Richard W. Wight* . . . New Haven, CT: Thomas H. Pease, 1855.

Miles, L. *Phrenology and the Moral Influence of Phrenology*. Philadelphia: Carey, Lea & Blanchard, 1835.

Morton, Samuel George. *Crania Americana; or, A Comparative View of the Skulls of Various Aboriginal Nations of North and South America*. Philadelphia: J. Dobson; London: Simpkin, Marshall & Co., 1839.

Nancy Farrer v. The State of Ohio, 2 Ohio St. 54. 1853.

New England Historic Genealogical Society. *Memorial Biographies of the New England Historic Genealogical Society*. Vol. 6. Boston: Stanhope Press, 1905.

Noble, Daniel. *The Brain and Its Physiology*. London: John Churchill, 1846.

Nott, Josiah Clark, and George R. Gliddon. *Indigenous Races of the Earth; or, New Chapters of Ethnological Inquiry*. Philadelphia: J. B. Lippincott & Co., 1857.

O'Dell, Stackpool E., and Geelossapuss E. O'Dell, eds. *Phrenology: Essays and Studies*. London: The London Phrenological Institution, 1899.

Otis, James F. *Report of the Trial of Major Mitchell, for Felonious Assault and Maiming, on the Person of David H. Crawford: Before the Supreme Judicial Court of the State of Maine, at the Term for the County of Cumberland, Held at Portland, on the First Tuesday of November, 1834; with the Arguments of Counsel*. Portland, ME: Colman & Chisholm, 1834.

Pinel, Ph. *A Treatise on Insanity*. Translated by D. D. Davis. Sheffield, UK: W. Todd, 1806.

Pitman, Benn. *The Assassination of President Lincoln and the Trial of the Conspirators*. New York: Moore, Wilstach & Baldwin, 1865.

Prichard, James Cowles. *Treatise on Insanity and Other Disorders Affecting the Mind*. London: Sherwood, Gilbert, and Piper, 1835.

Poe, Edgar Allan. *The Pit and the Pendulum and Other Tales*. Edited by David Van Leer. Oxford: Oxford University Press, 2018 [1998].

Randolf, J. *A Memoir on the Life and Character of Philip Syng Physick, M.D.* Philadelphia: T. K. & P. G. Collins, 1839.

Ray, I. "Hints to the Medical Witness in Questions of Insanity." *American Journal of Psychiatry* 8, no. 1 (April 1851): 53–67.

———. *A Treatise on the Medical Jurisprudence of Insanity*. Boston: Charles C. Little and James Brown, 1838.

Roget, P. M. *Outlines of Physiology: With an Appendix on Phrenology*. 1st American ed. Philadelphia: Lea and Blanchard, 1839.

Selpert, H. G. C. von. *D. Gall's Vorlesungen über die Verrichtungen des Gehirns und die Möglichkeit die Anlagen mehrerer Geistes und Gemüthseigenschaften aus dem Baue des Schädels der Menchen und Thiere zu erkennen*. Berlin: Johann Friedrich Unger, 1805.

Sewall, Thomas. *An Examination of Phrenology; in Two Lectures*. London: James S. Hodson, 1838.

Shufeldt, R. W. *America's Greatest Problem: The Negro*. Philadelphia: F. A. Davis Company, 1915.

Shurtleff, Nathaniel. *An Epitome of Phrenology: Being an Outline of the Science as Taught by Gall Spurzheim and Combe . . .* Boston: Marsh, Capen & Lyon, 1835.

Sizer, Nelson. *Forty Years in Phrenology; Embracing Recollections of History, Anecdote, and Experience*. New York: Fowler & Wells Co., 1888.

Spurzheim, J. G. *Observations on the Deranged Manifestations of the Mind, or Insanity*. London: Baldwin, Cradock, and Joy, 1817.

———. *Observations sur la folie*. Paris: Treuttel et Würtz, 1818.

———. *Outlines of Phrenology*. Boston: Marsh, Capen and Lyon, 1832.

———. *Philosophical Catechism of the Natural Laws of Man*. 2nd ed. Boston: Marsh, Capen and Lyon, 1832.

———. *Phrenology, in Connexion with the Study of Physiognomy*. Boston: Marsh, Capen & Lyon, 1833.

———. *Phrenology, or the Doctrine of the Mental Phenomena*. 2 vols. Boston: Marsh, Capen & Lyon, 1832.

———. *Phrenology, or, the Doctrine of the Mind; and of the Relations between its Manifestations and the Body*. 3rd ed. London: Charles Knight, 1835.

———. *The Physiognomical System of Drs. Gall and Spurzheim*. London: Baldwin, Cradock, and Joy, 1815.

———. *A View of the Elementary Principles of Education, Founded on the Study of the Nature of Man*. Boston: Marsh Capen and Lyon, 1832.

Stone, Thomas. *Observations on the Phrenological Development of Burke, Hare, and Other Atrocious Murderers; Measurements of the Heads of the Most Notorious Thieves Confined in the Edinburgh Jail and Bridewell, and of Various Individuals, English, Scotch, and Irish, Presenting an Extensive Series of Facts Subversive of Phrenology*. Edinburgh: Robert Buchanan; William Hunter; and John Stevenson; London: T. and G. Underwood; Glasgow: Robertson and Atkinson; Aberdeen: Alex. Brown & Co.; Dublin: J. Cuming, 1829.

———. *A Rejoinder to the Answer of George Combe, Esq., to "Observations on the Phrenological Development of Burke, Hare, and Other Atrocious Murderers."* Edinburgh: Robert Buchanan; William Hunter; and John Stevenson; London: T. and G. Underwood; Glasgow: Robertson and Atkinson; Aberdeen: Alex. Brown & Co., 1829.

Supplement to the Fourth, Fifth, and Sixth Editions of the Encyclopædia Britannica: With Preliminary Dissertations on the History of the Sciences. Vol. 3. Edinburgh: Archibald Constable and Company, 1824.

Testimonials on Behalf of George Combe as a Candidate for the Chair of Logic in the University of Edinburgh. Edinburgh: Anderson Jr.; London: Simpkin & Marshall, 1836.

The True Fortune-Teller, or, Guide to Knowledge: Discovering the Whole Art of Chiromancy, Physiognomy, Metoposcopy, and Astrology. London: E. Tracy, 1698.

Van Evrie, J. H. *Negroes and Negro "Slavery": The First an Inferior Race; The Latter Its Normal Condition*. New York: Van Evrie, Horton & Co., 1861.

Vaught, L. A. *Vaught's Practical Character Reader*. Chicago: L. A. Vaught, 1902.

Webb, R. T. *The Phrenologist; A Farce, in Two Acts: Containing a Popular Summary of that Pseudo, or Real Science*. London: Printed for the author, by C. Slater, 1824.

Wells, R. B. D. *A New Illustrated Hand-Book of Phrenology, Physiology, and Physiognomy*. London: H. Vickers, [1878?].

White's New Illustrated Melodeon Song Book. New York: H. Long & Brother, 1848.

Whiting, Bowen. *Report of the Trial of Henry Wyatt, a Convict in the State Prison at Auburn, Indicted for the Murder of James Gordon, Another Convict within the Prison.* New York: J. C. Derby & Co., 1846.

Secondary Sources

Ackerknecht, Erwin H. *Medicine at the Paris Hospital, 1794–1848.* Baltimore: Johns Hopkins University Press, 1967.

Ackerknecht, Erwin H., and Henri V. Vallois. *François Joseph Gall et sa collection.* Paris: Editions du Muséum, 1955.

Aharoni, Eyal, et al. "Neuroprediction of Future Rearrest." *Proceedings of the National Academy of Sciences of the United States of America* 110, no. 15 (2013): 6223–6228.

Alden, Andrea L. *Disorder in the Court: Morality, Myth, and the Insanity Defense.* Tuscaloosa: University of Alabama Press, 2018.

Apple, Rima D. "Constructing Mothers: Scientific Motherhood in the Nineteenth and Twentieth Centuries." *Social History of Medicine* 8, no. 2 (1995): 161–178.

———. *Perfect Motherhood: Science and Childrearing in America.* New Brunswick, NJ: Rutgers University Press, 2006.

Armstrong, Mary A. "Reading a Head: *Jane Eyre*, Phrenology, and the Homoerotics of Legibility." *Victorian Literature and Culture* 33, no. 1 (2005): 107–132.

Arpey, Andrew W. *The William Freeman Murder Trial: Insanity, Politics, and Race.* Syracuse, NY: Syracuse University Press, 2003.

Asher, Robert, Lawrence B. Goodheart, and Alan Rogers, eds. *Murder on Trial, 1620–2002.* Albany: State University of New York Press, 2005.

Bakan, David. "The Influence of Phrenology on American Psychology." *Journal of the History of the Behavioral Sciences* 2, no. 3 (1966): 200–220.

Baker, Robert, Dorothy Porter, and Roy Porter, eds. *The Codification of Medical Morality: Historical and Philosophical Studies of the Formalization of Western Medical Morality in the Eighteenth and Nineteenth Centuries.* Dordrecht: Kluwer Academic Publishers, 1993.

Baltzell, E. Digby. *Puritan Boston and Quaker Philadelphia.* New Brunswick, NJ: Transaction Publishers, 1996 [1979].

Banton, Michael. *Racial Theories.* 2nd ed. Cambridge: Cambridge University Press, 1998 [1987].

Beirne, Piers. *Inventing Criminology: Essays on the Rise of* Homo Criminalis. Albany: State University of New York Press, 1993.

Bell, Andrew McIlwaine. *Mosquito Soldiers: Malaria, Yellow Fever, and the Course of the American Civil War.* Baton Rouge: Louisiana State University Press, 2010.

Bell, Suzanne. *Crime and Circumstance: Investigating the History of Forensic Science.* Westport, CT: Praeger, 2008.

Beshara, Christopher J. "Moral Hospitals, Addled Brains and Cranial Conundrums: Rationalizations of the Criminal Mind in Antebellum America." *Australasian Journal of American Studies* 29, no. 1 (2010): 36–60.

Bindman, David. *Ape to Apollo: Aesthetics and the Idea of Race in the 18th Century.* Ithaca, NY: Cornell University Press, 2002.

Bittel, Carla. "Testing the Truth of Phrenology: Knowledge Experiments in Antebellum American Cultures of Science and Health." *Medical History* 63, no. 3 (2019): 352–374.

———. "Woman, Know Thyself: Producing and Using Phrenological Knowledge in Nineteenth-Century America." *Centaurus* 55, no. 2 (2013): 104–130.

Blomberg, Thomas G., and Karol Lucken. *American Penology: A History of Control.* 2nd ed. New Brunswick, NJ: Transaction Publishers, 2017.

Blum, Deborah. *The Poisoner's Handbook: Murder and the Birth of Forensic Medicine in Jazz Age New York.* New York: Penguin, 2010.

Blumenthal, Susanna L. *Law and the Modern Mind: Consciousness and Responsibility in American Legal Culture.* Cambridge, MA: Harvard University Press, 2016.

Bonner, Thomas Neville. *Becoming a Physician: Medical Education in Britain, France, Germany, and the United States, 1750–1945.* New York: Oxford University Press, 1995.

Boyer, Paul. *Urban Masses and Moral Order in America, 1820–1920.* Cambridge, MA: Harvard University Press, 1992 [1978].

Branson, Susan. "Phrenology and the Science of Race in Antebellum America." *Early American Studies* 15, no. 1 (2017): 164–193.

Brown, Jason W., and Karen L. Chobar. "Phrenological Studies of Aphasia before Broca: Broca's Aphasia or Gall's Aphasia?" *Brain and Language* 43, no. 3 (1992): 475–486.

Burkhead, Michael Dow. *The Search for the Causes of Crime: A History of Theory in Criminology.* Jefferson, NC: McFarland & Company, 2006.

Bynum, W. F. *Science and the Practice of Medicine in the Nineteenth Century.* New York: Cambridge University Press, 1994.

Cantor, G. N. "A Critique of Shapin's Social Interpretation of the Edinburgh Phrenology Debate." *Annals of Science* 32, no. 3 (1975): 245–256.

———. "The Edinburgh Phrenology Debate: 1803–1828." *Annals of Science* 32, no. 3 (1975): 195–218.

Carlino, Andrea. *Books of the Body: Anatomic Ritual and Renaissance Learning.* Chicago: University of Chicago Press, 1999.

Carlson, Eric T., and Norman Dain. "The Meaning of Moral Insanity." *Bulletin of the History of Medicine* 36, no. 2 (1962): 130–140.

Carré, Justin M., and Cheryl M. McCormick. "In Your Face: Facial Metrics Predict Aggressive Behaviour in the Laboratory and in Varsity and Professional Hockey Players." *Proceedings of the Royal Society B: Biological Sciences* 275, no. 1651 (2008): 2651–2656.

Carré, Justin M., Cheryl M. McCormick, and Catherine J. Mondloch. "Facial Structure Is a Reliable Cue for Aggressive Behavior." *Psychological Science* 20, no. 10 (2009): 1194–1198.

Carrington, Paul D. *Stewards of Democracy: Law as a Public Profession.* Boulder, CO: Westview Press, 1999.

Casper, Stephen T. *The Neurologists: A History of a Medical Specialty in Modern Britain, c. 1789–2000.* Manchester, UK: Manchester University Press, 2014.

Chaplin, Joyce E. *Subject Matter: Technology, the Body, and Science on the Anglo-American Frontier, 1500–1676.* Cambridge, MA: Harvard University Press, 2001.

Christianson, Scott. *With Liberty for Some: 500 Years of Imprisonment in America.* Boston: Northeastern University Press, 1998.

Claggett, Shalyn. "Putting Character First: The Narrative Construction of Innate Identity in Phrenological Texts." *VIJ: Victorians Institute Journal* 38 (2010): 103–126.

Clark, Michael, and Catherine Crawford, eds. *Legal Medicine in History.* Cambridge: Cambridge University Press, 1994.

Clothier, Anne A. "Prisons, Petticoats and Phrenology: Eliza Farnham and Reform at Sing Sing Prison, 1844–1848." MA thesis, State University of New York College at Oneonta, 2007.

Cohen, Patricia Cline. *A Calculating People: The Spread of Numeracy in Early America*. Chicago: University of Chicago Press, 1982.

Colbert, Charles. *A Measure of Perfection: Phrenology and the Fine Arts in America*. Chapel Hill: University of North Carolina Press, 1997.

Cole, Simon A. *Suspect Identities: A History of Fingerprinting and Criminal Identification*. Cambridge, MA: Harvard University Press, 2001.

Colvin, Mark. *Penitentiaries, Reformatories, and Chain Gangs: Social Theory and the History of Punishment in Nineteenth-Century America*. New York: St. Martin's Press, 1997.

Conklin, Alice L. *In the Museum of Man: Race, Anthropology, and Empire in France, 1850–1950*. Ithaca, NY: Cornell University Press, 2013.

Cook, James F. *The Governors of Georgia, 1754–2004*. 3rd ed. Macon, GA: Mercer University Press, 2005.

Cooter, Roger. *The Cultural Meaning of Popular Science: Phrenology and the Organization of Consent in Nineteenth-Century Britain*. Cambridge: Cambridge University Press, 1984.

———. "Phrenology and British Alienists, c. 1825–1845. Part I: Converts to a Doctrine." *Medical History* 20, no. 1 (1976): 1–21.

———. "Phrenology and British Alienists, c. 1825–1845. Part II: Doctrine and Practice." *Medical History* 20, no. 2 (1976): 135–151.

———. *Phrenology in the British Isles: An Annotated Historical Biobibliography and Index*. Metuchen, NJ: Scarecrow Press, 1989.

———. "Phrenology: The Provocation of Progress." *History of Science* 14, no. 4 (1976): 211–234.

Cornel, Tabea. "Something Old, Something New, Something Pseudo, Something True: Pejorative and Deferential References to Phrenology since 1840." *Proceedings of the American Philosophical Society* 161, no. 4 (2017): 299–332.

Critchley, Macdonald. "Neurology's Debt to F. J. Gall (1758–1828)." *British Medical Journal* 2, no. 5465 (1965): 775–781.

Cunningham, Andrew, and Perry Williams, eds. *The Laboratory Revolution in Medicine*. Cambridge: Cambridge University Press, 1992.

Curran, Andrew S. *The Anatomy of Blackness: Science & Slavery in an Age of Enlightenment*. Baltimore: Johns Hopkins University Press, 2011.

Dain, Bruce. *A Hideous Monster of the Mind: American Race Theory in the Early Republic*. Cambridge, MA: Harvard University Press, 2002.

Dames, Nicholas. "The Clinical Novel: Phrenology and *Villette*." *NOVEL: A Forum on Fiction* 29, no. 3 (1996): 367–390.

Davies, John D. *Phrenology: Fad and Science; A 19th-Century American Crusade*. Hamden, CT: Archon Books, 1971 [1955].

de Giustino, David. *Conquest of Mind: Phrenology and Victorian Social Thought*. London: Routledge, 2016 [1975].

Desmond, Adrian, and James Moore. *Darwin's Sacred Cause: How a Hatred of Slavery Shaped Darwin's Views on Human Evolution*. Boston: Houghton Mifflin Harcourt, 2009.

De Ville, Kenneth Allen. *Medical Malpractice in Nineteenth-Century America: Origins and Legacy*. New York: New York University Press, 1990.

Diamond, Bernard L. "Isaac Ray and the Trial of Daniel M'Naghten." *American Journal of Psychiatry* 112, no. 8 (1956): 651–656.

Downs, Jim. *Sick from Freedom: African-American Illness and Suffering During the Civil War and Reconstruction*. Oxford: Oxford University Press, 2012.

Eigen, Joel Peter. *Mad-Doctors in the Dock: Defending the Diagnosis, 1760–1913*. Baltimore: Johns Hopkins University Press, 2016).

———. *Unconscious Crime: Mental Absence and Criminal Responsibility in Victorian London*. Baltimore: Johns Hopkins University Press, 2003.

———. *Witnessing Insanity: Madness and Mad-Doctors in the English Court*. New Haven, CT: Yale University Press, 1995.

Eling, Paul, and Stanley Finger, eds. "Gall and Phrenology: New Perspectives." Special issue, *Journal of the History of the Neurosciences* 29, no. 1 (2020).

Erickson, Paul A. "Phrenology and Physical Anthropology: The George Combe Connection." *Current Anthropology* 18, no. 1 (1977): 92–93.

Fabian, Ann. *The Skull Collectors: Race, Science, and America's Unburied Dead*. Chicago: University of Chicago Press, 2010.

Falk, Pasi. *The Consuming Body*. London: Sage Publications, 1997 [1994].

Finger, Simon. *The Contagious City: The Politics of Public Health in Early Philadelphia*. Ithaca, NY: Cornell University Press, 2012.

Finger, Stanley. *Minds behind the Brain: A History of the Pioneers and Their Discoveries*. Oxford: Oxford University Press, 2000.

———. *Origins of Neuroscience: A History of Explorations into Brain Function*. New York: Oxford University Press, 1994.

Finger, Stanley, and Paul Eling. *Franz Joseph Gall: Naturalist of the Mind, Visionary of the Brain*. New York: New York University Press, 2019.

Fink, Arthur E. *Causes of Crime: Biological Theories in the United States, 1800–1915*. Philadelphia: University of Pennsylvania Press, 1938.

Finn, Jonathan. *Capturing the Criminal Image: From Mug Shot to Surveillance Society*. Minneapolis: University of Minnesota Press, 2009.

Floyd, Janet. "Dislocations of the Self: Eliza Farnham at Sing Sing Prison." *Journal of American Studies* 40, no. 2 (2006): 311–325.

Foucault, Michel. *The Birth of the Clinic: An Archeology of Medical Perception*. Translated by A. M. Sheridan Smith. New York: Vintage Books, 1994 [1973].

———. *Discipline and Punish: The Birth of the Prison*. Translated by Alan Sheridan. New York: Vintage Books, 1995 [1977].

Freedman, Estelle B. *Redefining Rape: Sexual Violence in the Era of Suffrage and Segregation*. Cambridge, MA: Harvard University Press, 2013.

Gay, Peter. *Freud: A Life for Our Time*. New York: W. W. Norton, 2006 [1998].

Geniole, Shawn N., et al. "Evidence from Meta-Analyses of the Facial Width-to-Height Ratio as an Evolved Cue of Threat." *PLOS One* 10, no. 7 (2015): e0132726, https://doi.org/10.1371/journal.pone.0132726.

Gerber, John C. *A Pictorial History of the University of Iowa*. Iowa City: University of Iowa Press, 2005.

Gibson, Mary. *Born to Crime: Cesare Lombroso and the Origins of Biological Criminology*. Westport, CT: Praeger, 2002.

Glickstein, Mitchell. *Neuroscience: A Historical Introduction*. Cambridge, MA: MIT Press, 2014.

Golan, Tal. *Laws of Men and Laws of Nature: The History of Scientific Expert Testimony in England in America*. Cambridge, MA: Harvard University Press, 2004.

Gómez-Valdés, Jorge, et al. "Lack of Support for the Association between Facial Shape and Aggression: A Reappraisal Based on a Worldwide Population Genetics Perspective." *PLOS One* 8, no. 1 (2013): e52317, https://doi.org/10.1371/journal.pone.0052317.

Goodheart, Lawrence B. "From Cure to Custodianship of the Insane Poor in Nineteenth-Century Connecticut." *Journal of the History of Medicine and Allied Sciences* 65, no. 1 (2010): 106–130.

———. *Mad Yankees: The Hartford Retreat for the Insane and Nineteenth-Century Psychiatry.* Amherst: University of Massachusetts Press, 2003.

Gordon, R. Michael. *The Infamous Burke and Hare: Serial Killers and Resurrectionists of Nineteenth Century Edinburgh.* Jefferson, NC: McFarland & Company, 2009.

Greenblatt, Samuel H. "Phrenology in the Science and Culture of the 19th Century." *Neurosurgery* 37, no. 4 (1995): 790–805.

Gregory, Sarah, et al. "The Antisocial Brain: Psychopathy Matters: A Structural MRI Investigation of Antisocial Male Violent Offenders." *Archives of General Psychiatry* 69, no. 9 (2012): 962–972.

Grob, Gerald N. *The Mad among Us: A History of the Care of America's Mentally Ill.* New York: Free Press, 1994.

Gross, Charles G. *Brain, Vision, Memory: Tales in the History of Neuroscience.* Cambridge, MA: MIT Press, 1998.

Gross, Robert A., and Mary Kelly, eds. *A History of the Book in America.* Vol. 2, *An Extensive Republic: Print, Culture, and Society in the New Nation, 1790–1840.* Chapel Hill: University of North Carolina Press, 2010.

Guenther, Katja. *Localization and Its Discontents: A Genealogy of Psychoanalysis & the Neuro Disciplines.* Chicago: University of Chicago Press, 2015.

Hall, Jason Y. "Gall's Phrenology: A Romantic Psychology." *Studies in Romanticism* 16, no. 3 (1977): 305–317.

Haller, John S., Jr. *American Medicine in Transition, 1840–1910.* Urbana: University of Illinois Press, 1981.

———. *The History of American Homeopathy: From Rational Medicine to Holistic Health Care.* New Brunswick, NJ: Rutgers University Press, 2009.

———. *Kindly Medicine: Physio-Medicalism in America, 1836–1911.* Kent, OH: Kent State University Press, 1997.

———. *The People's Doctor: Samuel Thomson and the American Botanical Movement.* Carbondale: Southern Illinois University Press, 2000.

Halttunen, Karen. *Confidence Men and Painted Women: A Study of Middle-Class Culture in America, 1830–1870.* New Haven, CT: Yale University Press, 1982.

———. *Murder Most Foul: The Killer and the American Gothic Imagination.* Cambridge, MA: Harvard University Press, 1998.

Hamilton, Cynthia S. "'Am I Not a Man and a Brother?' Phrenology and Anti-slavery." *Slavery and Abolition* 29, no. 2 (2008): 173–187.

Harring, Sidney L. *Policing a Class Society: The Experience of American Cities, 1865–1915.* New Brunswick, NJ: Rutgers University Press, 1983.

Harrington, Anne. *Medicine, Mind, and the Double Brain: A Study in Nineteenth-Century Social Thought.* Princeton, NJ: Princeton University Press, 1989 [1987].

Hartley, Lucy. *Physiognomy and the Meaning of Expression in Nineteenth-Century Culture.* Cambridge: Cambridge University Press, 2001.

Haselhuhn, Michael P., and Elaine M. Wong. "Bad to the Bone: Facial Structure Predicts Unethical Behavior." *Proceedings of the Royal Society B* 279, no. 1728 (2012): 571–576.

Haselhuhn, Michael P., Elaine M. Wong, and Margaret E. Ormiston. "Self-Fulfilling Prophecies as a Link between Men's Facial Width-to-Height Ratio and Behavior." *PLOS One* 8, no. 8 (2013): e72259, https://doi.org/10.1371/journal.pone.0072259.

Haselhuhn, Michael P., Margaret E. Ormiston, and Elaine M. Wong. "Men's Facial Width-to-Height Ratio Predicts Aggression: A Meta-Analysis." *PLOS One* 10, no. 4 (2015): e0122637, https://doi.org/10.1371/journal.pone.0122637.

Hilts, Victor L. "Obeying the Laws of Hereditary Descent: Phrenological Views on Inheritance and Eugenics." *Journal of the History of the Behavioral Sciences* 18, no. 1 (1982): 62–77.

Hinton, Elizabeth, and DeAnza Cook. "The Mass Criminalization of Black Americans: A Historical Overview." *Annual Review of Criminology* 4, no. 1 (January 2021; preprint June 22, 2020): 1–26.

Hogarth, Rana A. *Medicalizing Blackness: Making Racial Difference in the Atlantic World, 1780–1840.* Chapel Hill: University of North Carolina Press, 2017.

Horn, David G. *The Criminal Body: Lombroso and the Anatomy of Deviance.* New York: Routledge, 2003.

Horwitz, Morton J. *The Transformation of American Law, 1780–1860.* Cambridge, MA: Harvard University Press, 1977.

Hoyme, Lucile E. "Physical Anthropology and Its Instruments: An Historical Study." *Southwestern Journal of Anthropology* 9, no. 4 (1953): 408–430.

Hruschka, John. *How Books Came to America: The Rise of the American Book Trade.* University Park: Pennsylvania State University Press, 2012.

Hughes, John Starrett. *In the Law's Darkness: Isaac Ray and the Medical Jurisprudence of Insanity in Nineteenth-Century America.* New York: Oceana Publications, 1986.

Humphreys, Margaret. *Intensely Human: The Health of the Black Soldier in the American Civil War.* Baltimore: Johns Hopkins University Press, 2008.

———. *Marrow of Tragedy: The Health Crisis of the American Civil War.* Baltimore: Johns Hopkins University Press, 2013.

Hungerford, Edward. "Poe and Phrenology." *American Literature* 2, no. 3 (1930): 209–231.

Jacobson, Matthew Frye. *Whiteness of a Different Color: European Immigrants and the Alchemy of Race.* Cambridge, MA: Harvard University Press, 1998.

Jenkins, Bill. "Phrenology, Heredity and Progress in George Combe's *Constitution of Man.*" *British Journal for the History of Science* 48, no. 3 (2015): 455–473.

Johnson, David R. *Policing the Urban Underworld: The Impact of Crime on the Development of the American Police, 1800–1887.* Philadelphia: Temple University Press, 1979.

Johnston, Norman. *Forms of Constraint: A History of Prison Architecture.* Urbana: University of Illinois Press, 2000.

Jones, David A. *History of Criminology: A Philosophical Perspective.* Westport, CT: Greenwood Press, 1986.

Kahan, Paul. *Seminary of Virtue: The Ideology and Practice of Inmate Reform at Eastern State Penitentiary, 1829–1971.* New York: Peter Lang, 2012.

Kann, Mark E. *Punishment, Prisons, and Patriarchy: Liberty and Power in the Early American Republic.* New York: New York University Press, 2005.

Kaser, David, ed. *The Cost Book of Carey & Lea, 1825–1838.* Philadelphia: University of Pennsylvania Press, 1963.

———. *Messrs. Carey & Lea of Philadelphia: A Study in the History of the Booktrade.* Philadelphia: University of Pennsylvania Press, 1957.

Kimball, Bruce A. *The "True Professional Ideal" in America: A History.* Lanham, MD: Rowman & Littlefield, 1995.

Kohlstedt, Sally Gregory. "Curiosities and Cabinets: Natural History Museums and Education on the Antebellum Campus." *Isis* 79, no. 3 (1988): 405–426.

———. "Parlors, Primers, and Public Schooling: Education for Science in Nineteenth-Century America." *Isis* 81, no. 3 (1990): 424–445.

Lande, R. Gregory. *Abraham Man: Madness, Malingering and the Development of Medical Testimony.* New York: Algora Publishing, 2012.

LaPiana, William P. *Logic and Experience: The Origin of Modern American Legal Education.* Oxford: Oxford University Press, 1994.

LaPointe, Leonard L. *Paul Broca and the Origins of Language in the Brain.* San Diego: Plural Publishing, 2013.

Leaney, Enda. "Phrenology in Nineteenth-Century Ireland." *New Hibernia Review* 10, no. 3 (2006): 24–42.

Lewis, W. David. *From Newgate to Dannemora: The Rise of the Penitentiary in New York, 1796–1848.* Ithaca, NY: Cornell University Press, 1965.

Lightman, Bernard. *Victorian Popularizers of Science: Designing Nature for New Audiences.* Chicago: University of Chicago Press, 2007.

Lofland, Lyn H. *A World of Strangers: Order and Action in Urban Public Space.* New York: Basic Books, 1973.

Long, Lisa A. *Rehabilitating Bodies: Health, History, and the American Civil War.* Philadelphia: University of Pennsylvania Press, 2004.

Lukasik, Christopher J. *Discerning Characters: The Culture of Appearance in Early America.* Philadelphia: University of Pennsylvania Press, 2011.

Lyons, Sherrie Lynne. *Species, Serpents, Spirits, and Skulls: Science at the Margins in the Victorian Age.* Albany: State University of New York Press, 2009.

Macmillan, Malcolm. *An Odd Kind of Fame: Stories of Phineas Gage.* Cambridge, MA: MIT Press, 2000.

Magoun, Horace Winchell. *American Neuroscience in the Twentieth Century: Confluence of the Neural, Behavioral, and Communicative Streams.* Leiden: A. A. Balkema, 2003.

Marcus, Alan I. *Plague of Strangers: Social Groups and the Origins of City Services in Cincinnati, 1819–1870.* Columbus: Ohio State University Press, 1991.

Marshall, Jonathan W. *Performing Neurology: The Dramaturgy of Dr Jean-Martin Charcot.* New York: Palgrave Macmillan, 2016.

McCracken-Flesher, Caroline. *The Doctor Dissected: A Cultural Autopsy of the Burke and Hare Murders.* Oxford: Oxford University Press, 2012.

McCusker, John J. "How Much Is That in Real Money? A Historical Price Index for Use as a Deflator of Money Values in the Economy of the United States." *Proceedings of the American Antiquarian Society* 106, no. 2 (1997): 327–334.

McGlamery, Tom. *Protest and the Body in Melville, Dos Passos, and Hurston.* New York: Routledge, 2004.

McLaren, Angus. "A Prehistory of the Social Sciences: Phrenology in France." *Comparative Studies in Society and History* 23, no. 1 (1981): 3–22.

———. "Phrenology: Medium and Message." *Journal of Modern History* 46, no. 1 (1974): 86–97.

Meijer, Miriam Claude. *Race and Aesthetics in the Anthropology of Petrus Camper (1722–1789).* Amsterdam: Editions Rodopi bv, 1999.

Meranze, Michael. *Laboratories of Virtue: Punishment, Revolution, and Authority in Philadelphia, 1760–1835.* Williamsburg, VA: The Institute of Early American History and Culture, 1996.

Middleton, William Shainline. "Charles Caldwell, a Biographic Sketch." In *Annals of Medical History*, vol. 3, edited by Francis R. Packard, 156–178. New York: Paul B. Hoeber, 1921.

Miller, Edgar. "Idiocy in the Nineteenth Century." *History of Psychiatry* 7, no. 27 (1996): 361–373.

Miller, Martin B. "Sinking Gradually into the Proletariat: The Emergence of the Penitentiary in the United States." *Crime and Social Justice* 14 (1980): 37–43.

Miller, Zane L., and Patricia Mooney Melvin. *The Urbanization of Modern America: A Brief History*. 2nd ed. New York: Harcourt Brace Jovanovich, 1987 [1973].

Mintz, Steven. *Moralists and Modernizers: America's Pre–Civil War Reformers*. Baltimore: Johns Hopkins University Press, 1995.

Miron, Janet. *Prisons, Asylums, and the Public: Institutional Visiting in the Nineteenth Century*. Toronto: University of Toronto Press, 2011.

Mohr, James C. *Doctors and the Law: Medical Jurisprudence in Nineteenth-Century America*. Baltimore: Johns Hopkins University Press, 1996 [1993].

Moran, Richard. *Knowing Right from Wrong: The Insanity Defense of Daniel McNaughtan*. New York: Free Press, 1981.

———. "The Modern Foundation for the Insanity Defense: The Cases of James Hadfield (1800) and Daniel McNaughtan (1843)." *Annals of the American Academy of Political and Social Science* 477, no. 1 (1985): 31–42.

Morn, Frank. *"The Eye That Never Sleeps": A History of the Pinkerton National Detective Agency*. Bloomington: Indiana University Press, 1982.

———. *Forgotten Reformer: Robert McClaughry and Criminal Justice Reform in Nineteenth-Century America*. Lanham, MD: University Press of America, 2011.

Morris, Norval, and David J. Rothman, eds. *The Oxford History of the Prison: The Practice of Punishment in Western Society*. New York: Oxford University Press, 1998.

Muhammad, Khalil Gibran. *The Condemnation of Blackness: Race, Crime, and the Making of Modern Urban America*. Cambridge, MA: Harvard University Press, 2010.

Noel, Patricia S., and Eric T. Carlson. "Origins of the Word 'Phrenology.'" *American Journal of Psychiatry* 127, no. 5 (1970): 694–697.

O'Brien, James. *The Scientific Sherlock Holmes: Cracking the Case with Science and Forensics*. Oxford: Oxford University Press, 2013.

O'Connor, Thomas H. *The Athens of America: Boston, 1825–1845*. Amherst: University of Massachusetts Press, 2006.

Pandora, Katherine. "Popular Science in National and Transnational Perspective: Suggestions from the American Context." *Isis* 100, no. 2 (2009): 346–358.

Panek, LeRoy Lad. *Before Sherlock Holmes: How Magazines and Newspapers Invented the Detective Story*. Jefferson, NC: McFarland & Company, 2011.

Park, Katharine. "The Criminal and the Saintly Body: Autopsy and Dissection in Renaissance Italy." *Renaissance Quarterly* 47, no. 1 (1994): 1–33.

———. *Secrets of Women: Gender, Generation, and the Origins of Human Dissection*. New York: Zone Books, 2006.

Parssinen, T. M. "Popular Science and Society: The Phrenology Movement in Early Victorian Britain." *Journal of Social History* 8, no. 1 (1974): 1–20.

Pearl, Sharrona. *About Faces: Physiognomy in Nineteenth-Century Britain*. Cambridge, MA: Harvard University Press, 2010.

Penick, James Lal, Jr. *The Great Western Land Pirate: John A. Murrell in Legend and History*. Columbia: University of Missouri Press, 1981.

Penton-Voak, Ian S., et al. "Personality Judgments from Natural and Composite Facial Images: More Evidence for a 'Kernel of Truth' in Social Perception." *Social Cognition* 24, no. 5 (2006): 607–640.

Percival, Melissa. *The Appearance of Character: Physiognomy and Facial Expression in Eighteenth-Century France.* London: W. S. Maney & Son, 1999.

Porter, Theodore M. *Trust in Numbers: The Pursuit of Objectivity in Science and Public Life.* Princeton, NJ: Princeton University Press, 1995.

Poskett, James. *Materials of the Mind: Phrenology, Race, and the Global History of Science, 1815–1920.* Chicago: University of Chicago Press, 2019.

———. "Phrenology, Correspondence, and the Global Politics of Reform, 1815–1848." *The Historical Journal* 60, no. 2 (2017): 409–442.

Rafter, Nicole Hahn. *Creating Born Criminals.* Urbana: University of Illinois Press, 1997.

———. "The Murderous Dutch Fiddler: Criminology, History, and the Problem of Phrenology." *Theoretical Criminology* 9, no. 1 (2005): 65–96.

Ramsland, Katherine. *Beating the Devil's Game: A History of Forensic Science and Criminal Investigation.* New York: Berkley Books, 2007.

Ray, Angela G. *The Lyceum and Public Culture in the Nineteenth-Century United States.* East Lansing: Michigan State University Press, 2005.

Redman, Samuel J. *Bone Rooms: From Scientific Racism to Human Prehistory in Museums.* Cambridge, MA: Harvard University Press, 2016.

Reiss, Benjamin. *Theaters of Madness: Insane Asylums & Nineteenth-Century American Culture.* Chicago: University of Chicago Press, 2008.

Renneville, Marc. *Le langage des crânes: Une histoire de la phrénologie.* Paris: Institut d'Édition, Sanofi-Synthélabo, 2000.

Rennie, Ysabel. *The Search for Criminal Man: A Conceptual History of the Dangerous Offender.* Lexington, MA: Lexington Books, 1978.

Richardson, Ruth. *Death, Dissection and the Destitute.* 2nd ed. Chicago: University of Chicago Press, 2000 [1987].

Riegel, Robert E. "The Introduction of Phrenology to the United States." *American Historical Review* 39, no. 1 (1933): 73–78.

Robinson, Daniel N. *Wild Beasts & Idle Humours: The Insanity Defense from Antiquity to the Present.* Cambridge, MA: Harvard University Press, 1996.

Rosenberg, Charles E. *The Trial of the Assassin Guiteau: Psychiatry and the Law in the Gilded Age.* Chicago: University of Chicago Press, 1976 [1968].

Rosner, Lisa. *The Anatomy Murders: Being the True and Spectacular History of Edinburgh's Notorious Burke and Hare, and of the Man of Science Who Abetted Them in the Commission of Their Most Heinous Crimes.* Philadelphia: University of Pennsylvania Press, 2019.

Rothman, David J. *The Discovery of the Asylum: Social Order and Disorder in the New Republic.* New York: Aldine de Gruyter, 2002 [1971].

Rothstein, William G. *American Physicians in the Nineteenth Century: From Sects to Science.* Baltimore: Johns Hopkins University Press, 1992 [1972].

Rusert, Britt. *Fugitive Science: Empiricism and Freedom in Early African American Culture.* New York: New York University Press, 2017.

———. "The Science of Freedom: Counterarchives of Racial Science on the Antebellum Stage." *African American Review* 45, no. 3 (2012): 291–308.

Russett, Cynthia Eagle. *Sexual Science: The Victorian Construction of Womanhood.* Cambridge, MA: Harvard University Press, 1989.

Sappol, Michael. *A Traffic of Dead Bodies: Anatomy and Embodied Social Identity in Nineteenth-Century America.* Princeton, NJ: Princeton University Press, 2002.

Sawday, Jonathan. *The Body Emblazoned: Dissection and the Human Body in Renaissance Culture.* London: Routledge, 1995.

Schiebinger, Londa. *Nature's Body: Gender in the Making of Modern Science.* Boston: Beacon Press, 1993.

Schlag, Pierre. "Law and Phrenology." *Harvard Law Review* 110, no. 4 (1997): 877–921.

Schwartz, Harold. "Samuel Gridley Howe as Phrenologist." *The American Historical Review* 57, no. 3 (1952): 644–651.

Senior, Hereward. *Constabulary: The Rise of Police Institutions in Britain, the Commonwealth and the United States.* Toronto: Dundurn Press, 1997.

Seth, Suman. *Difference and Disease: Medicine, Race, and the Eighteenth-Century British Empire.* Cambridge: Cambridge University Press, 2018.

Shapin, Steven. "Phrenological Knowledge and the Social Structure of Early Nineteenth-Century Edinburgh." *Annals of Science* 32, no. 3 (1975): 219–243.

———. "The Politics of Observation: Cerebral Anatomy and Social Interests in the Edinburgh Phrenology Disputes." Special issue, *Sociological Review* 27 (May 1979): 139–178.

Shookman, Ellis, ed. *The Faces of Physiognomy: Interdisciplinary Approaches to Johann Caspar Lavater.* Columbia, SC: Camden House, 1993.

Shuttleworth, Sally. *Charlotte Brontë and Victorian Psychology.* Cambridge: Cambridge University Press, 1996.

Simpson, Donald. "Phrenology and the Neurosciences: Contributions of F. J. Gall and J. G. Spurzheim." *ANZ Journal of Surgery* 75, no. 6 (2005): 475–482.

Smith, Robert N. *An Evil Day in Georgia: The Killing of Coleman Osborn and the Death Penalty in the Progressive-Era South.* Knoxville: The University of Tennessee Press, 2015.

Smith, Roger. *Trial by Medicine: Insanity and Responsibility in Victorian Trials.* Edinburgh: Edinburgh University Press, 1981.

Sokal, Michael M. "Practical Phrenology as Psychological Counseling in the 19th-Century United States." In *The Transformation of Psychology: Influences of 19th-Century Philosophy, Technology, and Natural Science,* edited by Christopher D. Green, Marlene Shore, and Thomas Teo, 21–44. Washington, DC: American Psychological Association, 2001.

Stack, David. *Queen Victoria's Skull: George Combe and the Mid-Victorian Mind.* London: Hambledon Continuum, 2008.

Stanton, William. *The Leopard's Spots: Scientific Attitudes toward Race in America 1815–59.* Chicago: University of Chicago Press, 1960.

Staum, Martin. "Physiognomy and Phrenology at the Paris Athénée." *Journal of the History of Ideas* 56, no. 3 (1995): 443–462.

Stein, Melissa N. *Measuring Manhood: Race and the Science of Masculinity, 1830–1934.* Minneapolis: University of Minnesota Press, 2015.

Stepan, Nancy. *The Idea of Race in Science: Great Britain 1800–1960.* Hamden, CT: Archon Books, 1982.

Stern, Madeleine B. "Emerson and Phrenology." *Studies in the American Renaissance* (1984): 213–228.

———. *Heads & Headlines: The Phrenological Fowlers.* Norman: University of Oklahoma Press, 1971.

———. "Mark Twain Had His Head Examined." *American Literature* 41, no. 2 (1969): 207–218.

———. "Poe: 'The Mental Temperament' for Phrenologists." *American Literature* 40, no. 2 (1968): 155–163.

———. *Publishers for Mass Entertainment in Nineteenth Century America.* Boston: G. K. Hall, 1980.

Stiles, Anne, Stanley Finger, and François Boller, eds. *Literature, Neurology, and Neuroscience: Historical and Literary Connections.* Amsterdam: Elsevier, 2013.

Sysling, Fenneke. "Science and Self-Assessment: Phrenological Charts 1840–1940." *British Journal for the History of Science* 51, no. 2 (2018): 261–280.

Tarter, Michele Lise, and Richard Bell, eds. *Buried Lives: Incarcerated in Early America.* Athens: University of Georgia Press, 2012.

Teeters, Negley K., and John D. Shearer. *The Prison at Philadelphia, Cherry Hill: The Separate System of Penal Discipline, 1829–1913.* New York: Columbia University Press, 1957.

Temkin, Owsei. "Gall and the Phrenological Movement." *Bulletin of the History of Medicine* 21, no. 3 (1947): 275–321.

Teslow, Tracy. *Constructing Race: The Science of Bodies and Cultures in American Anthropology.* Cambridge: Cambridge University Press, 2014.

Thompson, Courtney E. "The Curious Case of Chastine Cox: Murder, Race, Medicine and the Media in the Gilded Age." *Social History of Medicine* 32, no. 3 (August 2019): 481–501.

Thurs, Daniel Patrick. *Science Talk: Changing Notions of Science in American Popular Culture.* New Brunswick, NJ: Rutgers University Press, 2007.

Tiihonen, J., et al. "Genetic Background of Extreme Violent Behavior." *Molecular Psychiatry* 20, no. 6 (2015): 792.

Tomes, Nancy. *A Generous Confidence: Thomas Story Kirkbride and the Art of Asylum-Keeping, 1840–1883.* Cambridge: Cambridge University Press, 1984.

Tomlinson, Stephen. *Head Masters: Phrenology, Secular Education, and Nineteenth-Century Social Thought.* Tuscaloosa: University of Alabama Press, 2005.

Twine, Richard. "Physiognomy, Phrenology and the Temporality of the Body." *Body & Society* 8, no. 1 (2002): 67–88.

van Wyhe, John. "The Authority of Human Nature: The *Schädellehre* of Franz Joseph Gall." *British Journal for the History of Science* 35, no. 1 (2002): 17–42.

———. *Phrenology and the Origins of Victorian Scientific Naturalism.* Aldershot, UK: Ashgate, 2004.

———. "Was Phrenology a Reform Science? Towards a New Generalization for Phrenology." *History of Science* 42, no. 3 (2004): 313–331.

Verstraete, Pieter. "The Taming of Disability: Phrenology and Bio-Power on the Road to the Destruction of Otherness in France (1800–60)." *Journal of the History of Education Society* 34, no. 2 (2005): 119–134.

Vidal, Fernando. *The Sciences of the Soul: The Early Modern Sciences of Psychology.* Translated by Saskia Brown. Chicago: University of Chicago Press, 2011.

Wadman, Robert C., and William Thomas Allison. *To Protect and Serve: A History of Police in America.* Upper Saddle River, NJ: Pearson Prentice Hall, 2004.

Walsh, Anthony A. "The American Tour of Dr. Spurzheim." *Journal of the History of Medicine and Allied Sciences* 27, no. 2 (1972): 187–205.

———. "Phrenology and the Boston Medical Community in the 1830s." *Bulletin of the History of Medicine* 50, no. 2 (1976): 261–273.

Walters, Ronald G. *American Reformers 1815–1860.* New York: Hill and Wang, 1978.

Warner, John Harley. *Against the Spirit of System: The French Impulse in Nineteenth-Century American Medicine.* Baltimore: Johns Hopkins University Press, 2003 [1998].

———. *The Therapeutic Perspective: Medical Practice, Knowledge, and Identity in America, 1820–1885.* Princeton, NJ: Princeton University Press, 1997 [1986].

Watts, Edward, and David J. Carlson, eds. *John Neal and Nineteenth-Century American Literature and Culture.* Lewisburg, PA: Bucknell University Press, 2012.

Weiss, Kenneth J. "Epilepsy and Homicide: Issac Ray [*sic*] on Mitigation." *Journal of Psychiatry & Law* 36, no. 2 (2008): 171–209.

———. "Isaac Ray at 200: Phrenology and Expert Testimony." *Journal of the American Academy of Psychiatry and Law* 35, no. 3 (2007): 339–345.

———. "Isaac Ray, Malpractice Defendant." *Journal of the American Academy of Psychiatry and Law* 41, no. 3 (2003): 382–390.

———. "Isaac Ray's Affair with Phrenology." *Journal of Psychiatry & Law* 34, no. 4 (2006): 455–459.

———. "Psychiatry for the General Practitioner: Isaac Ray's Jefferson Lectures, 1871 to 1873." *Journal of Nervous and Mental Disease* 200, no. 12 (2012): 1047–1053.

Weisz, George. *Divide and Conquer: A Comparative History of Medical Specialization*. Oxford: Oxford University Press, 2006.

Welter, Barbara. "The Cult of True Womanhood: 1820–1860." *American Quarterly* 18, no. 2 (1966): 151–174.

West, Donald J., and Alexander Walk, eds. *Daniel McNaughton: His Trial and the Aftermath*. Ashford, UK: Headley for the "British Journal of Psychiatry," 1977.

White, Christopher G. "Minds Intensely Unsettled: Phrenology, Experience, and the American Pursuit of Spiritual Assurance, 1830–1880." *Religion and American Culture* 16, no. 2 (2006): 227–261.

Whorton, James C. *Nature Cures: The History of Alternative Medicine in America*. Oxford: Oxford University Press, 2002.

Willoughby, Christopher D. "'His Native, Hot Country': Racial Science and Environment in Antebellum American Medical Thought." *Journal of the History of Medicine and Allied Sciences* 72, no. 3 (2017): 328–351.

———. "Running Away from Drapetomania: Samuel A. Cartwright, Medicine, and Race in the Antebellum South." *Journal of Southern History* 84, no. 3 (2018): 579–614.

Wilson, John B. "Phrenology and the Transcendentalists." *American Literature* 28, no. 2 (1956): 220–225.

Worthington, Heather. *The Rise of the Detective in Early Nineteenth-Century Popular Fiction*. New York: Palgrave Macmillan, 2005.

Wrobel, Arthur. "Orthodoxy and Respectability in Nineteenth-Century Phrenology." *Journal of Popular Culture* 9, no. 1 (1975): 38–50.

Wyatt-Brown, Bertram. *Southern Honor: Ethics & Behavior in the Old South*. Oxford: Oxford University Press, 1982.

Young, Robert M. *Mind, Brain, and Adaptation in the Nineteenth Century: Cerebral Localization and Its Biological Context from Gall to Ferrier*. New York: Oxford University Press, 1990 [1970].

Ziff, Katherine. *Asylum on the Hill: History of a Healing Landscape*. Athens: Ohio University Press, 2012.

Zola-Morgan, S. "Localization of Brain Function: The Legacy of Franz Joseph Gall (1758–1828)." *Annual Review of Neuroscience* 18, no. 1 (1995): 359–383.

Index

Note: Page numbers in *italics* indicate figures.

About the Author

Courtney E. Thompson is an assistant professor of the history of science and medicine and U.S. women's history at Mississippi State University.

Available titles in the Critical Issues in Health and Medicine series:

Emily K. Abel, *Prelude to Hospice: Florence Wald, Dying People, and Their Families*
Emily K. Abel, *Suffering in the Land of Sunshine: A Los Angeles Illness Narrative*
Emily K. Abel, *Tuberculosis and the Politics of Exclusion: A History of Public Health and Migration to Los Angeles*
Marilyn Aguirre-Molina, Luisa N. Borrell, and William Vega, eds., *Health Issues in Latino Males: A Social and Structural Approach*
Anne-Emanuelle Birn and Theodore M. Brown, eds., *Comrades in Health: U.S. Health Internationalists, Abroad and at Home*
Karen Buhler-Wilkerson, *False Dawn: The Rise and Decline of Public Health Nursing*
Susan M. Chambré, *Fighting for Our Lives: New York's AIDS Community and the Politics of Disease*
James Colgrove, Gerald Markowitz, and David Rosner, eds., *The Contested Boundaries of American Public Health*
Cynthia A. Connolly, *Children and Drug Safety: Balancing Risk and Protection in Twentieth-Century America*
Cynthia A. Connolly, *Saving Sickly Children: The Tuberculosis Preventorium in American Life, 1909–1970*
Brittany Cowgill, *Rest Uneasy: Sudden Infant Death Syndrome in Twentieth-Century America*
Patricia D'Antonio, *Nursing with a Message: Public Health Demonstration Projects in New York City*
Tasha N. Dubriwny, *The Vulnerable Empowered Woman: Feminism, Postfeminism, and Women's Health*
Edward J. Eckenfels, *Doctors Serving People: Restoring Humanism to Medicine through Student Community Service*
Julie Fairman, *Making Room in the Clinic: Nurse Practitioners and the Evolution of Modern Health Care*
Jill A. Fisher, *Medical Research for Hire: The Political Economy of Pharmaceutical Clinical Trials*
Charlene Galarneau, *Communities of Health Care Justice*
Alyshia Gálvez, *Patient Citizens, Immigrant Mothers: Mexican Women, Public Prenatal Care and the Birth Weight Paradox*
Janet Greenlees, *When the Air Became Important: A Social History of the New England and Lancashire Textile Industries*
Gerald N. Grob and Howard H. Goldman, *The Dilemma of Federal Mental Health Policy: Radical Reform or Incremental Change?*
Gerald N. Grob and Allan V. Horwitz, *Diagnosis, Therapy, and Evidence: Conundrums in Modern American Medicine*
Rachel Grob, *Testing Baby: The Transformation of Newborn Screening, Parenting, and Policymaking*
Mark A. Hall and Sara Rosenbaum, eds., *The Health Care "Safety Net" in a Post-Reform World*
Laura L. Heinemann, *Transplanting Care: Shifting Commitments in Health and Care in the United States*
Laura D. Hirshbein, *American Melancholy: Constructions of Depression in the Twentieth Century*
Laura D. Hirshbein, *Smoking Privileges: Psychiatry, the Mentally Ill, and the Tobacco Industry in America*

Timothy Hoff, *Practice under Pressure: Primary Care Physicians and Their Medicine in the Twenty-first Century*

Beatrix Hoffman, Nancy Tomes, Rachel N. Grob, and Mark Schlesinger, eds., *Patients as Policy Actors*

Ruth Horowitz, *Deciding the Public Interest: Medical Licensing and Discipline*

Powel Kazanjian, *Frederick Novy and the Development of Bacteriology in American Medicine*

Claas Kirchhelle, *Pyrrhic Progress: The History of Antibiotics in Anglo-American Food Production*

Rebecca M. Kluchin, *Fit to Be Tied: Sterilization and Reproductive Rights in America, 1950–1980*

Jennifer Lisa Koslow, *Cultivating Health: Los Angeles Women and Public Health Reform*

Jennifer Lisa Koslow, *Exhibiting Health: Public Health Displays in the Progressive Era*

Susan C. Lawrence, *Privacy and the Past: Research, Law, Archives, Ethics*

Bonnie Lefkowitz, *Community Health Centers: A Movement and the People Who Made It Happen*

Ellen Leopold, *Under the Radar: Cancer and the Cold War*

Barbara L. Ley, *From Pink to Green: Disease Prevention and the Environmental Breast Cancer Movement*

Sonja Mackenzie, *Structural Intimacies: Sexual Stories in the Black AIDS Epidemic*

Frank M. McClellan, *Healthcare and Human Dignity: Law Matters*

Michelle McClellan, *Lady Lushes: Gender, Alcohol, and Medicine in Modern America*

David Mechanic, *The Truth about Health Care: Why Reform Is Not Working in America*

Richard A. Meckel, *Classrooms and Clinics: Urban Schools and the Protection and Promotion of Child Health, 1870–1930*

Alyssa Picard, *Making the American Mouth: Dentists and Public Health in the Twentieth Century*

Heather Munro Prescott, *The Morning After: A History of Emergency Contraception in the United States*

Sarah B. Rodriguez, *The Love Surgeon: A Story of Trust, Harm, and the Limits of Medical Regulation*

Andrew R. Ruis, *Eating to Learn, Learning to Eat: School Lunches and Nutrition Policy in the United States*

James A. Schafer Jr., *The Business of Private Medical Practice: Doctors, Specialization, and Urban Change in Philadelphia, 1900–1940*

David G. Schuster, *Neurasthenic Nation: America's Search for Health, Happiness, and Comfort, 1869–1920*

Karen Seccombe and Kim A. Hoffman, *Just Don't Get Sick: Access to Health Care in the Aftermath of Welfare Reform*

Leo B. Slater, *War and Disease: Biomedical Research on Malaria in the Twentieth Century*

Dena T. Smith, *Medicine over Mind: Mental Health Practice in the Biomedical Era*

Kylie M. Smith, *Talking Therapy: Knowledge and Power in American Psychiatric Nursing*

Matthew Smith, *An Alternative History of Hyperactivity: Food Additives and the Feingold Diet*

Paige Hall Smith, Bernice L. Hausman, and Miriam Labbok, *Beyond Health, Beyond Choice: Breastfeeding Constraints and Realities*

Susan L. Smith, *Toxic Exposures: Mustard Gas and the Health Consequences of World War II in the United States*

Rosemary A. Stevens, Charles E. Rosenberg, and Lawton R. Burns, eds., *History and Health Policy in the United States: Putting the Past Back In*

Courtney E. Thompson, *An Organ of Murder: Crime, Violence, and Phrenology in Nineteenth-Century America*

Barbra Mann Wall, *American Catholic Hospitals: A Century of Changing Markets and Missions*

Frances Ward, *The Door of Last Resort: Memoirs of a Nurse Practitioner*

Shannon Withycombe, *Lost: Miscarriage in Nineteenth-Century America*